The Victorian
Vivisection Debate

# The Victorian Vivisection Debate

*Frances Power Cobbe, Experimental Science and the "Claims of Brutes"*

THEODORE G. OBENCHAIN

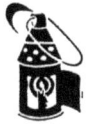

McFarland & Company, Inc., Publishers
*Jefferson, North Carolina, and London*

LIBRARY OF CONGRESS ONLINE CATALOG PUBLICATION DATA

Obenchain, Theodore G.
　　The Victorian vivisection debate : Frances Power Cobbe, experimental science and the "claims of brutes" / Theodore G. Obenchain.
　　　　p.　　cm.
　　Includes bibliographical references and index.

　　**ISBN 978-0-7864-7119-5**
　　softcover : acid free paper ∞

　　1. Vivisection—Great Britain—History—19th century.
　　2. Great Britain—Social life and customs—19th century.
　　　　　　　　　　　　　　　　　　　　　2012289597

BRITISH LIBRARY CATALOGUING DATA ARE AVAILABLE

© 2012 Theodore G. Obenchain. All rights reserved

*No part of this book may be reproduced or transmitted in any form or by any means, electronic or mechanical, including photocopying or recording, or by any information storage and retrieval system, without permission in writing from the publisher.*

On the cover: (left) illustration of vivesected dog from *Scientific American* Supplement, Vol. XVI, No. 415, December 15, 1883; (right) Frances Power Cobbe, 1894 (Wellcome Library, London)

Manufactured in the United States of America

*McFarland & Company, Inc., Publishers*
　*Box 611, Jefferson, North Carolina 28640*
　　*www.mcfarlandpub.com*

In the spring of 1960 when I was a sophomore medical student, three classmates and I were assigned a pharmacology project designed to evaluate the effects of various medications on the functions of the heart. The experimental setup consisted of one isolated dog's heart, connected, in series, to a large rectangular glass tube filled with blood donated by other euthanized dogs. In effect, we had an isolated circulatory system. No compensatory bodily functions could affect the heart or obscure the effects of our administered medications. Injection ports, pressure gauges and other monitoring devices made the physical setup quite elaborate. With three rehearsals and a final demonstration to the full class, we euthanized, in total, approximately 24 animals.

The dogs we used were all unclaimed strays donated by a local shelter to the medical school for research. We euthanized them very humanely by injecting an overdose of barbiturate medication into their veins. If the dog growled, bared his teeth or snapped at me while I was searching his foreleg for a vein, the process was not too difficult to complete. However, it could be emotionally draining if the dog proved to be friendly. I recall one spaniel mix in particular, sitting back on his haunches. As I knelt down to him, he offered me a trembling foreleg. I petted his head, said something soothing to him, shook his paw and placed a tourniquet just above it, hoping to raise a vein. With his head submissively lowered, he affectionately rolled his eyes up at me with a seemingly smiling face, meekly wagging his tail. As if my inner conflict were not yet sufficient, he licked my fingers as they searched for an avenue to his destruction. That image, forever emblazoned in my brain, still causes a disquiet within me decades later. My encounter with that unnamed waif, who made me pause and reflect upon my actions one memorable morning, serves as my motive for this effort. To him I dedicate this work.

# Contents

| | |
|---|---|
| *Acknowledgments* | ix |
| *Introduction* | 1 |
| **PART I: ORIGINS OF ANTIVIVISECTION** | 7 |
| 1. Frances Power Cobbe, the Great Sunbeam | 8 |
| 2. *The Rights of Man and the Claims of Brutes* | 21 |
| **PART II: GRATUITOUS VERSUS JUSTIFIED EXPLOITATION** | 35 |
| 3. The Early Vivisectors | 36 |
| **PART III: FERMENTATION AND SUPPURATION** | 48 |
| 4. Joseph Lister and Hospitalism: Is It Something in the Air? | 49 |
| 5. Louis Pasteur: Specific Microbes Cause Specific Conditions | 57 |
| 6. Lister: "It really charms me" | 66 |
| **PART IV: HER MAJESTY'S ROYAL COMMISSION** | 74 |
| 7. France Power Cobbe's Petition | 75 |
| 8. "This legislation is wholly uncalled for" | 85 |
| **PART V: GERM THEORY EXPANDED** | 97 |
| 9. Robert Koch: Templates of Hospitalism | 98 |
| 10. Louis Pasteur: The Infinitely Small Are Infinitely Great | 111 |
| 11. Showdown at Melun | 119 |
| **PART VI: THE INTERNATIONAL MEDICAL CONGRESS OF 1881** | 126 |
| 12. Portents of a Notable Decade | 127 |
| 13. Professor Ferrier and His Monkeys | 137 |
| 14. The Captain of All the Men of Death | 152 |

| | |
|---|---:|
| PART VII: RETREAT TO WALES | 166 |
| 15. Quitting London | 167 |
| PART VIII: SALVATION BY FILTH | 177 |
| 16. La Rage | 178 |
| 17. "Whither is Pasteurism to lead us?" | 193 |
| 18. Tuberculin: "Experiment Not Discovery" | 202 |
| PART IX: TRIUMPH AND DESCENT | 209 |
| 19. Nearly Universal | 210 |
| 20. Lister's Retrospective | 218 |
| 21. Descent | 226 |
| PART X: UPDATE | 235 |
| 22. Science Must Go On and On | 236 |
| *Epilogue* | 253 |
| *Chapter Notes* | 259 |
| *Bibliography* | 273 |
| *Index* | 281 |

# Acknowledgments

In *The Victorian Vivisection Debate*, I have portrayed the clash between experimental scientists and antivivisectionists by citing some critical primary sources and by utilizing the work of scholars in various fields, running the spectrum from medical science to feminism. While each scholar cited has elucidated their respective subjects' lives, such as that of Robert Koch, my objective was to tell a larger, overarching story of medicine's transition from medievalism to modernity within the context of the antivivisection movement. My intent also differed from the scholars' in that my comments have been aimed more at an enlightened general readership.

This biography of a conflict between two antipodal forces originated from two sources: First, I have held a longstanding desire to more clearly delineate the origins of both the scientific and the antivivisection movements in order to resolve my own ambiguities about the justification, or lack thereof, for animal experimentation. Second, the work was part of my master's dissertation in nonfiction writing at Lesley University. A special note of appreciation to the faculty at Lesley — in particular, Alexandra Johnson, Leah Hager Cohen and Katherine Russell Rich, all of whom offered much in the way of positive criticism.

Although this work is a complete narrative, it is not a complete history. So many individuals have contributed to the modernization of medicine that some, inevitably, had to be excluded — space did not allow for the fullest of expositions. As with most pioneering human endeavors, one could find a large number of individuals working in a particular scientific field in the Victorian era, often closing in on some major discovery. As some aspect of a scientific puzzle continued to evolve, such as a solution to the problems presented by anthrax, a flash point occurred, resulting in a scientific breakthrough. While many workers may have contributed significantly to that breakthrough, it was usually one or a small number of individuals who found themselves uniquely positioned to receive credit for the development, fairly or unfairly. This work excludes the contributions of some important medical movements as well, such as the German school of physiology, not because such groups were considered unimportant, but because they did not play a sufficiently critical role in the antivivisection confrontation. Similarly, this account covers only the birth of Western scientific medicine, not because Asian and Arabic contributions have been insignificant, but because little resistance to vivisection existed within those cultures.

I would like to acknowledge several works, exhaustive both in their scope and detail, which facilitated my research. I used them extensively, both to further the narrative and to make my own pro-vivisection argument. First, *Animal Welfare and Anti-Vivisection, 1870–1910*, edited by Susan Hamilton, contains much of Frances Cobbe's essays against vivisection, in addition to two other volumes representing both the antivivisection and pro-vivisection views. Lori Williamson's *Power and Protest: Frances Power Cobbe and Victorian Society* and *Frances Power Cobbe: Victorian Feminist, Journalist, Reformer* by Sally Mitchell are two biographies that prove to be as entertaining as they are scholarly. Richard French's 400-page work, *Antivivisection and Medical Science in Victorian Society*, is an exhaustive coverage of antivivisection, covering the spectrum from animal experimentation, to the agitation between both forces, and finally, to the antivivisectionists' ultimate descent. Published in 1975, it is still influential within the field because of its scope and quality of scholarship. Two biographies of Pasteur, one by Patrice Debré and another by Rene Dubose, plus a single narrative on Robert Koch by Thomas Brock, represent the principal amount of information available in the English language regarding these scientists. Being an Englishman, obviously more information was available in the native language on Joseph Lister, but Rickman Godlee's tome, which I cited liberally, was, by far, the most comprehensive.

I depended upon several great libraries with extensive holdings from the Victorian era for my research, including the Library of Congress and the National Library of Medicine, both in Washington, D.C. as well as the Rare Books and Special Collections division of the Francis A. Countway Library of Medicine, Harvard University, the Mutter Museum of the College of Physicians of Philadelphia, the New York Public Library, and the Huntington Library in Pasadena, California. I also relied heavily on the Library at Lesley University in Cambridge, Massachusetts, during my time there. Facilities that I consulted local to the Portland area included the Oregon Health Sciences University Medical Library, the Branford P. Millar Library of Portland State University, the Multnomah County Library, and the Fort Vancouver Public Library. The holdings at these quality institutions, supplemented by the utility of their inter-library loan programs, make such facilities great assets to their communities.

Finally, on a grammatical note concerning primary sources: Victorian writers notoriously salted their sentences with commas, capital letters and alternate spellings in a haphazard manner, as though no rules of grammar existed. I have preserved these antiquated conventions in any area where I made a direct quote. Otherwise, for information that I merely cited, modern rules of grammar have prevailed.

# Introduction

*The Victorian Vivisection Debate* is a biography illuminating the birth and development of two mutually repellant movements within Victorian England. Confrontation between the two was inevitable. Experimental scientists of that era, that is, physiologists, practiced the art of vivisection, a word derived from two Latin roots meaning, literally, to cut up or dissect an organism while it is still alive. In our modern time the word "vivisection" has become archaic and strongly pejorative. Through operative means, physiologists used, and still use, living animals to elucidate new facts concerning bodily function in both the normal and abnormal states. Until anesthetics were introduced in 1846, physiological operations were performed with the animal either fully awake or sedated with what was available at that time, alcohol or opium. Some experimental scientists, anxious to drag the field of medicine out of its medieval ways, heedlessly exploited lesser beings in pursuit of their goals, even if their acts did result in pain and suffering. Antivivisectionists, their polar opposites, viewed physiological acts of vivisection as so cruel, so repugnant, that they could never be justified, no matter how valuable the information gained. The costs, both to experimenter and animal, came at too high a price.

As with most social phenomena, sentiments surrounding animal experimentation have waxed and waned through the years, but the tension still exists, unresolved, 150 years later. Fueled by current animal rights activists, a concerted movement to stop all animal experimentation slowly gathers strength. It is not unusual to encounter contemporary newspaper articles in which some activist is making a charge against medical science. One such example, a May 2010 *Oregonian* article, featured Matt Rossell from an animal defense organization. He pondered how it was that animals do not suffer when, "in the name of science, animals are routinely injected with or forced to consume toxins, addicted to drugs, intentionally infected with disease, ... burned, shocked, starved, deprived of water, isolated and immobilized for hours, weeks, even months on end[?]."[1] Responding to such threats, the scientific community predictably offers rebuttals, justifying their activities in the name of medical progress.

Even modern philosophers align themselves against science. One, Nathan Nobis, declares that animal research is not "necessary to enter medical school or to practice or teach medicine.... Experience working in a clinic, assisting professionals, works very well."[2] He even declares it unethical to conduct such research to enhance humanity's "knowledge of life, to satisfy personal curiosity or spark scientific inspiration."[3] Nobis concludes by declaring animal dissection, "except for only some select aspects of veterinary curricula," to be indefensible, both from an educational and a moral perspective.[4]

In the last part of this work I offer a rebuttal to that argument. But first I must reveal my own background and what attitudes I may or may not bring to the subject of exploiting animals in the name of scientific research. I spent the majority of my professional life not in full-time research, but rather as a clinical neurosurgeon. However, as illustrated in the following paragraphs, I utilized animals through all stages of my career, as a medical student in the 1960s, specialty training in the 1970s and in my career spanning the remaining years of the millennium and beyond. Learning from animals added depth to my education. But my exploitation of other species does not mean that I am unsympathetic to animals. One of my earliest and, as a lover of animals, most wrenching encounters with dogs I have described in the dedication. Before my attention was directed towards humans in my junior year of medical school, I gained further experience with animals. As freshmen, my classmates and I surgically exposed spinal cords in cats, learning not only the elements of neurophysiology, but also the methodology of electrical recordings and the vagaries faced by scientists attempting to set up reliable experiments. A student of medicine can only gain a realistic grasp of science by working with the gadgetry and toiling with the difficulties encountered with experimentation. As sophomores, we learned anesthetic and operative techniques by surgically removing gall bladders, spleens, stomachs and other organs of dogs. Following them through their convalescence highlighted the importance of surgical technique and proper post-operative care.

In my years of neurosurgical specialty training, among other experiments upon animals, I rendered hydrocephalic (water on the brain) a group of monkeys through an operation at the base of the back of their heads. I then monitored the evolving pressure changes inside the brain over a continuous 24-hour epoch, maintaining light anesthesia the entire time.[5] The results added at least nominally to the general body of information concerning intracranial pressure dynamics.

In my early academic years I designed a laboratory exercise aimed at improving my own surgical technique for connecting microscopic blood vessels, a technique utilized in the treatment of certain stroke patients. The sutures required were so fine that one could not even feel them, leaving the surgeon devoid of the usual tactile cues of knot-tying. Part of the benefits realized for the surgeon was a re-programming of a part of his brain — the substitution of visual, instead of tactile, guides for the proficient completion of the knots. I operated on rats anesthetized with ether, first severing, then re-connecting, the minute femoral arteries in their groins. To better simulate the operative dimensions inside the depths of a human head, I operated though cardboard cones, with the small end directed towards the rat, forcing me to confine my movements within a very limited area, deep within the cone, all under magnification.

As my career progressed, experimentation with animals assumed a different form. Over a period of a decade I pursued a less invasive outpatient operative approach to the lumbar spine.[6] In search of this goal I first utilized isolated cattle spines, then the torsos of human cadavers. Finally, I used a series of live goats, which enabled me to deal with the unexpected, such as bleeding, variations of anatomy, or fogging of operative lenses with condensate, and so on. Experiencing the approach under battlefield conditions helps a surgeon better develop the kinesthetic skills required by a new technique.

To remain competent all surgeons must continue to develop new surgical skills and techniques. Becoming facile with laparoscopic techniques and new instrumentation, and learning new approaches to the spine or a novel approach to the brain are just a few of the procedures that one can learn in such a setting. Better that a surgeon hone his skills on animals than humans. An entire industry has emerged to serve these needs of surgeons. I participated in such courses many times over a period of 20 years, sometimes as part of the faculty, at other times, as one of the students. Various entities scattered across the country offer operative facilities and animals, with goats, pigs and sheep being the most popular subjects for learning the skills. In my years of visiting such facilities I have yet to find one that was poorly run. The animal care before, during and after these courses, including anesthesia administration, was handled very professionally by veterinarians and their staffs. Despite such exemplary care, these facilities were, on occasion, the targets for demonstrations by animal liberation forces.

The public is generally incognizant of activities such as these — medicine in transition, remodeling itself. People are similarly unaware of how medicine slowly evolved from medievalism into its modern state in less than a 200-year period. Whether one agrees with the practice of using animals in such a manner or not, it is undeniable that virtually all gains made in the march towards medical modernity have been earned at the hands of vivisectors working on animals. As a history of that evolution, this work is instructive.

*The Victorian Vivisection Debate* is organized into 10 parts. Part I introduces the principal antagonist, Frances Power Cobbe. In 1863, she came face to face with scientists purportedly mistreating animals in pursuit of science. Part II adds context to the narrative, first recounting the gratuitously cruel treatment of animals in the street. It then provides a picture of the origins of vivisection, putting the discipline of scientific medicine, with its emphasis on anatomy, into perspective — medicine as it existed prior to the advent of organized physiology. In the early 1800s, physicians learned the art of medicine through the study of anatomy. Before 1860, the average physician was virtually ignorant of physiology, that is, the mechanisms behind bodily function. Physiology was an appendage of anatomy, a mere adjunct, practiced only sporadically. By Part III we finally meet the full cast of characters, the protagonists who personified experimental science: English surgeon Joseph Lister and pure scientists Louis Pasteur and Robert Koch. In parts IV through X the confrontation develops to its full extent, ending with Cobbe's death in 1904. The final chapter brings the continuing debate surrounding experimental medicine and animal cruelty up to the present, into the 21st century.

Are experimental scientists warranted in their exploitation of animals — making some beings suffer in the present for a future, putative good? This work provides an answer from two different perspectives. The first is historical; the other my own. Since the work records the details of a confrontation that took place between two adversaries in Victorian England, it is historical. I have presented the narrative in as unbiased a manner as is humanly possible, keeping my own personal views entirely out of all 21 chapters. To my view, the revelations of history, as it evolves, serve as a self-evident argument in favor of using animals for experimentation. Scientists Lister, Pasteur and Koch could never have made their contributions without using animals. By examining their lives, it becomes evident that the work of each had to progress inevitably on to the exploitation of other species. Animals represented not just the best but the only available analogs of human disease states. As one reads of the scientists' accomplishments, the conclusion seems obvious: If medicine is to progress further, experimental science must continue to use animals in the pursuit of knowledge.

Finally, in the last chapter and epilogue I present a distillation of the main arguments proffered by the most prominent animal rights theorists, as well as my own answer to the central argument concerning the ethics of animal experimentation — to be accepted or rejected by the reader. After examining the major philosophical arguments, my position remains solidly on the side of experimental science.

This work not only adds to the history of medicine and the vivisection debate, it also delivers a social message, providing some guidance to anyone who remains confused or ambivalent about the current animal rights controversy. Given the emotional, sometimes inaccurate views expressed in the media, such ambivalence is not surprising. Having a better grasp of the origins of physiology and the antivivisection movement, as well as the manner in which the drama played out over time, provides one with a broader perspective concerning the roots of the problem. It adds context, allowing the reader to better understand the confrontation between the two camps, a conflict still raging today.

# I

# ORIGINS OF ANTIVIVISECTION

"Pain is the one supreme evil of the existence of the lower animals; an evil which (so far as we can see) has no countervailing good. As to Death — a painless one, so far from being the supreme evil to them, is often the truest mercy." — Frances Power Cobbe[1]

CHAPTER 1

# Frances Power Cobbe, the Great Sunbeam

The American writer Louisa May Alcott painted perhaps the most illuminating portrait of Frances Power Cobbe, whom she met at a friend's house in 1866. Alcott, while serving as traveling companion to Anna Weld, the melancholic, pampered daughter of a Boston shipping magnate, related the manner in which she unexpectedly made Cobbe's acquaintance:

> As I sat pouring over Gustave Dore's *Illustrations of Dante* one morning, the door suddenly flew open, and in rolled an immensely stout lady, with skirts kilted up, a cane in her hand, a fly-away green bonnet on her head, and a loud laugh issuing from her lips, as she cast herself upon the sofa, exclaiming breathlessly:
> "Me dear creature, if you love me, a glass of sherry!"
> The wine being ordered, I was called from my nook, and introduced to Miss Cobbe. I had imagined the author of *Intuitive Morals* to be a serious, severe lady, of the "Cornelia Blimber" school, and was much surprised to see this merry, witty, Falstaffian personage. For half an hour she entertained us with all manner of droll sayings, as full of sense as of humor, one minute talking earnestly and gravely on the suffrage question ... the next criticizing an amateur poem in a way that convulsed her hearers, and in the middle of it jumping up to admire a picture, or trot about the room, enthusiastically applauding some welcome bit of news about "our petition." Cheery, sensible, kindly, and keen she seemed; and when she went away, talking hard till out of the gate, and vanishing with a hearty laugh, it was as if a great sunbeam had left the room, so genial and friendly was the impression she made. I saw her several times afterward, and always found her the same wherever she was, people gathered about her, as if she was a social fire, and everyone seemed to find warmth and pleasure in the attractive circle which surrounded her. It was truly delightful to see a woman so useful, happy, wise, and beloved.[1]

With her analytical mind, classical self-education and natural talent for exposition, it was obvious that young Frances was destined for fame in some yet-to-be-determined pursuit. In a culture different from that of the Victorians, she could have been anything she wanted to be, from politician to theologian or academician. Cobbe might have earned millions as a barrister with her talent for turning a phrase, expertly playing the jurists' emotions like she plucked the strings of her harp. Instead, she chose a literary career, as an essayist, taking aim mainly at Victorian societal inequities. She was prolific, publishing more than 100 articles in periodicals and over 200 monographs on antivivisection. Additionally, between 1868 and 1875, she wrote well over 1,000 pieces for the London periodical *Echo* on politics, public issues and social causes, all anonymous and thereby genderless. She counted many notables as her friends, from cardinals, bishops, Parliamentarians, academicians, the literati and lesser nobility. Writer Elizabeth Cady Stanton called her "one of the most remarkable and genial women" in England, "frank and cordial and pronounced in all her views." It was Alcott who gave her the moniker "The Great Sunbeam." However, to her detractors Cobbe was "manly" or "strong-minded." To one observer, she had "a tone of the trousers."[2]

With her independent and unconquerable spirit, Frances Cobbe was a study of contrasts, defending some Victorian traditions, while inexplicably rejecting others. She challenged gender inequality throughout her life, but never questioned the peerage, or inherent class system of England. A snooty elitist, Cobbe considered it a given that Oxford and Cambridge graduates were morally superior to members of the artisan class. She fought mightily for women's access to education, including medicine, yet objected when such graduates took on signature attributes of the profession of which she did not approve. As a free thinker, she shed the shackles of her Evangelical upbringing to embrace Theism, only to later express anti–Semitic and anti–Catholic attitudes. In her early years, she delved into workhouse reform, never hesitating to allow the government to step in and separate families, if she considered it beneficial to the cause at hand. Later, however, she expressed indignation at a government that could separate loved ones based upon theories of contagion or disease prevention. She claimed intuitive ethics and morals as her guiding principles of life. Still, in the heat of polemic, she willingly stretched the truth if it served her own purposes. Charles Adams, Cobbe's estranged former employee, commented on her character late in her career:

> For superabounding energy, for absolute self-conviction, for magnificent unscrupulousness of assertion, for entire imperviousness alike to reason and ridicule, and for inextinguishable eloquence, especially in the direction of vituperation, she is, in these latter days, almost, if not quite, unsurpassed. And for a public agitation of any kind, these are the gifts required; the indispensable, if not the only, requirements for practical success.[3]

Cobbe applied her talents liberally. With her strong personality, her innate tenderness and protective sentiment towards animals, it was not so much that Cobbe became allied with the antivivisection movement. She practically birthed it in England. As she reminisced later,

> I have felt all of my life an irresistible impulse to rush in wherever anyone is "oppressed" and try to "deliver" him, her or it, as the case may be, from the "adversary"! In the case of beasts, their helplessness and speechlessness appeal, I think, to every spark of generosity in one's heart; and the command, "Open thy mouth for the dumb," seems the very echo of our consciences. Everything in us, manly or womanly (and the best in us all is both), answers it back.[4]

Such were Cobbe's sentiments, but the intriguing question remains: Why would she take on this battle against the vivisectionists, a fight that would consume most of her time and energy from 1875 until her death in 1904? As one of her biographers, Lori Williamson, noted, "Cobbe gave her time to Theists, to workhouse inmates and to women, but she gave herself to animals."[5] She had already become an established London literary figure with a productive, meaningful existence, public adulation, major victories in the feminist arena and a comfortable income. Why not just live the good life? Instead she nobly devoted most of her time and talents to confront this perceived evil.

## Origins

Cobbe's early up-bringing in a devoutly Evangelical Anglo-Irish family gives some valuable insights into her adult attitudes and activities regarding religion, feminine issues and animal rights. She claimed to have been "well born" in Newbridge, a large family estate in County Dublin, to indulgent parents, from an aristocratic line of predecessors dating back to 1323.[6] Although English in origin, Frances' family had resided in Ireland since 1717. She could count the archbishop of Dublin, several members of parliament, a field marshal, an admiral and the primate of Ireland in her lineage. Charles, Frances' father, had a military career as a member of the Light Dragoons, spending many years in India before retiring to farming and managing the 360-acre Newbridge estate. Fanny, as she was called as a child, had four brothers all between five to ten years her senior. Her siblings were either away at school or had already left in pursuit of their own lives by the time Fanny was old enough to interact with them, depriving her of the usual influences of older brothers. She suffered the solitude peculiar to an only child. Since education for a female was considered unnecessary, she received a home-based, informal schooling, studying all morning, each day. At noon she was free to spend the day as she wished, running through the woods with her dog, or riding her pony about the estate or over to the rocky Irish coast of Portrane, two miles away. Being surrounded by her beloved pets was a perfect setting for this future advocate of animals. Fanny had access to several personal libraries which enabled her to gain an excellent grounding in classical subjects. With her preference for works like Shelley, Plutarch and Gibbon, her precocious literary tastes were evident. She had even written some serious poetry by age 10.

Fanny's parents, believing that their corpulent and unrestrained 14-year-old tomboy could use some serious lessons in charm and femininity, sent her to Brighton, considered the best finishing school for women in all of England.[7] Her classmates were bright and capable, coming from some of the leading families of England. Frances developed nothing but disdain for the school, run by the Misses Runciman and Roberts, but, in deference to her parents, she mutely tolerated the banalities she encountered there.

The school's goal was the transformation of raw puerility into decorous young women. By the time the young ladies had completed training, they should be versed in literature and the arts, have some fluency in French, play the harp or piano, and know how to dress, sit, walk and converse with other cultured people. Setting a proper place at the dining table, knowing how to seat guests appropriately for any occasion and mastering the art of composing a formal letter should be second nature to the graduating young woman.

The courses offered there were, like the entire curriculum, at least in Fanny's eyes, bland and superficial. As she lamented years later in her autobiography, in reference to her classmates, "this fine human material was deplorably wasted."[8] Being too independent herself to ever consider spending life as some spouse's decoration, she merely bided her time, emerging essentially unchanged, at age 16. With the two years thankfully behind her, she could now return to her beloved Newbridge.

As Frances grew older, she found much in Victorian society with which she vehemently disagreed, Victorian women's expected behavior and manner of dress being two of them. Ladies' attire was designed to emphasize the helpless femininity of the wearer. That hourglass body was the ideal, never mind the discomfort one had to endure to acquire it. There were darts and hooks and stays and boney struts, all mercilessly applied in the name of beauty, aggressively laced down to achieve that vaunted shape. Necklines varied diurnally — high during the day and very low in the evening. One footman, accustomed to seeing fashionable ladies, noted, "The young ladies are nearly naked to the waist, only just a little bit of dress hanging on the shoulder, the breasts are quite exposed except a little bit coming up to hide the nipples."[9]

Frances, no slave to convention, felt that clothing should allow "liberty of action to all the organs of the body and freedom from pressure."[10] She dressed for function, wearing drab, loose, comfortable clothing that could easily accommodate her rotund frame. As one of her intimates observed, "My dear, it is not that you dress badly; you do not dress at all."[11]

Laughing was, in general, inadvisable; Frances with her ready laugh, easily audible in the adjacent room, had trouble with that dictate. At dinner parties a woman was never to eat more than a bird-like morsel, nor more than touch her lips to the glass when partaking of a toast.[12] Frances had always enjoyed a large appetite, reveling in good food and wine. Her acquaintance Lady Paget observed, "Miss Cobbe's bright blue eyes flamed when she spoke, but, to many, her huge size, her fine appetite, and rather mannish ways were repellant."[13] With her decidedly epicurean tastes, and unconcern for appearances, it was becoming clear that young Frances was not fitting into that Victorian mold. Her personality traits were emerging loud and clear. She had no time for the meaningless superficialities relating to fashionable conduct, food or sartorial expression.

Back home in Newbridge after Brighton school, she buried herself in intense study for the next four years, not due to some requirement but because she yearned for learning and wisdom. No casual learner, she immersed herself in Greek, mathematics and all of the great books. She studied Homer, Sophocles, Euripides, Thucydides, Horace, Pope, Dryden and Milton, to name but a few.[14]

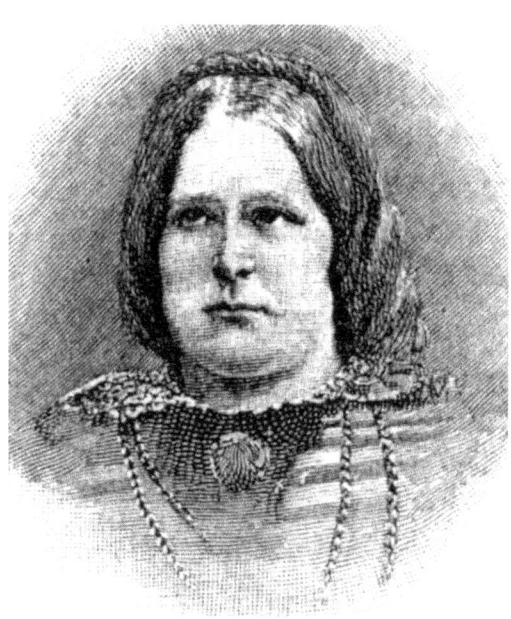

Frances Power Cobbe, age 20. Her habitus and sartorial tastes are already evident. *The Strand Magazine* 31 (1893).

Next came all of the philosophers from whom she hoped to gain answers to the great questions of the human soul. She was intense, making detailed charts, including all of the great scholars, theologians and philosophers, cataloguing their main views and teachings. Under philosophers, one could find Descartes, René, 1596–1650, Writings—*Discourse on Method, Treatise on Man*, and so on. She did the same for the entire line of succession of English royalty. For ease of access to this fount of information, she committed all of the catalogued material to memory. This labor of love provided a valuable storehouse for her later writings; she could draw from her quiver at will, shooting an arrow straight to the heart of the argument at hand.

## Heretical Thoughts

Frances admitted to being unusually devout for her age. Raised in a stern, Christian home, she grew up on a diet of traditional religious dogma which she accepted unquestioningly until her mid-teens. Her father, Charles, led daily family religious services. On Sundays, he allowed only activity related to religion. Being nurtured on religious readings, Frances was especially stirred by Bunyan's *Pilgrim's Progress* and the idea that one *could* progress towards heaven through a "vale of tears." She was reassured. Hard work, devotion and dedication may, after all, earn one a place in heaven. However, after reading Robert Chambers' *Vestiges of Creation*, and other works, doubts began creeping into to her mind. Her first ideological impasse occurred with the miracle of the loaves and fishes. "Did the fish grow? Did they multiply before being eaten? How was this miracle brought about? It's not possible. This is nonsense!"[15]

Then she would sink into a depression over each one of her successive irreverences. Over the years, the more she read, the more thorough her doubts. Distressed by her own heresy, she kept her views hidden from her parents, further burying herself in religious readings. When Frances turned 24, as her agnosticism peaked, her mother died, sending her into a deeper emotional tailspin. No longer believing in immortality, Frances could not handle the thought of her beloved mother—"the only one that truly loved me"—being gone forever—no thoughts of her mother benignly watching over her—no chance of meeting her on that other side.[16]

Frances would often walk through the woods or retreat to her favorite glen to read and contemplate in solitude. She was a soul lost in the wilderness, searching for anything to guide her to safety. She consumed religious, theosophical, philosophical readings, all to no avail. Finally, when she discovered the Boston theologian Theodore Parker's *Discourse on Religion*, it transformed her. Parker preached divine inspiration, an intuitive rather than doctrinal route to the acceptance of a Creator. His approach allowed Frances to gradually embrace the concept of immortality and still remain intellectually consistent. She was reborn—not as a Christian but as a Deist, rejecting not only the Trinity but the usual ecclesiastical accompaniments as well. Frances began an epistolary relationship with Parker until she finally met him in Florence, in 1860. In the terminal stages of tuberculosis, Parker died four days after Cobbe's arrival, but not before the two had forged a deep spiritual bond. That attachment proved so deep that Parker's descendants later requested that she edit his 14 volumes on religion.

Later, her beliefs evolved from Deism to Theism but to most, the differences were slight. Describing her beliefs as heterodox, Frances remained devout her entire life, religious principles guiding her every move. In her reconstructed faith, the Creator was a God of mercy and love, the guiding star that proved so important in her antivivisection battles. In her world, scientific principles must always be subordinated to religion. The absolute goodness of God was supreme; there could be no blemishes on His goodness. One cannot be good to some of God's creatures and not to others.[17] Her religious convictions remained anchored in bedrock throughout her life.

Despite her rebirth, however, Frances's troubles were not entirely behind her. She finally confronted her father with her heretical religious views. Charles was less than understanding. "Theism? It's not a religion — it's a word in the dictionary," he responded to her pleadings. He argued that if one rejects Christ and disbelieves the Bible, "a man is called upon to keep the plague of such opinions from his own house." With Charles's banning Frances from the comforts of Newbridge, she was forced to live with her brother on a farm "in the wilds of Donegal." While there she wrote "Essay on true Religion," one of her three major religious works. After 10 months in exile, her father summoned her home to manage the household. In an uneasy truce, they mutually agreed that she could meditate in her favorite retreats, instead of attending the more traditional daily devotions with her family.[18] Little did she know that soon she would be caring for him on his deathbed. Serving in the Indian campaign, Charles had contracted malaria, suffering periodic fevers throughout the rest of his life. Finally, in 1857 he died. In Victorian custom the eldest son inherited the estate, meaning Frances was suddenly without a home. With an inherited annuity of 200 pounds per year, Charles had left her at least some level of security.

## Essay on Intuitive Morals

With Charles' death, Frances' philosophical horizons broadened.[19] Her first book, *Essay on Intuitive Morals*, served as her credo concerning morals, science and religion. Although Frances wrote the book when she was 33, she waited until two years after Charles' death to publish it. In the 280-page work, Cobbe lucidly presented her views on philosophy and the subject of morals. Although much of it might be considered dated today, the book gives interesting insights into her sense of the cosmos, helping one better understand her motivations and her views on equality, justice and the defenseless. She argued that pure morals did not rest on any traditional philosophic or historical dogma, but on strong intuitions, as clear and true as the axioms of geometry. Just as a triangle *always* contains 180 degrees, once one has found her philosophic underpinnings, she could rely on them with the same level of certainty. These truths are necessary, not contingent; they are as stable and immutable as bedrock.

Cobbe believed that the human is a rational being, one who can freely choose right or wrong and may therefore be either virtuous or vicious. Although man might follow his sensations — intellectual, affectional or sensual — that route leads only to happiness.[20] The highest level of achievement, only available to rational souls, is not happiness but virtue — the voluntary but disinterested obedience of a free, rational intelligence.[21] This act must be carried out with no hope of any sort of reward — a purely selfless, beneficent act. Animals, on the other hand, being neither rational nor freely choosing, cannot attain virtue; their highest level of achievement is happiness. Being amoral, animals are neither virtuous nor vicious.

Cobbe took issue with the late Jeremy Bentham and other philosophers of the Utilitarian school who placed happiness as the highest level of attainment for the human soul. To them, virtue and happiness are as inseparable as a body and its shadow — virtue is the judicious pursuit of happiness. Their school placed a premium on the sensual, affectional and intellectual senses; these are the stair steps to happiness. Cobbe decried their ideal of "the greatest good (happiness) for the greatest number." She felt that one must renounce happiness as a goal; the soul progresses only through virtue. As though she were foreshadowing her future vivisectional trials, she believed that without trials, one's soul stands still. The soul leaps forward with giant strides when Providence hands it extraordinary trials.[22] Any suffering inflicted on man through these trials is just — it helps one attain virtue and is therefore "absolutely Good."[23] So needful are self-denial and self-sacrifice to the "hardihood" of the soul that, if not present, they must be created.[24]

This heavy load to carry through life was consistent with Frances' later free contributions of time and talent to egalitarian and humane causes. Certainly her aim was higher than that of the utilitarians, who could be accused of selfishly pursuing the senses. With her views on life now fully crystallized, valuable insights to her psyche are gained, explaining her future actions. Her grand exegesis completed in 1859, and with no formal home, Cobbe decided to broaden her perspective by taking the great international tour, something traditional for the British male upon completing his education.

With her habit of defying convention, Frances traveled alone for one year, something considered inappropriate for a proper lady. She traveled through Italy, France, Egypt and the Middle East, which was beneficial on two counts. It not only helped her build self-confidence, but seeing other women living independently in differing lifestyles made her desire the same situation for herself. On her return trip, she visited her Florentine friend Isa Blagden in her feminist enclave of English, French and American ex-patriots. Others, such as the Brownings and the Trollopes, lived close by, nursing their consumptive conditions. Feeling a great comfort in this cultural community, Frances returned here periodically over her lifetime.

## Social Pursuits

Upon her return to England, Cobbe hoped to pursue some activity addressing a social ill. Through Lady Byron, she arranged an interview with Mary Carpenter, a social activist who ran two ragged schools in Bristol. These schools, much like reformatories, were run by each parish and named for the tattered and wayward youth that attended them. Benefactors designed these schools for children who were creatures of the streets, similar to wharf rats, eking out an existence by scavenging. They crept barefoot along the pavement's edge, tattered, filthy, "pursuing the passer-by with a shrill, persistent beggar's whine."[25] Carpenter hoped to change these unemployable youngsters into well-behaved people with some rudimentary social skills, some self-respect and a chance to escape the only life they had ever known — crime and poverty.

Writer Jo Manton's description of Cobbe arriving for the interview is revelatory. "She was already hugely stout, with multiple chins and a booming jolly laugh. She now squeezed herself, along with her Pomeranian bitch, up the narrow stairs to meet her [future] landlady."[26] Although the two would remain friends for years, it was far from a perfect match. The Spartan Carpenter, used to working 16-hour days, was content to eat some ham for dinner and retire early, after preparing for her next day. Frances, despite her ascetic philosophical views, wanted lavish meals, wine, and long, meaningful conversations about religion. While Cobbe was also desirous of finding a life partner, the single-minded, indefatigable Carpenter had neither time nor interest in any such arrangement. Making matters worse, Cobbe found that she had little rapport with the young students. Surely, her future must lie elsewhere.

Remaining in Bristol, Cobbe taught at the reformatory Red Lodge School. There she met fellow teacher, Margaret Elliot, an impassioned advocate for workhouse improvement. Cobbe was vaguely aware of workhouses, where the most unfortunate of society were sequestered, pushed out of sight, but she had never harbored any interest in visiting one. Just as with ragged schools, each parish had to provide workhouses. The destitute entered here only when all other options, such as staying with family or friends, had run out. Spouses, married for years, would be split into wards of male and female paupers, while their younger children, separated from their families, received an education in a trade. Each floor housed people with different diagnoses, such as the "insane lunatics" and epileptics, but most moving was the floor that held those with incurable illnesses.

When Elliot finally persuaded Cobbe to visit a sick friend in St. Peter's Workhouse, she was appalled. Intense suffering and desperation were everywhere. Nursing care was rendered by fellow inmates, often inebriated, since they were compensated in gin for their efforts. Stirred by her encounter, Cobbe felt compelled to "put in my oar" for the workhouse reform waters.[27]

She and Elliot began lobbying the government for improvements. Cobbe raised money to support the facilities and penned an article in *Macmillan's* magazine entitled, "Workhouse Sketches." She advocated three points for the government to enact: First, if people are forced into workhouses, they should be treated as patients, not paupers. Second, the orphans there were supposed to be educated and made fit "to earn their bread honestly." Finally, the workhouse should provide for the sick, disabled, aged, helpless and suffering "a shelter which should partake of none of the penal elements which belong to the treatment of the idle and vicious pauper."[28] Cobbe's essay and her lobbying, along with the work of Florence Nightingale and others, launched a movement which resulted in improvement to all workhouses.[29]

One seemingly unremarkable event occurred in October 1862 that not only brought Cobbe's Bristol workhouse labors to an end, but shaded her views of science and physicians for a lifetime. While stepping out of a train in Bath, she lost her footing when she miscalculated the height of the platform, severely spraining her ankle. Faced with swelling, unremitting pain and disability, she consulted multiple physicians over the course of several months. Each one offered different advice, "elevate it, bear weight on it, don't bear weight on it, use heat, use ice, use a splint." Disgusted, she persevered, using crutches for nearly four years. Interestingly, a similar malady had rendered her mother an invalid years before, again with medical treatment being ineffective. Not surprisingly, Cobbe held physicians in contempt for the rest of her days. Several years later, when she had improved enough to climb Cader Idris, a mountain in Wales, she placed a sign at the summit, "Hang the Doctors," as a token of her unflagging contempt.[30]

Cobbe's ankle strain forced her away from social causes requiring any significant physical activity, pushing her more into literary pursuits. Before her Florence trip, while still in London, she had become a prolific writer, publishing essays in *Macmillan's*, *Fraser's* and other periodicals, sometimes using her name, sometimes anonymously. Her subjects varied from religion, to travel, to various aspects of equal rights — economic, political and legal.[31]

Given the Victorian attitudes towards women, she had entered fertile grounds. In "Criminals, Idiots, Women and Minors: Is This Classification Sound?," she wondered about marital law as it might appear to a visitor from another planet. "Why is the property of the woman who commits murder, and the property of the woman who commits Matrimony, dealt with alike by your law?" she inquired.[32] Cobbe argued in favor of women for the pulpit in "The Fitness of Women for the Ministry of Religion." In *The Final Cause of Women*, she contended that women should be defined in their own right. The concept of woman can only be acceptable by standing independently as noun; not woman as adjective, defined in terms of others.[33]

Cobbe was dismayed by the countless examples of women's disadvantaged state in society. It spurred her further into the field of women's rights. Early in her career she recognized the root cause for feminine powerlessness: Society as a whole considered women inferior to men. In her own Victorian view, men were likely smarter than their feminine counterparts, but women were more sympathetic than, more religious than and morally superior to men.[34] As such, they had a special task in this world that could be summed up in one word: Reform. She passionately carried the flag for social, political and economic equality of the sexes.

One area ripe for reform was women's suffrage. Accomplished, educated, taxpaying women had no voice in government whereas some ill-bred men of no means voted just because they possessed that appropriate appendage. According to Cobbe, the woman had a congenital defect that she could never hope to overcome. And for a "proud and gifted woman to be told that she is in every possible respect inferior to the footman who stands behind her chair, can hardly be thought pleasing intelligence."[35]

In marriage, the situation was even worse. Not only did the bride's dowry become the husband's possession immediately upon completion of the ceremony; he owned the bride herself. By custom, the husband had the right to "chastise" his wife, much as he might his horse or dog. Even though, in practice, this often included physical beatings, the general public seemed little bothered by it. If the man were brought to court because of serious injury or death of his wife, the judge typically handed down a lenient sentence, further piquing feminists' ire. In an 1878 *Contemporary Review* article, "Wife-Torture in England," Cobbe vented her righteous anger.

> How does it happen that the same generous-hearted gentlemen, who would themselves fly to render succor to a lady in distress, yet read of the beatings, burnings, kicking, and "cloggings" of *poor* women well-nigh every morning in their newspapers without once setting their teeth, and saying, "This must be stopped! We can stand it no longer!"[36]

Cobbe, of course, had earlier chafed at her first exposure to gender bias as an innocent teenager at Brighton school. As dictated by society — woman as adjective — young ladies were shaped into decorous ornaments for a masculine household. Whether as a teenager or later, Frances began to realize just how pervasive were the cultural restraints placed upon women. These restrictions produced in the young woman an excruciating disconnection from life, suffering in the midst of happiness, starvation at the core of plenty. The malady, peculiar to middle- and upper-class American and British women, persisted unnamed for decades. Many Victorian homes had a special room or attic set aside for the queer aunt or the strange sister, suffering from an affliction with no name. Initially, few physicians, social critics or even philosophers addressed the problem in any comprehensive manner.

The apparent lack of concern stemmed from lingering medieval attitudes about disease causation in general. Humors that boiled within a person, causing his disease, originated from within the bowels of the earth, far removed from human control. Many physicians and some women held similarly antiquated views concerning feminine behavior. Those supernatural forces dictating such conduct originated from a different planet, empowered by some mysterious interplay of lunar and endocrine cycles. Women were the fragile, passive victims of these powerful forces. Prominent Victorian gynecologist Dr. Edward Tilt contended that menstruation was so disruptive to the young woman's nervous system that menarche should be postponed as long as practical. Delay could be accomplished through such simple practices as avoiding feather beds, taking cold showers and wearing drawers. Tilt reckoned that it was this delay of menarche throughout Victorian culture that was "the principle cause of the pre-eminence of English women, in vigour of constitution, soundness of judgment, and ... rectitude of moral principle."[37]

Finally, in 1880, the affliction gained a name when American George Beard detailed his experience with the disease, writing *A Practical Treatise on Nervous Exhaustion* (Neurasthenia). Symptoms ran the psychological gamut, from tenderness of the scalp, loss of energy, noises in the ears, lack of concentration, depression, insomnia and morbid fears or phobias. Suicidal ideation was not uncommon. Treatments rendered were about as nonspecific as the symptoms, ranging from tonics, strychnine, arsenic, electrical stimulation, massage and even cannabis. Physicians agreed that rest, both physical and mental, constituted the most important part of the regimen. Patients were to give up all activities such as seeing friends, communicating, writing and keeping diaries.[38] Women, unsurprisingly, often deteriorated further under such regimens with consequent mental impairments ranging from neurasthenia, to hysteria, to full-blown insanity. Treating what ails one with a bigger dose of the same medicine could only eventuate in a more severe state of what ailed one in the first place. Suffering patients came to that realization earlier than did their doctors.

Along with other assertive women such as Charlotte Bronte and Florence Nightingale, Cobbe had become concerned with the spread of this feminine fragility. In one of her essays, "The Little Health of Ladies," she confronted the problem, bemoaning a society that had canonized "bodily and mental feebleness, cowardice, and helplessness among women."[39] Later, she lamented:

> That the Creator should have planned a whole sex of Patients — that the normal condition of the female of the human species should be to have legs which walk not, and brains which can only work on pain of disturbing the rest of the ill-adjusted machine — this to me is simply incredible.[40]

Much of the blame for this sad state of affairs Cobbe placed directly on practicing physicians — like their ulterior motives in encouraging valetudinarianism in women. In Cobbe's view, these women represented the ideal patient for the avaricious physician to recruit. Coming from the wealthier classes, and never improving clinically, such women were ever dependent on their doctors, paying for interminable care — an unending monetary fount to the physicians' livelihood. Cobbe's remedy made eminent sense:

> Let women have larger interests and nobler pursuits, and their affections will become not less strong and deep, but less sickly, less craving for demonstrative tenderness in return, less variable in their manifestations. Let women have sounder mental culture, and their emotions — so long exclusively fostered — will return to the calmness of health, and we shall hear no more of the intermittent feverish spirits, the causeless depressions, and all the long train of symptoms which belong to Protean-formed Hysteria, and open the way to madness on one side and to sin on the other.[41]

Cobbe persisted in her consciousness-raising efforts on behalf of women. In her writing and campaigning, she proposed legislation to protect women from different forms of prejudice. In one such effort she was instrumental in Parliament's passing the Matrimonial Causes Act of 1878, an act that strengthened the woman's position against a physically abusive husband.[42] Cobbe's efforts even influenced legislation 20 years later in the Summary Jurisdiction Act of 1895. This act not only allowed women to leave an abusive relationship but even to occasionally gain custody of her children.[43]

With her vigilance, acerbic wit and trenchant insights, Cobbe rose to great popularity with women in general. When it came to the spectrum of feminist concerns from suffrage, to educational opportunities, to matrimonial problems, women knew their interests would be forcefully voiced whenever Frances Cobbe approached the dais.

CHAPTER 2

# *The Rights of Man and the Claims of Brutes*

In 1862, Cobbe delivered a speech at the National Association for the Promotion of Social Science (NAPSS), advocating that women be admitted to the university examination system in London. With her reputation growing, her speech, while well received by women, was vilified in the press. The *Spectator* thought that such an action would put half the young women in the country in brain fever or a lunatic asylum. Or the "enlightened" opinion expressed by a writer in the *Saturday Review* who would have been more likely to listen to speeches by women if they did not have *Miss* before their names: "an unmarried woman is only half a woman, and therefore can only deliver half-truths."[1]

Several events further sharpened Cobbe's nascent feminist views, the first being her own upbringing. With her "decorous" Brighton education and her feeling of dependency and vulnerability at her father's death, she saw a need for practical feminine education and independence. In addition, her experience in Bristol workhouses convinced her that she had the ability to make a difference through both writing and agitation. In 1861 she wrote "Celibacy v. Marriage," for *Fraser's* magazine, validating the single woman and arguing again for feminine education.

Until 1863, Cobbe had virtually no experience with physiologists or their methods of experimentation. While nursing her ankle sprain at Aix-les-Bains, a spa in southeastern France, she read an article concerning teaching methods used at a prestigious veterinary school in Alfort, France. In these Napoleonic times, horses were still instruments of war. As the animals grew infirm and too old for military purposes, the government sent them to Alfort, so that students might gain greater operative dexterity operating on them. It was a common, 100-year practice to have eight veterinary students operating in "musical chairs" fashion on eight un-anesthetized horses over a 10-hour period.

The students learned operative exposure of the chest and abdomen, operations on the hooves and legs, and other parts. Appalled by such practices, the Royal Society for the Protection of Animals (RSPCA) first petitioned the emperor in 1861 to stop the practice. Their plea fell upon deaf Napoleonic ears. Two years later, the editors of *Lancet* initiated their own agitation, further exposing the Alfort problem. As Cobbe read the *Lancet* article, she became increasingly disturbed by the gratuitous cruelty of such a practice.

This *Lancet* revelation inspired the creation of her seminal essay on animal welfare, *The Rights of Man and the Claims of Brutes*. In it she wondered how people could allow such atrocious activity to go on. With likely hyperbole, she described "the mangled creatures, hoofless, eyeless, burned, gashed, eviscerated, skinned, mutilated in every conceivable way."[2] Cobbe composed her entire essay while receiving treatment at the spa. Her piece became a virtual manifesto of vivisectional ethics as of 1863, an analysis of her principles of human behavior towards beasts. In an essay of tedious reasoning she poses three questions. First, what constitutes cruelty to animals? Second, what are man's duties to "the brute"? And last, how does that duty rank in comparison to duties to his fellow man?

Certain aspects of her attitudes and opinions expressed in this essay would echo throughout her subsequent writings, such as her declaration that all higher animals are sentient beings, and as such, are capable of enjoying happiness and pleasure. Happiness is their highest state of attainment. Since man is not only sentient but rational and moral, he is capable of a higher attainment — that of virtue. In a natural order, the rational being takes precedence over the merely sentient one. Man, being of moral character, must not only avoid cruelty, but must ensure the happiness of the lower being. Additionally, "everything which could be fairly interpreted to be a 'want' for man must have precedence over even the life of the animal."[3] It is therefore permissible to kill animals for legitimate "wants" such as food or clothing but not for wantonness — that is, an illegitimate or gratuitous desire. Likewise, man can inflict pain if it is towards a legitimate purpose, but not for sheer wantonness.

Next Cobbe argued that man may take an animal's life if it is for a legitimate scientific need. However, there must be no needless infliction of pain. Since anesthetics had been introduced in 1847, vivisectors could not now justify the infliction of pain unless they were investigating phenomena in which the anesthetic might interfere with the results of the experiment. In short, by Cobbe's reasoning, if animals could speak, they would say, "Respect Our Lives!" In her final pages, Cobbe concludes in prayerful but preachy eloquence:

> If there be one moral offense which more than another seems directly an offence against God, it is this wanton infliction of pain upon His creatures.... In a word, He places them absolutely in our charge.... Surely as sins of the flesh sink man

below humanity, so sins of cruelty throw him into the very converse and antagonism of Diety; he becomes not a mere Brute but a Fiend.[4]

It would be hard to argue that her views were anything but rational and moderate at this point in her life.

As a humanitarian, Cobbe was frequently criticized for eating meat but her views, as expressed above, are entirely consistent with that position. People accused her of having a double standard. Why was she so hard on vivisectionists when she made excuses for the fox hunter and cock fighter? But she defended the sportsmen by stating,

> The men ... may plead at least the excuses of custom and of partial ignorance. Turn we, on the other hand, to those boasted motives of lofty and far-sighted philanthropy which are alleged to spur the vivisector to his ugly work in his laboratory, where no fern brakes or heathery hills, no fresh breezes or dancing streams such as throw enchantment round the pursuits of the sportsman, are present to cast any glamour over the process of torture, and where no chance of escape on the part of the brute, or risk to his own person, may stir his pulse with the manly struggle for victory.[5]

In 1863, with her first animal protection article behind her, and her ankle still giving her grief, Cobbe made a fateful trip to Villa Brichieri in Florence, to visit her old friend Isa Blagden. Drawn to this enclave of cohabiting women, Cobbe hoped to find a life partner. She envisioned such a relationship as more equal and spiritually ideal than the usual heterosexual one, unless the latter relationship was based entirely on love. She had already seen too much of the usual male-dominated marriage. Settling in Florence, she mingled with Robert and Elizabeth Barrett Browning, American actress Charlotte Cushman, Harriet Beecher Stowe and the retired mathematician Mary Somerville, who had become a surrogate mother to her. Somerville introduced Cobbe to the Welsh sculptor Mary Lloyd, Cobbe's eventual life partner.

Honoring Mary's request for privacy, Frances never publicly offered any description or details of her while she was alive, only referring to her as "my dear friend." In Cobbe's 1904 autobiography, published seven years after Mary's death, Cobbe described her as a gifted sculptor and artist, with a self-effacing manner, a quick sense of humor and a "keen, highly-cultivated intellect."[6] Acquaintances, however, offered a different picture, describing Mary as dark, moody, and pessimistic, bordering on anti-social. Cobbe was understandably mum about the details of their relationship, but in conversation and letters she referred to Mary in spousal terms. Also in her autobiography written at age eighty, Cobbe proclaimed:

> God has given me two priceless benedictions in life,—in my youth a perfect mother; in my later years a perfect Friend. No other gifts, had I possessed them,

Genius or beauty, or fame, or the wealth of the Indies, would have been worthy to compare with the joy of those affections.[7]

While still in Florence, Cobbe and Miss Blagden were holding a reception in Villa Brichieri when an interesting visitor, Dr. Appleton of Harvard University, approached her. Earlier, in 1860, Appleton had accompanied the terminally consumptive Theodore Parker to Italy, attending to him during his final days. On this visit the doctor described some animal cruelty that he had witnessed firsthand in the Specola, run by Professor Mauritz Schiff, physiologist, trained by the eminent Parisian Claude Bernard. In her autobiography, Cobbe later claimed that Appleton had personally seen atrocities carried out on dogs, pigeons and other animals, putting them in a "frightfully mangled and suffering state." A Tuscan officer had reportedly seen a cat so mistreated that he forced Schiff to kill it.[8] Not only did Schiff reportedly sacrifice 700 dogs annually during the course of his experiments, but neighbors had also complained to authorities about the nocturnal howls and moans emanating from his laboratory.

Cobbe apparently never knew about the nature of Schiff's experiments. She never mentioned it in her writings. As early as 1859, he had reported on the effects of removing the thyroid glands from both guinea pigs and dogs. He observed a consistent picture in such animals of anemia, tremulousness, swelling of the soft tissues, and progressive mental dullness culminating in death at six weeks. If he implanted the animals' own excised glands in their abdomens, he could extend their lives for several more months. Concluding that some vital element resided within the thyroid gland, Schiff even suggested treating the human condition with an emulsion of the gland.[9] Unfortunately, the results of his research languished, neglected for nearly 30 years until resurrected by others, such as Victor Horsley.

Incensed by the inherent cruelty she perceived in Schiff's experiments, Cobbe felt that she must immediately oppose his activities. She sprang into action, first writing an anonymous letter to the English-speaking *Daily News* describing his atrocities. She also composed a petition to the scientist, requesting that he stop such cruel activities. Friends eagerly circulated her petition, gathering 783 signatures, including nearly all of the old Florentine aristocracy. Schiff responded, first to the *Daily News* letter, demanding to know its author and denying the charges. He stated that such petitions were "absolutely useless."[10] Claiming to believe in the "holy cause of protecting animals," he denied ever treating them unkindly. Some of Schiff's co-workers came to his defense as well, attesting to his humanity in subsequent newspaper articles. In January 1864, an observer of Schiff, Fabio Uccelli of Pisa University, recalled, "with real pleasure seeing some puppies whose spleens had been removed running happily to brush affectionately against the distinguished scientist's feet."[11]

Schiff performed most of his experiments on dead animals. Those performed on live subjects, whether dogs, cats, rabbits and even frogs, were always performed under ether anesthesia.[12] Schiff invited Cobbe and her protesters to his laboratory to observe physiological experimentation themselves, but no one accepted his offer. In fact, there is no evidence that Cobbe, at any time during her antivivisection years, ever visited the physiological laboratories that she so hated.

Cobbe wrote a rebuttal to Schiff's article in *La Nazione*, but the editors would not grant her free space. Determined to get her feelings known, she finally purchased space in the advertising section. But her article enjoyed popularity only among her friends. The regular Italian citizens resented an English woman coming to their country and putting her non-scientific nose into scientific business. Italians loved animals but looked upon them more as utilitarian creatures. Cobbe and her friends attributed human traits to dogs, pampering and expressing excessive love for them. By Italian standards, such anthropomorphism was very strange, indeed.

On the other hand, Cobbe put much of the blame for this Italian tolerance of cruelty on the Catholic Church's anthropocentric views of animals. The Church's *Summa Theologica* stated that animals are not rational and are created for man's use.[13] The Church later made its position clear in the *Catholic Encyclopedia*. Vivisection is permissible when it is done for scientific purposes. Similarly, animal protection societies were considered proper so long as they did not incorporate animal rights, a sense of charitable duty, or include "sentimental love for inferior creatures."[14] Disgusted with the lack of respect given animals in Florence, Cobbe departed with her new mate, Mary, for the more compatible London scene.

Schiff continued his work in Florence for more than a decade, his dual reputation unchanged. Students considered his courses in physiology exemplary, feeling fortunate to be able to attend them. In 1873, Schiff, who believed in the humanitarian treatment of animals, became one of the founding members of the Society for the Protection of Animals in Florence. A large number of foreign members belonged to the society, including one unnamed, rotund spinster from London who had become a formidable force in her own right.

In September 1873, responding to some agitators who wanted to keep pressure on Schiff, three aristocratic Florentine residents brought suit against him. The charges were for disturbances caused by "the heart-rending howls of animals in pain, caused by the operation to which they are subjected night and day."[15] Then, just prior to trial, one of the plaintiffs, Marquis Capponi, suddenly withdrew his complaint. Not satisfied, Schiff insisted that the trial proceed, to demonstrate to the community just how baseless were the charges in the first place. Although Schiff's protest was in vain, he did receive a statement from the Marquis stating, "I have never believed, nor do I believe now, that the howling that disturbed me was caused by his methods of experimentation."[16] Evidently, other parties had pressured the plaintiffs to initiate the suit. Cobbe revealed in 1894 that she and others of the Florentine society had led this skirmish against Schiff from the beginning.[17] Schiff ultimately grew tired of the vendetta against him and his work. In 1876, the scientist Carl Vogt invited him to carry on his work at the University of Geneva. Schiff quickly accepted—a great loss to the city of Florence. In Geneva he worked in a peaceful environment for the rest of his career.

## From Dead to Living Tissue

The activity in Florence that Cobbe found so atrocious was practiced only sporadically by a few even though vivisection was an old form of scientific inquiry. In the first half of the 19th century, particularly in England, anatomical dissection, not physiology, represented the *sine qua non* of medical education. But England's near-exclusive reliance on anatomical inquiry revealed a

Frances Power Cobbe, age 55. She considered this her favorite photograph, since it enhanced her image as "a formidable old woman." (Reproduced with permission of Mary Evans Picture Library/The Woman's Library.)

deeper dilemma: Medical science had never developed beyond the study of structure. Physicians' understanding of anatomy and disease causation was simplistic and often erroneous, little changed from ancient and Renaissance times. Unlike other contemporary disciplines, such as geology or botany, medicine was still practiced more by artisans than scientists. Physicians had little idea of how the body actually functioned, either in the normal or pathologic state.

Some of the more visionary scientists recognized the advantages of superceding structure by advancing to the study of bodily function. While anatomy is passive—the study of static, dead tissue—experimental science (physiology) is dynamic, the assertive study of living tissue. Here the scientist could pose a question, formulate a hypothesis, and set up an experiment with all variables controlled. He could repeat the experiment as many times as necessary to ensure the proper conclusion.

With ignorance of bodily function the norm, areas for inquiry for even a minimally inquisitive physician were virtually endless. During an operation a surgeon might observe that, while the blood leaving the heart en route to the lungs was dark, when it exited the lungs, returning to the heart, it was bright red. How and why do such changes occur? How do the heart and lungs interact? Is blood flowing in a large artery subject to the same principles of physics as is water flowing inside of a pipe? How do diseases begin within the body? How do they develop? In how many different ways might they manifest themselves as the face of disease before spontaneously resolving or leading to death?

Anatomy was still important to physiology. Young physicians and scientists learned to understand physical and chemical processes in the context of bodily structure. Famed experimental scientist Claude Bernard stated it best, several decades later, when he declared:

> [Physiologists] follow a different idea from the anatomists. The latter, as we have seen, try to infer the source of life from anatomy: they therefore adopt an anatomical plan. Physiologists adopt another plan and follow a different conception: instead of proceeding from the organ to the function, they start from the physiological phenomenon and seek its explanation in the organism.[18]

Physiology, of necessity, is closely structured around the parts of the body where the actions take place, the functioning cells, blood vessels and associated nerves.[19] In the days before modern chemistry and physics, function of tissue was the physiologist's lowest common denominator.

This ideological leap from anatomy to the study of function had not happened in England for a reason. An old Roman attitude persisted there— an exalted view of things cerebral coupled with a disdain for manual pursuits.[20] Surgeons were apprentice-trained, while physicians held university degrees. It was inadvisable for physicians to actually get their hands dirty operating on humans because of the stigma associated with it. Even when a doctor ordered bloodletting, it was an apprentice-trained apothecary who actually withdrew the blood. In addition, natural theology reigned supreme, with medicine subordinate to it. Medical leaders did not possess the necessary vision, temerity or ideological autonomy to head off in a new direction without the accompaniment of theologians.

Transformation had to materialize in France, where the proper nutritional stew had been simmering for decades. It was the French Revolution and the crucial decade of the 1790s that facilitated such changes. Up to that time, medical educators had approached learning much like a religion. Students studied, memorized and regurgitated a catechism — the study of medical doctrines — theories handed down from authorities based not upon science but upon their individual musings. Disease causation was still explained within a context of the four humors. Students spent more time in the library than they did with sleeves rolled up, observing medical problems directly. Recognizing the weaknesses of such a method, the new French regime put a stop to that scheme by centering learning within the large public hospitals. A student at the bedside learned about disease by dealing directly with the suffering patient and the autopsied corpse. Additionally, research, always valued in France, grew stronger under the new political regime. Consequently vivisection ascended naturally as research flourished.

## Necessary Inhumanity

Were vivisectors really as evil and cruel as portrayed by humanitarians? Many anatomists and experimental scientists in the early stages of physiology were often called cruel or unfeeling. Was that image accurate or was there some other explanation? Around 1780, William Hunter, English anatomist and midwife, while lecturing to medical students, claimed that anatomy "informs the Head, guides the hand, and familiarizes the heart to a kind of necessary Inhumanity."[21] Such emotional distancing from the task at hand was vital. It helped the practitioner cope, whether dealing with dead flesh, whining animals, bleeding bodies or grieving families. Now well recognized as a defense mechanism that deliberately objectifies the subject, "clinical detachment" allows the practitioner to function — to view or perform acts on the living or the dead, human or animal, that in other contexts would be considered an atrocity — unbearably repugnant. In some situations the practitioner might appear merely professionally objective, while in others, he may seem uncaring or even cruel. When does one's behavior cross over that line into abnormality?

## England Is the Hell of Dumb Animals

But to be fair, one has to first judge the behavior of these vivisectors within the context from which they arose. In England gratuitous animal torment had a long and perversely rich tradition. A young William Shakespeare was no stranger to such cruelty. He spent the majority of his working years outside the jurisdiction of London's officials, immersed in the urban areas of entertainment where people engaged in fisticuffs, danced, guzzled beer or just loitered about while pickpockets and prostitutes worked the crowds. He drew his inspiration from the carnival-like atmosphere, the Elizabethan sports and the cruel competitions. Henry VIII and Queen Elizabeth both brought visiting dignitaries to the omnipresent bull- or bearbaiting contests adjacent to Shakespeare's theater.[22] Cockpits might host a dogfight, a cockfight or feature a solitary dog systematically killing rats as they were released from a sack. The audience placed bets on how quickly the dog might decimate the pack.[23] In another variety of entertainment, the operators tied a monkey on to the back of a pony while releasing a pack of attack dogs. "To see the animal kicking amongst the dogs, with the screams of the ape, beholding the curs hanging from the ears and neck of the pony is very laughable," wrote one visitor.[24]

But institutional cruelty began 400 years before Shakespeare's time. In 1204, the Earl of Warren, traveling through England as an emissary of King John, happened upon a game of animal harassment called bull running. In such a game, the bull's owner released the animal into a confined area of a village, forcing the bull to seek cover from the villagers who were intent upon injuring him with clubs, rocks, knives or other sharp objects. The earl thought the spectacle such fun that he convinced the king to officially sanction the activity. His royal edict provided meadows to the commoners enabling the sport to flourish.[25]

The object of such contests was simple — either kill the bull or weaken it to a level that brought some sense of satisfaction to the tormentor. In one of the other more popular forms of bullbaiting, organizers tethered the animal to a rope connected to a stake in the ground. The rope, perhaps 20 feet in length, was just long enough to allow the animal some maneuverability. Otherwise he was left to his own devices. Specially bred bulldogs were unleashed, usually several at a time, attacking the bull from all angles. Endowed with prominent underbite and wide nostrils, such dogs could continue breathing while hanging on. The bull kept his head low in an attempt to snag the most threatening dog with a horn to the belly, throwing him into the air. A veteran bull developed skills for trampling any dog that ended underfoot, usually ending with the dog's death. With multiple dogs attacking, one would sooner or later find its target — the bull's neck, snout, lip or tongue — hanging on forever with all the might of his tenacious grip. Once the dog attached himself, the bull's defenses were reduced to ineffective attempts at shaking the dog loose with upper-body movements.

With the roar of the crowd, moans of anguish, clouds of dust and pools of blood, the bull might finally fall, bleeding, too exhausted to continue the fight. More often the aggressor dogs received the worst in the exchange, being thrown in the air, spines or legs broken upon landing — or bellies ripped open, entrails sliding out. In smaller towns animal baiting, be it bull, bear, badger or monkey, was often the main feature of a festival, accompanied by beer, betting and a general good time. Bullbaiting was so popular that some townships had ordinances declaring that all bulls must be baited before they could be butchered. A theory circulated that the juices stirred up in the process of the fight preceding an animal's dying in distress, sweetened the meat — a sort of pre-mortem marinade. For jaded and overworked factory employees the fights provided a respite from their bleak, miasmatic, slum-dwelling existence.

Cock throwing was another popular sport, in which the losing bird from a one-on-one cockfight was the singular target — his moral retribution for losing. Participants, working within a pit or some restricted portion of a neighborhood, threw anything convenient such as cudgels, stones or pieces of wood at the poor bird. Breaking some bones was the object of the game. The spectacle continued until someone finally delivered the fatal blow. If birds were in short supply, people discovered that they could extend the life of their current crop by greasing them. Now, objects thrown at the bird would glance off more easily, prolonging the pleasures of the game. Since the birds were small, young boys often played the game in the schoolyard before the bell.

In 1825, one frustrated journalist, witnessing the ubiquity of animal cruelty, had to regretfully agree with the old proverb "England is the hell of dumb animals."[26] Early humanists, as well, looked on aghast, repulsed by such barbaric forms of public entertainment. Sometimes they raised their voices in protest, but they generally went unheeded. In an attitude reminiscent of Rome, the early 18th century public cultivated cruelty rather than discouraged it. If the sport involved youth, one could rationalize their actions. These young men had to be fierce for future sea battles, or to put down insurrections in some territorial colony. Dealing with blood and cruelty was almost a rite of passage. No laws of consequence existed against such acts.

## Humane Origins

Western religion has been relatively silent regarding man's relationship with animals as fellow occupants of the world. The Bible contains sporadic references to man's treatment of animals but no encompassing doctrine has ever been expounded. Around A.D. 400, the theologian and philosopher St. Augustine asserted that humans were preeminent. Man had no right to rule over other men but he did have the right to rule over animals. In his grand scheme, it was God over man, man over animals and animals over plants.

In the 1200s, the great theologian and educator St. Thomas Aquinas recognized a hierarchical order much like St. Augustine had envisioned. Humans were immortal because they possessed the ability to reason. Since animals cannot reason, they cannot be immortal. Furthermore, animals were created for use by man and that use is unlimited. However, these rules come with some caveats: One must not misuse animals, because in doing so, one also misuses man. Aquinas' views therefore provided a theological basis not only for experimentation on animals but also for utilizing them for food, clothing, motive powers and whatever other use man deemed necessary, so long as that use was not abusive.

Generally, philosophers were more vocal than theologians on the matter of animal cruelty. In the 17th century René Descartes, with his polarizing theory separating mind from body, often spoke about human and animal relationships. He viewed animals, including the dog, as insensate mechanisms, only capable of reflex activity. Since animals could not reason, they possessed no soul. They were in effect, automatons. His views, so antithetical to the later humane movement, were readily accepted by vivisectionists.[27]

In the early 1700s, a gradual elevation of social consciousness occurred concerning the subject of animal cruelty. One of the first of the humanitarians to give voice to this evolving sentiment was an obscure minister, Reverend Humphry Primatt. Sensing that his views might resonate with some enlightened minds, Primatt, in 1776, wrote *A Dissertation on the Duty of Mercy and Sin of Cruelty to Brute Animals*. His book is considered the cornerstone of the present-day Royal Society for the Prevention of Cruelty to Animals (RSPCA). His treatise is a vivid religious plea for mercy towards lesser beings. In God's and Primatt's world, both man and animals are part of the grand design. Although man may sit at the top of the heap, he must still treat all beings below him with the utmost of respect:

> Now, if amongst men, the differences of their powers of the mind, and of their complexion, stature and accidents of fortune, do not give any one man a right to abuse or insult any other man on account of these differences, for the same reason, a man can have no natural right to abuse and torment a beast, merely because a beast has not the mental powers of a man.[28]

To Primatt, cruelty, the wanton infliction of pain on another being, is the great evil, the worst of heresies. Cruelty is atheism itself. "Pain is pain ... and the creature that suffers it, whether man or beast, being sensible of the misery of it whilst it lasts, suffers *evil*."[29] Cobbe often quoted this sentiment in the heat of her debates against science. It still resonates with contemporary animal welfare theorists.[30]

Since God has granted man dominion over all creatures, humans have a right to eat the flesh of animals for their own sustenance, Primatt reasoned.

However, in the animal's preparation, one must not cause a lingering death or unnecessary pain. As Primatt stated, "I ought to dispatch him suddenly and with the least degree of pain."[31]

As the English populace moved from country to city with the industrial revolution, people's attitudes towards animals became progressively more enlightened. Still, it was hard to discern any improvement in everyday scenes of life. Filth and cruelty on the street were ever present, especially in larger metropolitan areas. London was crowded with dogs, horses and cattle. Ducks and geese were driven by the hundreds through the streets to market. Cowsheds, dairies and abattoirs were scattered randomly throughout urban areas. At mid-century, Smithfield stock market, sitting in the middle of London, sold on average 5,000 cattle, 30,000 sheep and 2,000 pigs per week.[32] Farmers typically drove their livestock from farm to market, a journey of several days, without any food or water. Sheep or cattle, too exhausted to continue the trek were commonly flogged as they lay in the spot where they fell.

Beginning in the early 19th century, humanitarians, gaining in both numbers and savvy, began strategizing. In an effort to improve their effectiveness, they examined some of the more successful aspects of the abolitionist movement which had begun in 1787.[33] Just as abolitionists had done before them, humanitarians began using pamphlets and town hall meetings to voice their concerns. They also appropriated an iconic phrase attributed to Josiah Wedgewood, renowned ceramicist and grandfather to Charles Darwin. Earlier, Wedgewood had requested his artisans to create a seal suitable for the stamping of wax on envelopes. The seal featured an African male, kneeling in chains, with uplifted hands asking, "Am I not a Man and a Brother?" The image proved so poignant that it set off an explosion of replications, spreading enlightenment on cuff links, snuff boxes and sundry items.[34] Humanitarians modified the phrase to "Are not dumb beasts, man's *animal* slaves, worthy of compassion too?" The impact proved similarly evocative, giving further voice to abused animals, long suffering in silence.[35]

Certain public spectacles, carried out by sadistic profiteers, further stoked public sentiment against animal cruelty. In one such event, festival organizers in Surrey scheduled a bull for celebratory baiting on Guy Fawkes Day. Since the animal's attendants considered the bull to be insufficiently fearsome, they enraged him by repeatedly pricking him with knives. Just prior to releasing the bull into the ring, the men resorted to another not uncommon tactic — cutting off all four hooves. The pathos of watching a gang of bulldogs released on an animal that could barely get up on all fours was more than most in the crowd could stand, resulting in a huge public outcry. A local paper, *The Bury Post*, editorialized, "Good God! In what age, in what country, do we live?... The beast is tortured merely for the diversion of savages."[36] Such events, meant to heighten entertainment, had the opposite effect, repulsing and angering the public.

Inevitably, legislation came. In 1822, the year of Cobbe's birth, Parliamentarian Richard Martin, a colorful Irishman from Galway, became the first to succeed in passing a law protecting animals from cruelty. His bill prevented the ill treatment of horses and cattle, but through some legislative sleight of hand, bullbaiting escaped the ban. Despite the bill's weaknesses, it represented a milestone — the first legislative act in the world to address the general subject of animal cruelty.

In June 1824, partly as a result of the Martin Act, another seminal event took place in London's ironically named Old Slaughter Coffee House. It was a meeting "for a Society instituted for the purpose of preventing cruelty to animals" (SPCA). Brandishing a fresh copy of Primatt's treatise, founder Rev. Arthur Broome used it as his guide and inspiration throughout the formative years of the Society. After some early financial difficulties the Society finally began to flourish, broadening its membership and prestige over the ensuing decades. In 1840 the SPCA gained the queen's imprimatur, becoming the RSPCA.[37]

Initially the RSPCA carried out widespread educational programs with the aim of minimizing wanton street cruelty. As the Society gained a better financial foothold, its strategy added another feature — policing and enforcing the Martin Act of 1822. In 1835, Parliament extended the law to protect all domestic and farm animals from wanton cruelty, increasing opportunities for the prosecution of offenders. As the RSPCA gained financial strength, it acquired a private force of constables to carry out the arrests, working in cooperation with city police forces.

The Society published an annual report of litigated cases, giving details of the incident in factual but predictable, formulaic prose designed to emphasize the cruelty involved. The abused were described as "noble, suffering or exhausted," while the abusers were "filthy, rough or of low character."[38] Cruelty to draught horses constituted over eighty percent of all cases prosecuted. Pulling wagons was typically the last job given to elderly horses before they were assigned to the knacker's yard, where their meat was rendered into dog food and their bones into a variety of products. Near the end of their journey, such horses were commonly weak, under-nourished, and suffering from ailments such as injured fetlocks or ulcerated hide from ill-fitting harnesses. As the horses' monetary worth sank commensurate with their inability to pull their load, they were ripe for abuse. Seeing a drover venting his frustrations on the back of a horse with a whip, cudgel, stick or iron bar was all too common a spectacle. In the first year of the program's existence, 147 successful prosecutions were completed. The number later plateaued at approximately

8,000 cases annually, until the engine replaced the horse as the primary means of locomotion.[39]

As the major embodiment of the general humanitarian cause, the RSPCA became its major enforcer. But that vexing problem, vivisection, caused a schism within its ranks. In the 1860s, when physiology was not yet a significant force in England, the RSPCA chose to ignore isolated reports of vivisectional atrocities. Most prosecutions for cruelty brought by the RSPCA were against the poor, since they were the drovers, costermongers and farm hands — the ones dealing with the older, struggling animals on a daily basis.

Staunch humanitarians, such as Martin, were completely set against vivisection, since it was "too revolting to be palliated by any excuse that Science may be enlarged or improved by so detestable a means."[40] But to many, this group of well educated, pioneering scientists known as physiologists represented a different moral category.[41] The majority of RSPCA members considered the scientists' activities acceptable so long as their efforts were guided by a true sense of scientific inquiry. That was the prevalent attitude at midcentury near the time of Cobbe's entrance upon the scene.

Cobbe's attitude towards these two groups was just the opposite. She excused the English public and their gratuitous cruelty. But, with some level of credence, she charged the vivisectors' indulgences in such animal atrocities as inexcusable. They were miscreants, posing behind a façade of science. But one diligent and idealistic young medical student, Joseph Lister, introduced a different perspective to the debate. Lister was strongly influenced by his revered professor of physiology, William Sharpey, a man who served as a link to the physiological past. Sharpey's own youthful Parisian experiences provide an elucidating glimpse at those who founded modern physiology in France — the most direct link to England. It was these early French physiologists who gave Frances Cobbe her ominous sense of foreboding, and who initially fueled her righteous indignation.

# II

# GRATUITOUS VERSUS JUSTIFIED EXPLOITATION

"Turning from nation to classes, we find as a rule that the most cultivated are the most merciful.... In France, alas! It is men of science — men belonging to the learned professions — who disembowel living horses and open the brains of dogs." — Frances Power Cobbe[1]

CHAPTER 3

# The Early Vivisectors

If one were to select a person possessing the characteristics necessary to lead a revolutionary movement against some great scourge in medicine, Joseph Lister would hardly have been that man. He was born into wealth in 1827, to a genteel Quaker family at Upton House, in London. All Friends, as they were called, were expected to lead simple, frugal lives, free of ostentation in both dress and habits. Pursuit of such self-indulgent pastimes as theater, music and dance was discouraged. Proper Quakers used the appellations "thee and thou," not only when conversing among themselves but even with family members. Young Joseph revered his father both for his success and his sober dependability. He was not only a successful wine merchant, but an acclaimed microscopist, who contributed greatly to the science of optics by introducing the achromatic lens into the field. Such lenses improved image quality by minimizing any mal-alignment of light rays. Through this accomplishment the elder Lister gained acceptance into the prestigious Royal Society in 1832. After Joseph left home in pursuit of his becoming a surgeon, he sent detailed letters chronicling his thoughts and accomplishments along the way. His father served as both Joseph's confidant and sounding board. Cursed with less than robust health for much of his life, Joseph the son suffered from a congenital stammer as well. With the anxiety of public speaking, his impediment invariably increased, leaving him further embarrassed and humiliated. However, with practice and increasing success, he slowly conquered his problem, maturing into an accomplished speaker.

As a Quaker, Joseph could attend neither Oxford nor Cambridge Universities, since both institutions were reserved for members of the Anglican faith. He enrolled at University College, London, where he excelled in science and the classics. At 21, however, he passed into an unexplainable period of depression and hyper-religiosity, finally suffering a full "nervous breakdown" in March 1848. He could do nothing but rest and travel for more than one year. As his recovery ensued, friends noted a certain flattening of his affect, a permanent loss of his prior youthful spontaneity. As a result, Lister's interpersonal relationships were forever marred by a certain emotional stiffness. Another vestige of his mental breakdown involved a lifelong aversion to direct confrontation, as though the mental strife involved in debate would be too emotionally taxing for him. Instead, he preferred to carry out disagreements in written form. Sufficiently improved by the autumn of 1849, he re-enrolled at University College, registering for botany and pre-clinical studies.[1] Despite such questionable traits, Lister's intelligence and strong sense of conviction would serve to carry him through his pioneering role in medicine.

In medical school Lister was heavily influenced by William Sharpey, the first British professor to teach a course dedicated purely to physiology. In the early 1850s, physiology was still considered a developmental appendage of anatomy.[2] As his tenure at University College endured, Sharpey became known as the Father of Physiology in Britain. He was venerated not so much as a scientist, but as a lecturer and as one who took great personal interest in his students. Half of Sharpey's career transpired before the advent of anesthesia in 1846, but he still believed, unlike some physiologists from his past, that most experimental science could be practiced satisfactorily while avoiding atrocious acts on animals.

## François Magendie, the French Butcher

In 1821, after the young William Sharpey had just completed his London education, he visited Paris to study anatomy for one year under the famous surgeon, Guillaume Dupuytren.[3] While in Paris he encountered two important individuals. The first was fellow student and Parisian visitor, James Syme, future iconic Professor of Surgery at Edinburgh University. Syme would, as well, loom large both personally and professionally in the life of Joseph Lister.[4] Sharpey and Syme became lifelong friends as they later headed back to Great Britain. While in Paris, Sharpey attended a series of lectures given by physiologist François Magendie at the College de France. Sharpey later recalled being "so utterly repelled by what I witnessed that I never went back again."[5] Magendie seemed to take great pleasure in causing pain, cutting into the skin of rabbits in front of students just to confirm the obvious: Rabbit skin was sensitive. He often repeated painful experiments unnecessarily, well after the point of his lecture had been made. One demonstration Sharpey found especially abhorrent involved a study on the mechanism of vomiting. Magendie surgically replaced a dog's stomach with a pig's bladder. After filling the implanted bladder with water, he induced vomiting in the dog by injecting a powerful emetic, thereby demonstrating that the stomach, despite having muscles in its wall, was only passively involved in the act of vomiting. The stomach contents were emptied through pressure transmitted from the diaphragm and muscles in the abdomen and chest wall.[6] To Sharpey, the information gained by the experiment was not at all worth the pain and suffering involved in setting it up. Sharpey retained such a simmering dislike for Magendie that he made him the object of barbed comments during the course of his own 38-year physiology lectureship at University College. To Sharpey, Magendie was the personification of physiological cruelty.

Undoubtedly, Magendie did symbolize a newer blend of early–19th-century physiology — prodigious, competent and cruel. Firmly ensconced at the College de France, his experimentation was wide ranging and often groundbreaking. With more than a little feigned humility, he claimed, "I am a mere street scavenger of science with my hook in my hand and my basket on my back. I go about the streets of science, collecting what I find."[7]

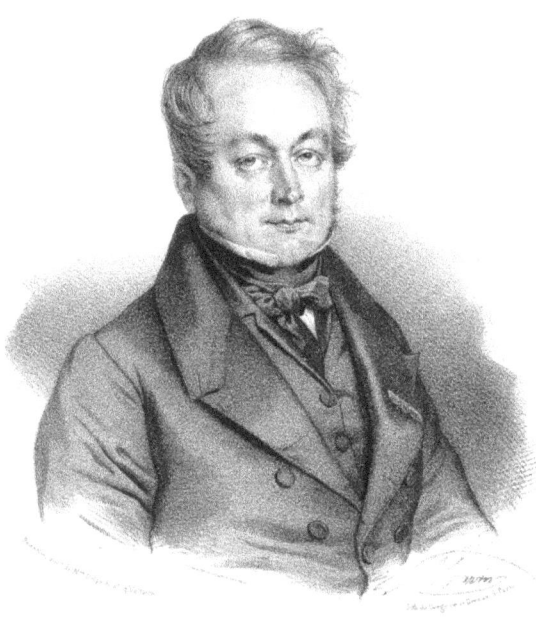

François Magendie, early icon of French physiology. To many British citizens he was "the French Butcher." Lithograph by N.E. Maurin. (Reproduced by permission of the Wellcome Library, London.)

Magendie, with his sneering, sarcastic mien, would have made a fascinating character study. Despite his positive contributions, he thrived on conflict and confrontation, all too eager to denigrate fellow physicians. He typically joked as he provoked pain in un-anesthetized or sedated animals. Many of his students recognized that some pain was unavoidable but Magendie's reveling in it was inexcusable. More than one observer bolted his demonstrations, filled with enough anger, disgust and hate to last a lifetime. Buttressing the claims of Sharpey, an unnamed American physician studying under Magendie in 1840 expressed his own mixed reactions to the professor:

This surgeon's spring course in experimental physiology commenced in the beginning of April. I seldom fail of "assisting" at his murders. At his first lecture a basketful of live rabbits, a glass receiver full of frogs, two pigeons, an owl, several tortoises and a pup were the victims ready to lay down their lives for the good of science!... Monsieur M. has not only lost all feeling for the victims he tortures, but he really likes his business. When the animal squeaks a little, the operator grins; when loud screams are uttered, he sometimes laughs outright.... Living dissection is as effectual a mode of teaching as it is revolting, and in many cases the experiments are unnecessarily cruel and too frequently reiterated; but so long as the thing is going on, I shall not fail to profit by it, although I never wish to see such experiments repeated.[8]

In 1824, British physicians invited Magendie to London to give a public demonstration on the differing functions of the anterior (front) and posterior (back) nerve roots in the neck. Organizers presented him with a greyhound that had been specially procured for the event. To secure the animal for the dissection, Magendie used an old trick he had learned at Alfort Veterinary School, where he frequently vivisected. He fixed both front and hind legs to a board by pounding large, dull nails into all four of the dog's feet. Otherwise, he claimed, the dog might have pulled loose from sharper nails during its mid-experimental agony. Then, using the same type of nails, he folded over the dog's long ears and nailed them to the board for better immobility. Magendie then cut into the dog's upper neck, dissecting out the nerves on one side. Upon concluding his dissection, Magendie announced to the audience that, assuming the dog makes it through the night, he would then continue the operation the following day. However, "I shall have the opportunity of cutting him up alive, and showing you the motion of the heart" the following morning if the animal does not display much vitality.[9] This one event not only repulsed many in his audience, but provoked heated articles in the London newspapers and even in Parliament. It marked the beginning of Magendie's infamy in England.

Most physiologists adopted the use of anesthesia after its introduction in 1846, markedly diminishing the specter of pain. But Magendie resisted the trend, arguing that such agents were unnatural. Even their mere presence might interfere with experimental results.

Still, the man did make many positive contributions in his field, such as the introduction of new drugs into the medical armamentarium. For centuries, the elders of Java and Borneo handed down through generations an art for conquering their enemies with a single consummate act. One shot of an arrow, previously dipped in *upas tiute*, and a horrible death visited the victim within minutes. In the early 1800s, Magendie studied the toxic effects of *upas* in various experimental permutations with dogs, putting each animal through the same horrible death. Magendie concluded that the alkaloid, a crude form of strychnine, acted directly on the spinal cord.[10]

By such studies, Magendie set France off on a pioneering course. Over a 12-year period, he thoroughly analyzed the effects of many drugs on the body, similar to that of *upas*. Compiling all of those results, he published his *Formulaire* in 1821, providing physicians with vital information on the effects and dosages of many drugs. He collaborated with pharmacists Joseph Pelletier and Joseph Caventou, studying the physiological effects of crude plant extracts, the alkaloids. The product of their work proved to be a major advance, steering medicine away from drugs laced with heavy metals—a holdover from the medieval days of alchemy when physicians searched for that panacea, much as alchemists sought to synthesize gold. The work of Magendie and the pharmacists shifted the emphasis from heavy metals to alkaloid extracts, eventuating in such drugs as strychnine, morphine, codeine, curare and digitalis. In the process they helped give birth to a new field, pharmacology—the physiology of drugs.[11]

Magendie devoted much of his vivisectional activity to the nervous system. He studied the function of nerves exiting the spinal cord in the neck, eventuating in the Bell-Magendie Law: Nerves exiting from the back half (posterior) of the spinal canal serve sensation, while those in the front half are motor in function. Magendie, through four years of research, also correctly identified cerebrospinal fluid existing inside the nervous system. Fellow scientists had considered this fluid to be merely an abnormal collection in response to various diseases.

Contrasting Magendie's original contributions with his strong negatives, he remained an enigmatic figure—the revered professor at the College de France, even as his name evoked scorn in the halls of Parliament. Inside France, he was the paternal icon of physiology, the official interface of his specialty with France's Academy of Science, promulgating policy and setting standards for the new science. In England, he was the sadist, one who reveled in animal suffering. These two faces of Magendie endured well after his death in 1855.

## Claude Bernard, Prince of Vivisection

In 1841, a young, aspiring physiologist, Claude Bernard, became Magendie's *preparateur*, beginning a productive collaborative relationship lasting nearly a decade. Bernard adopted his mentor's interests by taking on the study of poisons, digestion, and nervous supply to the digestive glands and intestinal tract. However, once Bernard was on his own, his style of research became more systematic than that of his old chief, studying various problems for years at a time until he felt he had accomplished as much as possible. With Magendie's death, Bernard assumed his position at the College de France.

Bernard devoted his entire life to physiology, having virtually no outside interests. As a committed materialist philosophically, he coined the term "scientific determinism" to explain his view. He positioned himself firmly on the side against the vitalists, those nihilistic physiologists who believed that the undefinable, life-giving force could not be controlled, making it impossible to study bodily functions. Bernard insisted that if all aspects of an experiment could be controlled, then scientifically reproducible results were not only possible but to be expected. Conversely, if identical results were not obtained, it was not because of vital forces. Something in the experiment must have been set up wrong. That was his scientific determinism; every natural phenomenon is determined by some antecedent cause. Through his meticulousness and dogged determination over the years, he proved that scientific determinism in physiology did in fact exist. Bernard thus helped usher in an intellectual revolution in his own lifetime by extinguishing the debilitating concept of vitalism.[12]

Bernard wanted to further the influence of experimental science as well as improve on the sad state of clinical medicine. He hoped to make medicine more scientific stating, "we are not yet in the habit of believing that he [a physician] needs a laboratory; we think that hospitals and books should suffice. That is a mistake; clinical information no more suffices for physicians than knowledge of minerals suffices for chemists and physicists."[13] As a strong proponent of experimental medicine, Bernard worked hard to ensure that antivivisectionists did not impede vivisection in the same manner that the church had held back the study of anatomy.

Antivivisectionists accused him of being indifferent to animal suffering. It was true that, when demonstrating a scientific principle before a crowd, Bernard's laconic manner gave him an exaggerated air of indifference. He was well aware of his critics, but being absorbed with the work at hand, he did not let emotions rule. As he proclaimed, "A physiologist is not a man of fashion, he is a man of sci-

French physiologist Claude Bernard. He succeeded Magendie in 1855. (Reproduced by permission of the Wellcome Library, London.)

ence, absorbed by the scientific idea which he pursues: he no longer hears the cry of the animals, he no longer sees the blood that flows, he sees only his idea and perceives only organisms concealing problems which he intends to solve."[14]

According to some of his students Bernard was fond of animals despite his apparent indifference. It was not unusual to see dogs gamboling about his laboratory, tails wagging, rubbing up against his leg. An American visitor, Dr. Francis Donaldson, wrote:

> It was curious to see walking about the amphitheatre of the College de France dogs and rabbits, unconscious contributors to science, with five or six orifices in their bodies from which, at a moment's warning, there could be produced any secretion of the body, including that of the several salivary glands, the stomach, the liver, and the pancreas.[15]

The animals seemed to feel at home in his laboratory and he appeared to enjoy their presence.

Bernard outraged antivivisectionists with his practice of producing fistulas (artificial communications or drainage of glandular secretions to the outside via surgical openings in the skin) in animals, to further carry out studies on digestion — a continuation of Magendie's interests. He became adept at creating fistulas surgically, so that he might better examine the effects of food on glandular secretions. There were fistulas of salivary glands, stomach, duodenum, gall bladder and pancreas. For over one year he worked diligently on safely creating pancreatic fistulas in dogs. Dogs proved very sensitive to duodenal injury with a high operative death rate. Finally, in 1848, with his technique perfected, he could produce a fistula with only a two inch operative incision.[16] This surgical feat led to two big breakthroughs: First, at a time when the stomach was considered the only organ of digestion, Bernard proved that the small intestine played an important role as well. Second, properly functioning pancreatic fistulas provided him with a ready supply of pancreatic juices. By immersing specimens of meat and fat in pancreatic juices outside of the body, he discovered that the fat was completely emulsified within hours, converted to fatty acids and the carbohydrate glycerol, both ready for absorption into the body.

In another experimental plan Bernard began a study of the liver. Before his time, scientists believed that only plants could produce sugars. Humans were thought to be dependent upon external sources for nutritional sugars. But Bernard found high quantities of glucose in the liver and in the vessels draining it. Through a methodical series of experiments, he ligated (tied off) various combinations of hepatic vessels, followed by removal of the liver and washing it clear of metabolites. Curiously, he still found consistently high quantities of glucose in the liver after such maneuvers. Ultimately, he discovered that glucose was not only produced within the liver, but also stored there in its space-saving form, glycogen. He announced the isolation of pure glycogen in 1857.[17]

Bernard was beginning to realize not only how dependent the human body was for this primary fuel, glucose, but also how important was the maintenance of sugar at a constant level within the body. He recognized that the liver released glucose into the circulation to be consumed as fuel for the body's metabolic activities, working via a production-utilization-depletion-production cycle that continuously furnished the body with nutrition. Through elucidation of this cycle, Bernard conceived of a feedback mechanism at its most nascent level. He postulated that opposing mechanisms, termed "nerf assimilateur" and "nerf deassimilateur," worked against each other, alternately synthesizing or metabolizing glucose in a push-pull fashion, resulting in that critical constancy of blood sugar maintenance. He thought, incorrectly, that the autonomic nervous system carried out this function. After Bernard's death, other researchers found the process to be hormonally controlled, but Bernard's concept of a feedback mechanism still held true.[18]

Despite all of his work with the pancreas, Bernard never discovered the important role the organ played in blood sugar regulation. Still, he had hit upon a critical concept: The body was capable of maintaining its internal environment through integrated regulatory mechanisms, hierarchically organized. This was truly a revolutionary concept based on scientific discovery — a far cry from those medieval theories of boiling, excessive humors, considered by many physicians just a few years before to be the determinants of normalcy and disease.

As Bernard's knowledge grew, he visualized a grander scheme. Some of the regulators of the body were glandular, possessing drainage ducts, such as the pancreas, liver (gall bladder) and salivary glands, secreting their products into the external world via the intestinal tract. Then he described the internal secretions — glands that emptied directly into the blood stream, exemplified by the liver, the thyroid, the adrenals and the spleen. At first Bernard believed that only the plasma represented the internal environment, but as he gained more knowledge his view of the milieu expanded to include the red blood cells, interstitial fluids and the lymph. After his death, of course, others demonstrated that it included cellular and sub-cellular sites as well.

The importance of maintaining other conditions besides glucose levels soon became apparent. In Bernard's day, the level of sophistication of pH determination was limited to using litmus paper, but acid/base balance was still recognized as important to the internal milieu. So too was water balance, body heat, internal glandular secretions and even serum osmolality, that is, the concentration of all solutes within body fluids.

Despite barely scratching the surface on the subject of maintenance of the internal environment, Bernard had opened a wide panorama for his successors — a rich heritage of paths for exploration. He was arguably the progenitor of endocrinology, a subsequent area of specialization undreamed of before Bernard's pioneering work. Harvard physiologist Walter B. Cannon further developed Bernard's concept of the internal milieu. In his 1932 book *The Wisdom of the Body*, Cannon coined the term "homeostasis," while illustrating the role that the endocrine secretions, hormones, played in maintaining that internal milieu.[19] Cannon gave full attribution to Bernard's seminal efforts.

Bernard was responsible for other miscellaneous works, too numerous to describe in detail. He discovered the reason that carbon monoxide is poisonous to man. It replaces the oxygen molecule at the site where it ordinarily combines with hemoglobin, rendering the red blood cell, and therefore the person, anoxic. Prior to that, scientists thought that oxygen was bound within the plasma, rather than the red blood cell.[20]

He discovered the site of action of curare, a drug incorrectly considered to be an anesthetic. Used by Amazon Indians to coat their blow-gun darts, curare caused death within minutes by muscular paralysis, earning it the moniker "Flying Death." In 1595, Sir Walter Raleigh introduced the alkaloid to Europeans upon his return from Guiana.[21] When physiologists used curare, the animal, usually a dog, remained fully conscious, feeling everything while being utterly unable to react to the pain. Some unscrupulous vivisectors used it purely for their own convenience. An animal that was unable to move stood no chance of jeopardizing their experiment. But most physiologists agreed; this was the worst kind of agony — a fully sentient animal that has no way to react to pain or even signal that it was suffering. To antivivisectionists, curare was more heartless than no anesthetic at all — it was the height of sadism. Bernard made a systematic study of the drug in his laboratory, finally elucidating its site of action at the neuro-muscular junction — that interface where the finest of nerve fibers terminate within the muscle spindles.

Bernard devoted a large part of his career to the study of the autonomic nervous system — an automated electrified grid that naturally regulates the body's infrastructure. This system ensures that the heart, lungs, breathing, blood pressure, and glandular and bowel functions all continue automatically, irrespective of mental input or state of wakefulness. Bernard elucidated the function of the vaso-motor nerves — fine nerve filaments within the autonomic system that supply the smooth muscles within the vessel walls, giving muscular tone to the vessel. If the nerve is cut, the arterial wall becomes flaccid as the vessel dilates, making all tissues in its area of supply red and warm.

Bernard was a prolific writer, producing well over 100 articles and books on physiology. In 1865, he published *An Introduction to the Study of Experi-

*mental Medicine*, summarizing his work and views on physiology. It was immediately proclaimed worldwide as a masterpiece. As late as 1957 Professor Bernard Cohen of Harvard stated that the book was "as splendid a statement of the basic features of scientific research as has ever been written."[22] In it Bernard proclaimed that vivisectors had the right "wholly and absolutely" to use animals, just as mankind can use them for food, transportation, clothing and even sport.[23]

## The Torture Chamber of Science

One layman supporting the opposite point of view, who provided vivid imagery against the likes of Bernard, was Baron Ernst von Weber, a wealthy, young German writer, given more to travel and adventure than anything of a serious nature. He made a resounding, widespread impact on public consciousness after making an unauthorized visit to a "palace-like building," the physiological laboratories of Professor Carl Ludwig in Leipzig. His friend, a dissident employee of the laboratory, arranged the trip on a vacation day, when no vivisectionist was working.

As they roamed about, the blood-stained surfaces, surgical instruments, metal cages, iron restraints and breathing machines repulsed him. Moving to the cellar, von Weber was reminded of a prison, by the high, cold, gray stone walls enclosing multiple cells for holding imprisoned lab animals. Heavy entry doors were firmly shuttered. Elevated windows covered with iron bars were set high above the floor, preventing any possibility of escape. The wooden parts of the cage doors revealed evidence of gnawing by their canine occupants. If one strolled by the cages, he could not help but notice that this was not just some friendly kennel. While some dogs might stand at the front of their cages, lustfully barking, pacing back and forth, wagging their tails, looking for friendly attention, others remained at the back of their pens, lying on their stomachs, snout resting on forelegs, body trembling, eyes nervously rolled upward, trained on the attendant. Von Weber recalled, "In the most melancholy frame of mind I took leave of these chambers of horrors in this palace of scientific cruelty."[24]

So moved was von Weber that he formed his own German antivivisection society. Like Cobbe, he proactively perused physiological journals collecting any cases he considered cruel. He featured physiologists from all parts of Europe performing experiments involving suffocation, drowning, baking, burning and open operations on most organs of the body. From his experience he compiled a book, *The Torture Chamber of Science*, which caused an immediate sensation. The tract was so educational to the public and so successful that it was eventually translated from German into English, Polish, Italian, Danish, Swedish and French, raising the consciousness of much of the Western world. Although the majority of the atrocities occurred outside of England, the work was still relevant because of the enormity of its reaction and the specific practices uncovered. The starkness of his imagery spoke to people of all countries.

Von Weber's book took the public inside the laboratory with a detailed accounting of the physiologists' activities. First was the standardized process for moving dogs from cage to the vivisection room. If the animals were friendly, they could be handled manually and taken straight to the demonstration area. For the more recalcitrant dogs, especially those seized with terror, the handlers had a novel device. A cage-like frame could be lowered over the animal and pincers utilized to grab the dog by the neck, at which time the handler placed an encompassing muzzle around the dog's snout, nearly completing its submission. Next he secured the animal's legs, completing the most dangerous part of the procurement. With legs bound, dog and cart were off to the auditorium where the vivisecting professor awaited.

The animal next encountered a large tabletop with an elongated experimentation device attached to it, designed to hold the animal in position for the procedure. Its base had a long trough for catching blood, water and bodily fluids, which accounted for Cobbe's favorite moniker, "torture trough." The dog's legs were now merely tied down to the frame in differing positions, depending upon whether the operation required prone or supine placement.

Vivisectors used many different kinds of animals for experimentation, from dogs and cats to rabbits, guinea pigs, frogs and even snakes. While a hierarchy may have existed based on the animal's degree of sentience, humanitarian interests likely had little to do with choice of animals. The dog and frog were most utilized; the former because of its ubiquity and the latter because of its low cost and ease of handling. Still, it was undeniably easier to put down a frog that lacked sensitive, trusting eyes, licking tongue and wagging tail that could tug at the experimenter's conscience.

According to the antivivisectionist, Dr. George Hoggan, who had earlier worked in Claude Bernard's laboratory, some animals were more readily put to sleep than others. He claimed that the rabbit was the most heedless animal in existence. When lifted to the table, the rabbit was more concerned about getting one more bite of the carrot than the impending restraints. The cat, on the other hand, was more likely to eye the experimenter with a suspicious glance that says, "'I know what you're up to and I'll resist you and hate you for it till the end.' But the dog comes up sometimes with an air of trustful curiosity and enquiry, 'Well, friends, what have we met here for?'— or else with a frightened appeal for help in his eyes and gestures."[25]

Doctor John Anthony, an English physician who had been a student in Paris, attested to the general cruelty of vivisectionists. He alleged that most physiologists seemed indifferent about what happened to the animal once it had served its scientific purpose. It was merely cast aside, to crawl into a corner and die. "The men there seemed to care no more for the pain of the creature being operated upon than if it were so much organic matter."[26] Tales of atrocities against animals were not unusual. Whether allegations against them were true or not, experimental physiologists Mantagazza, Spallanzani and Schiff in Italy, Karl Ludwig in Germany and others in Eastern European countries were notorious.

Still, France seemed a special place for cruelty. Physiologists there were free to carry out nearly any form of experiment they desired with little chance of professional or public rebuke. One researcher inflicted multiple gunshot wounds in dogs' abdomens to better understand the agonal changes accompanying death. In another, a scientist removed the breasts of a nursing dog to evaluate the strength of the maternal instinct for feeding her young. Other workers placed small animals, such as mice and birds, in bell jars and evacuated the air to better understand, in a crude manner, the vital connection between air and breathing. In yet another scheme, scientists shaved, and then varnished the bodies of a series of dogs, resulting in a slow death — performed to more thoroughly appreciate the role of skin in metabolism.

While it is true that some other physiologists on the Continent made contributions to the field, Magendie and Bernard were the two most revered and influential scientists. They set the standard for France at mid-century. Since Magendie died in 1855, eight years before Cobbe entered the animal welfare debate, she could view him only in retrospect. As Bernard's career faded in the 1860s, their mutual involvement on opposite sides of experimental science overlapped by a mere 10 years. Throughout her career Cobbe never gave such esteemed scientists their due, even early, when her views were moderate. Such recognition never seemed to enter her mind. She paid less attention to the other continental physiologists. In her eyes Magendie and Bernard, plus the activities at Alfort Veterinary School, were the fountainheads of this evil being perpetrated on animals, even at a time when physiology in England still languished in its infancy. Preemptive action seemed to her a prudent strategy — prevent this evil practice from crossing the channel into England.

# III

# FERMENTATION AND SUPPURATION

"I come to the conclusion in my own mind that pyaemia, if it does not find its birth-place, does find its natural home and resting-place in hospitals; and although a hospital may not be the mother of pyaemia, it is its nurse."—Sir John Erichsen

CHAPTER 4

# Joseph Lister and Hospitalism: Is It Something in the Air?

Given the influence of his father, the young Joseph Lister was an accomplished microscopist, producing papers on the microscopic analysis of smooth muscle in the iris and skin while still in medical school.[1] After earning his degree in 1852, he worked briefly in London. Being a freshly minted physician and the most junior house officer, one of his superiors assigned to him the "trivial," disagreeable and dirty task of cleansing (debriding), daily, all pus-filled (purulent) wounds on the ward. Lister was well aware that, microscopically, pus was composed of white blood cells and tissue debris. When he examined these wounds microscopically, he noted a consistent presence of small bodies, particles which he considered to be parasitic in nature. From his undesirable task, Lister came away with something positive. After many of these debrided wounds were well on their way towards healing, Lister was struck by the conspicuous absence of suppuration. On reflection, perhaps this pus was not so necessary to the process of healing, after all.[2]

In 1853, Professor Sharpey formally introduced Lister, the new graduate, to his old friend James Syme, Professor of Surgery at Edinburgh University. As a result, Lister moved to Edinburgh intending to study under Syme for one month. He found such a comfortable niche in his house surgeoncy at the Royal Infirmary that the month turned into years. Not only did Syme remain a major influence in Lister's professional life, but, in 1856, Lister married his daughter, Agnes, as well.[3] She served as both his faithful partner and amanuensis until her death in 1893.

As Lister became established in Edinburgh, he entered into one of his most important eras of research. With the nascent ideas developed there he had unwittingly set the stage for his later revolutionary work in clinical disease.

He became a student of inflammation, at a time when the process was considered to be a disease entity itself rather than a general manifestation of disease. Experimenting in his own house at night, Lister and an assistant placed frogs, anesthetized with chloroform, under his microscope, to better study the vessels in the web spaces of their feet. Here he could see arteries dividing into capillaries, as well as the veins on the other side of the circulation, that received the spent blood. Under controlled conditions, Lister placed heated water onto the web space, each experiment devoted to a progressively hotter dose, ascending from 80° to nearly 200°C (176°–392°F.) In other experiments he studied the effects of irritants, such as mustard, on the frogs' feet.

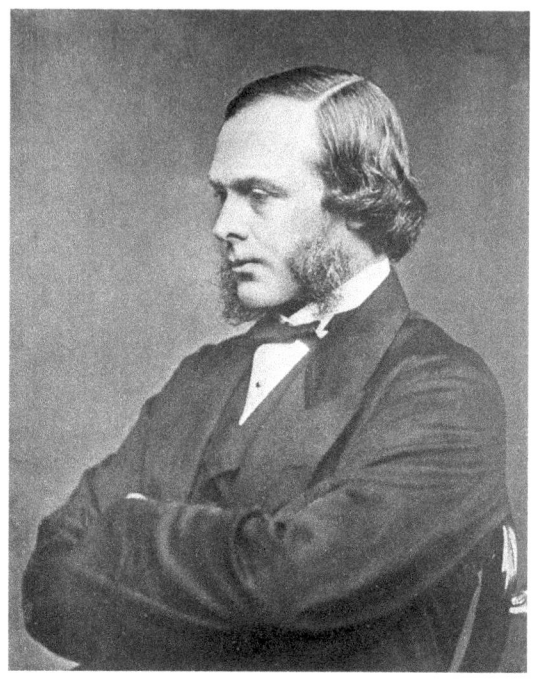

Joseph Lister around age 40, when he had just become aware of Pasteur's pioneering work in fermentation. (Reproduced by permission of the Wellcome Library, London.)

Lister noted that with increasing heat, the vessels dilated and the tissues became red. Capillaries that ordinarily allow the passage of one red blood cell at a time became so flaccid and dilated that three to four red blood cells could pass through, side by side. He also observed both red and white blood cells aggregating, sticking to each other and to the vessel walls. As the inflammatory process worsened with heat, movement of blood cells stagnated until obstruction finally occurred. In a letter to his father, Lister recounted these exciting new phenomena playing out before his eyes. He described what must have been, for a man plagued with his repressed feelings, a raucous display of emotion, stating, "I often uttered involuntary exclamations of delight during the time."[4] Lister made further original discoveries, finding that the minute smooth muscles in the vessel walls became extremely elongated and flat with visible nuclei. Under nervous control these muscles governed the amount of blood that flowed through the tissues. Had Lister carried his work into later stages of inflam-

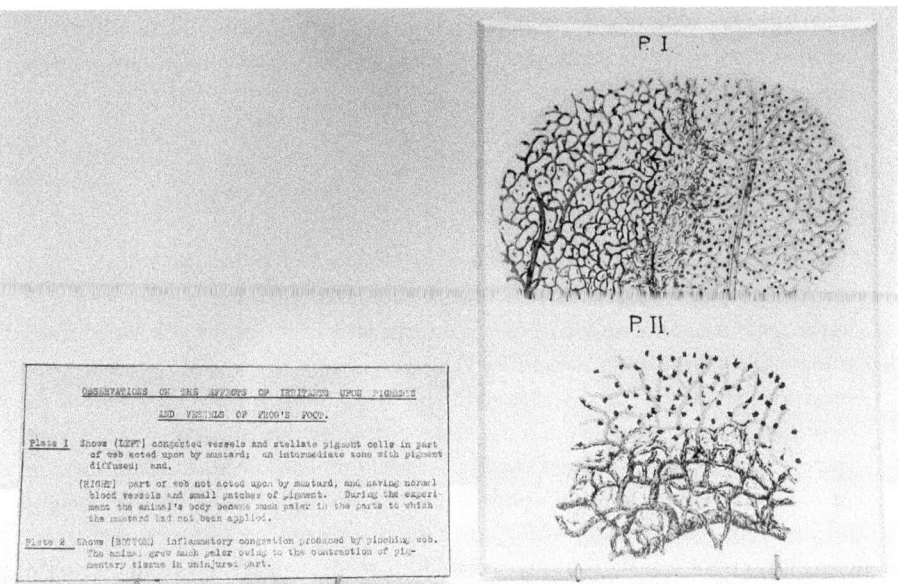

Web of frog's foot. The legend states, "*Plate 1.* Shows *(left)* congested vessels and stellate pigment cells in part of web acted upon by mustard; an intermediate zone with pigment diffused and; *(right)* part of web not acted upon by mustard and having normal blood vessels and small patches of pigment. *Plate 2.* Shows *(bottom)* inflammatory congestion produced by pinching web. The animal grew much paler owing to the contraction of pigmentary tissue in uninjured part." (Reproduced by permission of the Wellcome Library, London.)

mation, he would have also discovered that the white blood cells actually escaped through the vessel walls into the tissues, the formation of pus at its very fountainhead. Julius Cohnheim made that discovery in 1876.

This work, by far the most important of Lister's early efforts, covered the years 1855 through 1858. He presented his findings over these years to the Royal Societies of Edinburgh and London. Destined to become classics, he published them in their *Transactions* as well.[5] By 1859, Lister was firmly entrenched in Edinburgh, having not only gained the reputation as a first-rate researcher, but he had elucidated the essentials of the inflammatory process as well — now equipped with information that proved helpful in later clinical challenges.[6]

In 1859, a Dr. Lawrie, Professor of Surgery at Glasgow University, was forced to resign his position due to ill health. When the university made enquiries of Mr. Syme regarding potential candidates, Syme immediately volunteered the name of Lister for the position, claiming that Lister possessed "remarkably sound judgment, united to uncommon manual dexterity and a practical turn of mind."[7] After receiving the appointment, Lister embarked on the Glasgow leg of his academic journey in 1860, accompanied by his wife Agnes.

## Hospitalism

If the images evoked by vivisection offended large portions of the Victorian citizenry, the state of their hospitals proved even more repugnant to a larger segment. One only had to stroll through any active, overcrowded ward to have his senses overpowered by the sweetish, fetid stink of infection permeating the air. Hospital wards were at least as dangerous as they were malodorous. In fact, mortality rates in the major urban institutions were so high that the public often viewed them as places one entered to die, rather than be cured. It was an age-old conundrum but the problem reached its height in the 1860s. Sanitarians, who studied such phenomena, claimed that overcrowding, poor ventilation and general filth accounted for its origins. Certain hygienists treated hospital environments with the same principles of cleansing the air, the water and the physical plant that they had used in urban settings. But such moves proved ineffective.[8] Less tangible factors such as medical ignorance and persisting medieval attitudes towards illness played a role as well.

Since Lister carried a light clinical load while in Edinburgh, he had enjoyed a several-year hiatus from the daily strain of this debilitating situation, but the wards he encountered with his move to Glasgow represented some of the worst. Still, the problem was far from unique to Glasgow. It plagued all major hospitals in the Western world, as well as the physicians who worked in them. Surgeons dared not operate on any person with a problem such as a broken leg or inflamed appendix unless it was in desperation to save a life. Mortality rates after leg amputations at some of the larger and finest institutions such as the Edinburgh Infirmary hovered around 43 percent; Vienna's Allgemeines Krankenhaus, 43 percent; Paris' Hotel Dieu, 58 percent. In some military hospitals mortality rates ran as high as 75–90 percent.[9] Infections were not unique to surgical wards; they ran rampant among patients with medical conditions as well. The problem was so pervasive in Britain and the Continent that it earned the moniker "hospitalism"—a term signifying the invasion of a wound or the entire human body by a contaminant. If sufficiently severe, this condition led to sepsis. Since germ theory was not yet established, sepsis was not viewed as an infection per se, but rather as a life-threatening condition of unknown or non-specific origin. Professor John Erichsen, one of Lister's early mentors and author of a book on hospitalism, gave some insight into its mysterious nature when he stated, "I come to the conclusion in my own mind that pyaemia, if it does not find its birth-place, does find its natural home and resting-place in hospitals; and although a hospital may not be the mother of pyaemia, it is its nurse."[10] A major hospital might be saturated with sepsis while the town proper remained inexplicably unaffected. Once sepsis permeated the wards, no measures could rid the hospital of the problem. Some cities resorted to razing their hospitals, building anew on a different site. While that solved the problem temporarily, it proved an expensive and impractical solution.

Hospitalism could take one of several different forms. Pyemia (pus in the blood) was the most common manifestation. Another type, gangrene, was the most feared in that it had the highest mortality rate. Septicemia, a less specific term, included such maladies as childbed (puerperal) fever, also highly fatal. Physicians later found other septicemic forms, such as erysipelas and cellulitis, to be caused, like puerperal fever, by the newly described organism, streptococcus. Abscess, the last form of hospitalism, was usually caused by blood-borne staphylococci, but that specific organism was not yet known in early Victorian times. Since no effective treatment existed for infections, the natural sequel was "blood poisoning" or sepsis, as bacteria invaded the bloodstream. First the affected area became hot, swollen, red, and very painful. Then the scenario of high fever, flushed face with parched lips, shaking chills, rapid heartbeat, delirium and death ensued, something all too familiar to treating physicians. With such fulminating conditions, they had little to offer besides comfort.

Before the 1860s, physicians recognized sepsis when they saw it develop in a patient, but they were at a loss to explain it. Pus was still considered laudable. To those physicians still clinging to the humoral theory, the appearance of pus meant that excessive humors were beginning to drain properly from the body — a good sign. To others, pus was just a natural sequel in the healing of a wound — no need for any change. Since cleanliness was not considered all that important, physicians and nurses paid it little respect. Patients with openly draining, purulent wounds were commonly placed adjacent to others without infections. As one of Lister's assistants recalled about physicians' attitudes, "When almost every wound was foul with suppuration, it seemed natural ... to postpone the cleansing of [our] hands and instruments, until the progress of dressings and probing had been finished."[11] Why should it be necessary to replace bed sheets just because someone died or was discharged from the hospital? The next patient would just soil them again. Buckets were commonly placed by each bedside, like ashtrays in a household of smokers. They were convenient receptacles for catching that sudden effluent escaping from a wound or abscess. With similar insouciance, hospital planners placed mortuaries and anatomy laboratories adjacent to the operating room. When coming from dissecting room to operating theatre, doctors and students seldom bothered to wash off their anatomical grime before joining an operation. They operated with their bare hands until William Halstead introduced rubber gloves in 1894. Surgeons rarely changed their black gowns, heavily encrusted with human debris. They often carried surgical instruments in their pockets, handy for immediate use should the need arise. Hospital staff members were blithely unaware that they were the principle purveyors of hospitalism.

## Lister's Approach

As a newly appointed Professor of Surgery at Glasgow University in 1860, Lister could now exercise his own full independence, taking those first steps down the path that more clearly defined his life's work. Tormented with the high incidence of hospital diseases, Lister observed that several of the wards in Glasgow were "some of the most-unhealthy in the kingdom."[12] He lamented, "I had too ample opportunity for studying hospital diseases, of which the most fearful was pyaemia."[13] Faced with this cloud hanging over all surgical endeavors, Lister turned further to animal experimentation, hoping to solve this problem by focusing more intensely on suppuration. In one line of inquiry, he implanted contaminated material into jugular veins of donkeys in hopes of gaining a fuller understanding of inflammation. He then removed the inflamed areas at varying time intervals for microscopic examination, tracing how a contaminated coagulum of blood evolved into the thick yellow liquid known as pus.[14]

Most surgeons just accepted poor wound healing as the norm, something inevitable. But Lister, like some of his colleagues, was convinced that something in the air caused these morbid conditions. Still, he was at a loss to know what it was. Was it oxygen or some other sort of particle that resided in the air? In any environment as contaminated as hospitals, surgical and traumatic wounds typically healed with the wound gaping open. Healing granulation tissue filled up the wound from its depths, requiring several months. Such healing left a wide, unattractive scar. Surgeons using stitches were forced to leave them long enough to protrude from the wound, serving as wicks for drainage of pus. In the rare wound that did heal without infection, its sides were nicely coapted. Granulation tissue bridged the wound from side to side rather than upwards from below. Healing only took a week, leaving a razor-thin scar.

Lister agreed with the general tenets put forth by the sanitarians. Cleanliness of the patient, the ward and hospital personnel were important. He enacted certain rituals, such as hand-washing in between patients, using clean towels and increasing the square footage allotted to each bed. Based upon the recommendations of an Italian professor, he had even begun using sulfite of potash as a type of general wound cleanser, even though he had little scientific justification for it.[15] Unfortunately all of his efforts proved fruitless in diminishing the scourge of sepsis. Lister, already prone to depression, passed into a state of chronic melancholy, mired in a swamp of fecklessness. His early ambition to be an innovative surgeon seemed pointless when many of his cases ended in death or infection after surgery.

Louis Pasteur, the rising scientific star, had a favorite saying regarding the act of discovery: "In the fields of observation, chance only favors the mind which is prepared."[16] Although Lister may have been discouraged by the insolubility of this problem of suppuration, his mind was primed not only by past and present researches but also by his daily struggles with sepsis, his eyes open for potential solutions.

## A Revelation

One late afternoon in 1864, Lister was walking home across the gloomy city of Glasgow, accompanied by Thomas Anderson, professor of chemistry. As Lister expounded on his struggles with sepsis, Anderson offered him a suggestion that he might find helpful. He urged Lister to read two articles published by the French chemist Louis Pasteur addressing the subjects of fermentation and putrefaction. Pasteur's 1861 paper appeared in *The Annals of Natural Science*, the other in the French Academy of Science's own literary arm in June 1863.[17] Although such esoteric subjects as fermentation and putrefaction might have been of great interest to chemists, vintners, brewers and others in the trade, it was certainly not a subject that would ordinarily spark the interest of a surgeon such as Lister.

After acquiring the articles, Lister digested their contents with great interest, already sensing a welcome ray of light into his darkness. In essence, Pasteur's papers were an articulation of his new theory about germs and their role in fermentation. He described these minute beings, invisible to the naked eye, which regulated natural processes. Pasteur asserted that fermentation was not just a chemical reaction; it was a living, biological process, brought about by the activity of some poorly understood reproducing microscopic beings. Since these organisms resided on dust particles, they can range far and wide with movements of the air. One can only get rid of such microbes through heat, filtration or by the use of tortuous, swan-necked flasks. Finally, Pasteur claimed that putrefaction, the decomposition of organic matter through anaerobic means, was but one additional type of ferment.[18]

Lister was entranced by such pronouncements, especially Pasteur's reference to air. So it was not the oxygen or some other gas in the air, but germs living on particulate matter that were responsible for the spread of disease. Lister immediately recognized the parallels between fermentation and septic wounds.

If Pasteur's claims were true, they held the key to solving one of the greatest scourges of humankind. How had this Frenchman been able to draw such conclusions?

CHAPTER 5

# Louis Pasteur: Specific Microbes Cause Specific Conditions

Pasteur was only 35 when he announced the essential tenets of the germ theory. Born in December 1822, he and Frances Cobbe were the same age. His origins were just as rural and middle-class as Cobbe's were of the privileged Anglo-Irish landed gentry. Under the influence of his father, an old Napoleonic army sergeant, young Louis received a spirited dose of patriotism, a powerful sense of nationalism that helped define him for a lifetime. He was an indifferent student, preferring to be out of doors, perhaps fishing in a nearby river. Until early high school he was not even competitive academically. Finally, after gaining entrance into the famed Ecole Normale in Paris, he completed dissertations in both chemistry and physics. In 1847, Pasteur received two doctorates. During the latter years of his education, he came under the influence of Jean-Baptist Biot, physicist, and Jean-Baptiste Dumas, founder of organic chemistry. Both proved deeply inspirational to the young student, serving as his intellectual mentors for decades.

Initially, Pasteur's research interests centered on the analysis of organic crystals, seemingly far removed from microbiological matters. However, as his career advanced he moved progressively from the study of organic matter, to fermentation, to spontaneous generation, to diseases of the silkworm, to veterinary diseases, and finally to the ultimate — the study of human diseases, as though guided by some providential hand. Each of these steps would make its own contribution to the establishment of microbiology as a discipline. Within the first several years of his career he won acclaim by solving a complex riddle concerning the light-rotating ability of certain isomers (substances that differ physically despite their identical molecular structure) that had confounded established scientists for decades. While Pasteur's feat contributed little of a practical nature to his future research in fermentation, it provided a foretaste of the young scientist's attention to detail, his powers of observation, and his inductive abilities.[1] At the age of 26 he had already entered into the highest ranks of French scientists.

## Sour Fermentations

In December 1848, Pasteur moved to the University of Strasbourg, his first academic post, where he continued his research in crystallography. More significantly, he met his future wife there, Marie Laurent, daughter of the rector of the University. Their marriage, in 1849, began a long and happy partnership, with Marie being her husband's faithful confidant and supporter of his onerous work load. Throughout his career Pasteur pursued his work agenda like a man possessed, aiming to bring honor both to his country and to his family.

In 1854, at the age of 32, he was offered the chair in chemistry at the Faculty of Sciences as well as Deanship of the University in Lille. In two short years at Lille his involvement in fermentation slowly eclipsed his crystallographic work while he simultaneously transformed the school into the finest of all the French provincial universities.

Stories differ as to why Pasteur changed course from the pursuit of organic crystalline structure to the subject of fermentation. In the more common narrative, a prominent wine merchant, M. Bigo, manufacturer of beetroot alcohol, approached Pasteur

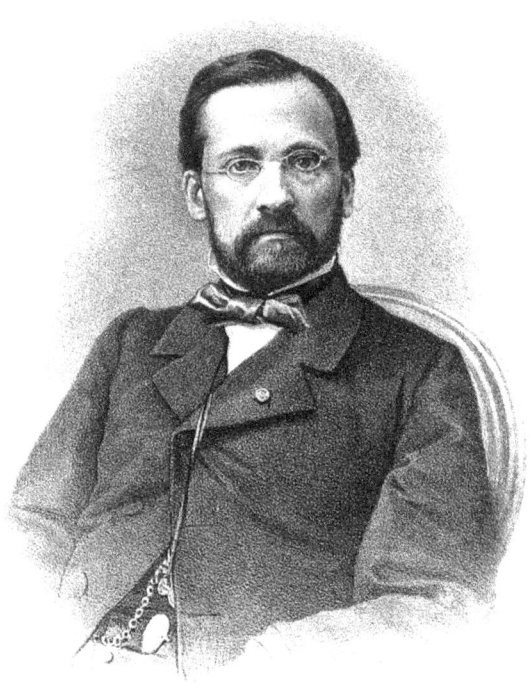

Lithograph by P. Petit of Louis Pasteur at age 35 while at his second academic post in Lille. It was at this time, August 1857, that he presented his work on fermentation, now considered the birthdate of germ theory. (Reproduced by permission of the Wellcome Library, London.)

in 1856 complaining that he and his colleagues were being financially threatened by sour fermentations.² Something bad was happening to the ferments but no one had any idea why. This was the 1850s, when workers within the industry were still pure artisans. They knew that grapes produced wine and malt produced beer, but they had little scientific understanding of the underlying processes. Families merely handed down, from one generation to the next, methods to be blindly followed in the production of wine, cheese, sourdough, beer or any other product of fermentation.

Pasteur's scholarly modern biographer, Gerald Gieson, gives a more credible reason for Pasteur's pursuit of fermentation. It was related not so much to the request of M. Bigo as it was to Pasteur's desire to better understand the production of amyl alcohol — a natural extension of the science of molecular asymmetry.³ Whatever his motivations, Pasteur became increasingly intrigued with the scientific potential of fermentation, per se, essentially placing the study of molecular structure on hold. As he investigated further, he discovered that Bigo's vats with the good beets produced a clear, dark fluid with robust foam and a pleasant aroma. In contrast, the barrels in which the beets had soured contained a malodorous gray slime. He examined samples of both specimens under his microscope. In the properly fermenting juices he found small globules growing and reproducing before his eyes — they were alive. He sensed intuitively that these reproducing buds represented the essence of fermentation. Moving to the rancid ferment, he put a bit of slime to the tip of his tongue. It was bitterly acidic — confirmed as he watched his litmus paper turn from blue to red. Under the microscope, he noted not only a conspicuous absence of the globules, but also a predominance of tiny rods arranged like strings of sausage. Clearly these microbes were different than those that produced alcohol. Pasteur postulated that these were the infesting microbes, interlopers hijacking the fermentative process, taking it off in an unwanted direction. As this ferment fragmented into its more elemental parts, lactic acid appeared instead of the expected alcohol. By studying in a similar manner, multiple types of fermentation from alcoholic, to lactic, to acetic, to butyric, Pasteur gained a greater perspective. It allowed him to generalize what was occurring on a larger scale. In some cases he was witnessing normal fermentations while in others the reactions were waylaid or "infected," biological processes usurped by unexpected and unwanted microorganisms.

Pasteur also observed that, no matter how different the ferment, a living organism was always part of the process. If he boiled the stew to kill the microbes, no fermentation occurred. Microorganisms were necessary for the process to take place. In another experiment, he added cultivated microbes specific to a particular ferment, then observed as the ferment developed into the predicted product. In still another special setup, he prepared a solution of mineral substances and sugar. He then demonstrated how he could, by using the same solutions, produce either lactic or alcoholic products by merely inoculating the solution with the "proper" organism.[4] Each strain of microbe demonstrated specificity of action. Organisms necessary to the fermentation of milk exerted no effect when placed in a fermenting environment that produced alcohol. Finally, fermentation was a living process, a biological phenomenon — not just chemical. Without living organisms, fermentation could not take place.[5]

On 3 August 1857, Pasteur presented his work on lactic fermentation, first to the Agricultural Society of Lille, followed by a second address on alcoholic fermentation to the Academy of Sciences in November. Historians consider these two addresses as his formal enunciation of the germ theory — the birth of microbiology.

Pasteur realized that his theories about fermentation and germs both flew in the face of orthodoxy. Since most scientists in the Academy still adhered to older theories about fermentation and the contagiousness of diseases, they were not at all receptive to this new idea about germs. Chemists themselves knew little about fermentation until the 19th century. Justus von Leibig, the demigod of German chemistry, maintained that fermentation was a purely chemical reaction. It had nothing to do with living matter. Although yeast could always be seen in the process, only its dead parts were necessary to fermentation. When Pasteur and his contemporaries were students, they had almost certainly learned Leibig's theories on fermentation. His was the orthodox scheme and his view was gospel. Even as late as 1860, Liebig still taught that fermentation was set in motion by means of an inorganic catalyst which he called a "zyme." Fermentations and contagious diseases were both a consequence of chemical contact with this poisonous zyme. If microbes were in the mix at all, they were a mere byproduct — an epiphenomenon.[6] When Liebig heard of Pasteur's new theory about germs, he predictably voiced strong disagreement.

When it came to contagious diseases Leibig's theory tied in nicely with people's attitude about miasmatic air, that acrid, foul air choking the streets of cities like London. If one found himself in the middle of such dirty air and the zyme touched him, disease could result. Now this irreverent Pasteur disagreed not only with Leibig's theory of contagion but with his views on fermentation as well. When Pasteur received word that Leibig rejected his new theory, Pasteur naively invited the master to Paris for a friendly interchange of ideas. Upon further reflection Leibig must have recognized that his views on fermentation were out of date. With no valid counterargument to offer, the imperious Liebig did not respond to Pasteur, in effect forfeiting the controversy.

Pasteur worked prodigiously, usually highlighting each major step along the way by either presenting his work to the Academy of Science or publishing it in scientific journals. His subjects ranged from the discovery of anaerobic life, to spontaneous generation, to organisms residing in the air, to acetic fermentation (vinegar), all in 1861. In 1863, he published a major paper on putrefaction — the destruction of plant and animal matter after death.[7] He was intrigued by the existence of anaerobic life, a condition in which organisms thrived in the absence of oxygen in the air. In butyric (butter) fermentation the microorganisms' oxygen source came not from ambient oxygen, but from the organic matter that they decompose. An entire class of anaerobic microbes existed which were integral to the process of putrefaction. Pasteur's reports on putrefaction, the anaerobic fermentation of organic matter, added further support to his germ theory.

## Spontaneous Generation

In 1858, Pasteur assumed the position of Director of Scientific Studies at École Normale in Paris where he remained for the rest of his career. His victory over Leibig caused an atypical lull in his work — one major confrontation aborted. It allowed him time to direct his attention towards another looming problem — spontaneous generation. With those billions of microorganisms teeming under the microscope it was only natural, philosophically and practically, to question their origin. Are these microbes replicated through direct parentage, or do they generate spontaneously? Pasteur realized that, if people were to be receptive to his theories about germs, this impasse had to be resolved. Even as late as 1870, most of the influential people were on the side of spontaneous generation. Reputable scientists, such as Virchow, Huxley and Burdon Sanderson, still believed that these small "particles" which accompanied sepsis and waylaid ferments were the products of spontaneous generation. Even among physicians, those encountering infectious diseases on a regular basis, opinions varied. Some rejected the germ theory outright, while others just did not understand it. If they knew about bacteria at all, they considered them microscopic curiosities. Their attitudes about infection were understandably nihilistic. If infections originated in filthy air or from deep within the body, what could anyone do about it?

Professor Félix-Archimède Pouchet, physician and Director of the Museum of Natural History in Rouen, was the strongest advocate for spontaneous generation. In an 1858 lecture to the French Academy of Science, he "proved" its existence by placing some hay and nutrient solution in a flask, heating it to 100°C (212°F) and then suctioning all air out of the flask with a vacuum pump. After each such experiment, he consistently witnessed germs coming to life inside the flask within hours after cooling. Since no organisms could survive that kind of heat, those new bacteria had to have arisen *de novo*, proving that spontaneous generation was the case.

Pasteur's fermentation studies had already led him to conclude that Pouchet's theory was likely false. He wisely sensed that the professor had made a mistake somewhere in his study — an error needing correction. Pasteur already knew that germs of putrefaction resided on particles of dust, and that they could be destroyed by heat, filtering through cotton or "filtered" through long, tortuous swan-necked flasks, in which air, but not dust, could negotiate all of the curves. In such cases, the liquid in the flasks remained sterile and translucent. The same claim could be made for any bodily fluid naturally free of organisms, such as blood and urine. If stored properly in a flask, they could be kept sterile indefinitely.[8] Armed with this information, Pasteur carried out many ingenious experiments, mainly with the swan-necked flasks, demonstrating that the fluids in the flasks remained sterile, independent of elevation or the filth of ambient air, so long as one followed the proper rules of sterility. If such were the case, how then could spontaneous generation exist? Would not organisms arise *de novo* within the flasks, contaminating these sterile solutions?

Coming as close as anyone could to proving a negative, Pasteur concluded that spontaneous generation has never been observed to occur and "thus may be regarded as a chimera."[9] In France, Pasteur had demolished the myth of spontaneous generation about as completely as humanly possible.

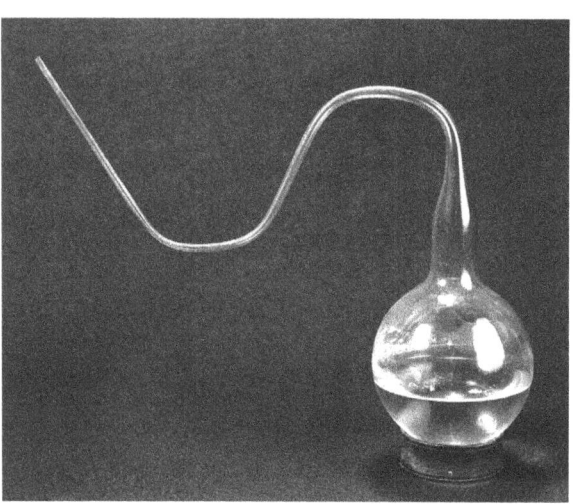

Swan-necked flask. Pasteur exploited the tortuosity of the glass necks to demonstrate a fact. Microbes, residing in the air, could not negotiate the curves to gain entrance into the flask. Such flasks helped him demonstrate that spontaneous generation was a chimera. (Reproduced by permission of the Wellcome Library, London.)

What of Pouchet's convincing demonstration with the hay infusions before the Academy? It would take Ferdinand Cohn, in 1876, well after resolution of the confrontation, to discover the reason for Pouchet's erroneous conclusion. The profuse bacterial growth that he had encountered after heating the flask was due to the persistence of spores, heat resistant well above 100°C, ultimately rendering Pouchet's experiments erroneous and worthless.[10]

So far, Pasteur had not made one sentient animal suffer or die in the name of science. But that would change as his methods and subjects of study evolved. He abhorred vivisection in its traditional sense, open operations on alert animals. However, for Pasteur to continue pursuing his research interests, taking up the art of vivisection was inevitable. His vivisections were, for the most part, performed in a different manner — a "mere" sticking of animals with needles. But the ethically significant part of this form of vivisection played out over hours or days as the diseases evolved, all within the confines of Pasteur's laboratory. Such suffering generally occurred out of public view. Virtually all of his animals died, either from the disease inflicted upon them or by being euthanized after they had fulfilled his purposes. In the mid–1860s, Frances Cobbe was probably already aware of such a celebrated scientist as Pasteur, but she was busy in her pursuits of journalism and social justice in London. Pasteur was now fully invested in the study of microorganisms, but in the 1860s his experience was limited to diseases of plants. With fragments of the germ theory and his inchoate ideas of infection filling his brain, he was anxious to bring his special insights to the study of human disease. Even though in his next step he would graduate from flora to fauna, he would first have to settle for the study of animal life significantly below that of human beings.

## Ailing Silkworms

In 1865, Jean-Baptist Dumas, Pasteur's old idol, was now a senator representing an area hard hit by the silkworm disease, a malady threatening the silk industry, both locally and worldwide. Since an epidemic was building in Dumas' district, he naturally thought of his brilliant pupil as the industry's potential savior. Paying a visit to Pasteur, he implored his former student to accept the job of solving this dilemma, but Pasteur was not at all interested. He knew nothing about silk production and had never so much as touched a silkworm. Dumas left, defeated. Reflecting further and wracked with guilt over refusing his old master, Pasteur acquiesced, deciding that he would take on the silkworm after all.[11]

Pasteur entered the fight to save an ailing silkworm industry in 1864. Although he had elucidated the major parts of his germ theory by the early 1860s, his silkworm studies enabled him to make two more substantial contributions to it. One disease, pebrine, caused "corpuscular" black spots on the bodies of silkworms, seriously hampering silk production by devastating newer generations of silkworms. In preparation for the silkworm task, Pasteur the chemist enrolled in an elementary physiology class under Claude Bernard. When he peered into a microscope, he needed to know what it was that he was looking at. In addition, he could improve upon his skills at dissection since, as a chemist, he had little expertise in that art, either. Pasteur also consulted famed entomologist Jean Henry Fabre, confessing his ignorance about silkworms, seeking his guidance, wishing for some specimens. Fabre later told of his encounter with Pasteur:

> He examines [the pupa].... He shakes it in front of his ear. "It makes a sound," he says, surprised, "Is there something inside?" "Of course there is." "Well, what is it?" "The pupa...." I was struck by his magnificent self assurance. Knowing nothing about caterpillars, cocoons, pupae or metamorphoses, Pasteur had come to regenerate the silkworm.... He came to the battle naked, that is, without even the simplest notion concerning the insect he was to rescue. I was dumbfounded; better than that, I was enchanted.[12]

Pasteur tackled the problem with his usual zeal. Setting up a laboratory in the heart of the silkworm activity, he was soon engulfed by mulberry leaves and silkworms. He first proved that the disease was contagious by feeding contaminated mulberry leaves to healthy silkworms — then watching them develop the disease. The solution to pebrine seemed simple enough: For the next breeding season, he instructed the silkworm breeders to select only the healthy batches of worms and dispose of the infected ones.

However, at the start of the next breeding season Pasteur found that problems remained; silk production still lagged. Although the black spots of pebrine were no longer evident, the silkworms remained unhealthy and their numbers small. Pasteur rededicated himself to this enigma, spending 18-hour days in his laboratory. Finally he discovered the reason; a second disease, flacherie, had co-existed all along, masked by the presence of pebrine. Ultimately it was his nose that led to the solution to the problem. He detected a smell of fermentation in the diseased silkworms leading him to dissect and examine their intestinal tracts microscopically. There he found flacherie organisms residing within the intestines of the silkworms. For this second disease Pasteur had a solution. He instructed the silkworm cultivators in the use of the microscope, enabling them to competently examine the silkworm entrails as well. When he found the workers less than enthusiastic about this part of the solution, he had his own 10-year-old daughter Marie-Louise demonstrate the ease with which the microscopic dissection could be performed, in effect, shaming them into its use. If the workers found flacherie microbes in the intestines of a particular batch of worms, Pasteur instructed them to destroy the entire batch. Only those worms free of the infestation should be saved for reproduction. Pasteur knew that his solution had been effective when the new breeding season came around. He found the silkworms and the industry restored to their prior vigor. Pebrine and flacherie provided two new examples of his germ theory axiom: One specific organism causes one specific disease.

## Pasteur's Stroke

On 19 October 1868, the 46-year-old Pasteur entered a time of great personal trial. Scheduled to deliver an update on his silkworm project to the Academy of Science, he noted, upon arising, a general malaise and a tingling in the entire left side of his body. He persevered, delivering an uneventful address before the Academy. However, by bedtime he was profoundly weak in his left arm and leg, and no longer able to speak. His family summoned the renowned Dr. Andral of the Academy of Medicine to the home. Andral applied leeches behind both of Pasteur's ears, an antiquated practice still used by contemporary physicians. Pasteur made a minor rally, but even days later his muteness and left-sided paralysis persisted. He remained lucid through the entire ordeal. Having suffered a cerebral hemorrhage in the medically medieval 1860s, he was fortunate to have survived. Within one week he rallied, beginning to speak once again, even dictating technical notes a few days later. Slowly strength returned to his arm and leg and he became ambulatory a few weeks later. Being Pasteur, he returned briefly to another silkworm laboratory at Saint-Hippolyte-du-Fort.[13] Next, at the invitation of Napoleon III, he further recuperated, supervising an experimental silkworm farm at an imperial estate, Villa Vincentina near Trieste.[14] By late 1869 Pasteur was sorely distressed with the slowness of his recovery. With "only one good hand and a sick brain," he had decided that his career would be reduced to observing and supervising his assistants.[15] Still, he made good use of his time at the Villa, not only solving a pebrine epidemic that had plagued the local farmers, but also by completing his two-volume work, *Diseases of Silkworms*. This work proved so successful in later years that he frequently advised aspiring microbiologists to read it as a primer on the germ theory as applied to plants and invertebrates.

After Pasteur completed his work at the Villa in June 1870, he traveled home with his family via Strasbourg, receiving the most recent and troubling news of the impending Franco-Prussian war.[16] Pasteur had entered the chronic phase of his stroke, never again to be neurologically normal. For the rest of his life he dragged his leg when walking. Since his left hand and arm were spastically contracted, making bimanual tasks difficult, he delegated simpler laboratory chores to his assistants. As a result he developed his well-known penchant for standing to the side of and a foot behind the nervous laboratory assistant, watching his every move.

With his neurological condition stabilized and *Diseases of Silkworms* completed, Pasteur could now move on to other pursuits.

CHAPTER 6

# Lister: "It really charms me"

The germ theory papers that Lister so eagerly digested represented all of Pasteur's points of argumentation up to but excluding his work with silkworm diseases — a sort of watershed. As Lister confronted the problems of wound infections, he again pondered the major points of germ theory. Pasteur asserted that an entire invisible world of microscopic life existed and that these small organisms were responsible for fermentation and putrefaction. Fermentation cannot occur without these microbes. In order to survive, each type of organism residing within these stews competed for the existing nutrients of fermentation. It was the action of a unique microorganism feeding off of a particular organic aliment that determined the final product of each ferment. If the wrong group of organisms happened to invade the fermenting pot and won the competition for nutrients, they became the dominant growth, waylaying the ferment in the process. Now, instead of producing a desired product such as wine or beer, the mix eventuated in something unexpected and unwanted. Putrefaction is a type of anaerobic fermentation. Anaerobic organisms extract their oxygen from the organic material they are decomposing, not from ambient air. Furthermore, organisms of fermentation reside on dust particles in ambient air as well as on surfaces of liquids and solids. Finally, these microbes can not only be purified through cultivation, but the newly cultured generation can even be used in a manner identical to the first.[1]

## The Antiseptic Principle

As Lister saw it, both processes, fermentation and sepsis, involved microorganisms. They only differed in their substrates — one involved the decomposition of human tissue while in fermentation it was other, disparate types of organic material, running the gamut from grapes, to cabbage, to malt. Lister recognized a therapeutic opportunity in Pasteur's assertion that the septic properties of the atmosphere originated, not from oxygen per se, but rather from the microorganisms suspended within it. Lister would base his scheme on the preemptive treatment of air and microorganisms, that is, treat the wound before putrefaction has a chance to set in. If human sepsis is the organic equivalent of "infected" fermentations, then one should be able to avoid infestations of organisms by employing principles of cleanliness. First, irrigate the wounds immediately after an injury to cleanse them of in driven microbes. Then, apply an antiseptic compound directly on the wound to keep it free of organisms. Finally, minimize further exposure to contaminated air by applying a thick dressing to the injured area.

Lister needed a proper cleansing agent, or antiseptic — some compound that would prove more harmful to the microorganisms than to the surrounding tissues. He soon learned of a program in which the residents of Carlisle Township had used carbolic acid, creosote, to cleanse their sewage system. The chemical reportedly not only killed the bacteria in the sewage, but also freed the town of its offensive odor.[2] Lister's work space soon began resembling a chemical laboratory as he experimented with different compounds, varying concentrations and states of viscosity, from putty-like to liquid. In 1865, after experimenting on animals, to better understand the toxicity of carbolic acid on living tissue, he was ready to employ his scheme.

One of the most serious aspects of hospital sepsis, and one that bothered Lister greatly, involved the care of patients with compound leg fractures, injuries in which bone fragments had penetrated the overlying skin. While simple breaks with intact skin healed uneventfully, compound fractures with their protruding bones posed a constant threat of blood poisoning. Leg fractures, complicated by in-driven dirt, debris and bacteria, were more serious than were fractures of the arm. Although not yet appreciated by surgeons, further oozing of serum into the fluids already stagnated at the fracture site created an ideal culture medium for bacteria. After setting such fractures, doctors anxiously monitored the skin puncture sites, concerned that sepsis might set in. At the very first suggestion of redness and swelling, they amputated the leg in hopes preventing sepsis. But often they were too late. Even after such surgery, mortality rates from sepsis still ranged between 25 percent and 50 percent.[3]

Lister believed that such compound leg fractures, with their constant threat of sepsis, represented the ideal clinical condition for first testing his treatment scheme. Such cases would constitute his first treatment series. If the antiseptic method worked, the patient's leg would be saved. If it failed, he could still resort to amputation, so the patient would be none the worse for the effort.

## "It really charms me"

In August 1865, 11-year-old James Greenlees presented to the hospital. He had been run over by a heavy wagon, sustaining a compound fracture just below his left knee. After setting the boy's leg under chloroform anesthesia, Lister irrigated his wound with carbolic acid suspended in linseed oil. Next, he placed carbolic putty widely over the wound and covered it with tinfoil to keep the compound in contact with the wound. Finally, he applied a thick dressing, incorporating a splint into the dressing to stabilize the fracture site. Lister waited four days before he changed the dressing, bursting with curiosity as to what he would encounter. Would it be the usual smelly purulence, or something even worse? As he peeled back the dressing on day four, he was gratified to see the skin defect filled not with pus but clear, serous fluid surrounded by dried blood — a clean wound with only the expected amount of tenderness. No odors of putrefaction. Lister was clearly pleased with this early observation. In a letter to his father he related, "And, what I really could not have expected, the original crust of clotted blood, lint and carbolic acid which was over the wound the day after the accident still remains there without a drop of matter (pus) having as yet formed beneath it."[4] He re-examined the wound five days later. Now when he inspected the wound it remained clean save for some minor tissue burns from the carbolic acid. When Lister changed the dressing more than two weeks after Greenlees' injury, well beyond the critical time for infection, the wound was well on its path to healing. The boy left the hospital six weeks after his accident with two intact and functional legs.

Encouraged, Lister continued this regimen for all patients presenting to the hospital with compound fractures. Increasingly confident with his early successes, he expanded his regimen to include abscesses in soft tissues. Treating such pockets of purulence proved to be even more gratifying than leg fractures. In another report to his father he stated, "The course run by cases of abscess treated in this way is so *beautifully* in harmony with the theory of the whole subject of suppuration, and besides the treatment is now rendered so simple and easy for *any* one [sic] to put in practice, that it really charms me."[5] Between March and July 1867, Lister published his early experience with antisepsis in a series of *Lancet* articles titled, "On a New Method of Treating Compound Fracture, Abscess, Etc., With Observations on the Conditions of Suppuration." Of 11 cases of fracture (nine legs, two arms), two developed gangrene. One patient required amputation and another died — not from sepsis but from delayed hemorrhage.[6] Although his sample was too small for any sweeping conclusions, these results were better than most surgeons had ever experienced.

Encouraged with his early results, Lister reported in a Dublin speech in April 1867:

> Since the antiseptic treatment has been brought into full operation, and wounds and abscesses no longer poison the atmosphere with putrid exhalations, my wards, though in other respects under the same circumstances as before, have completely changed their character; so that during the past nine months not a single instance of pyaemia, hospital gangrene or erysipelas has occurred in them.[7]

In a letter to his father in October 1867, one could even detect a mood change from depressed to elevated, now that the antiseptic method was measuring up to his expectations, "I now perform an operation for the removal of a tumor, etc., with a totally different feeling from what I used to have; in fact, surgery is becoming a different thing altogether."[8]

With his early successes, Lister quickly recognized that he was on to something that, if properly prosecuted to its full potential, would be of revolutionary proportions. His campaign to gain further exposure of his treatment method to physicians pursued various avenues. Many visited his wards in Glasgow and later in Edinburgh, curious about his scheme. Most left inspired enough to consider bringing the program to their own hospitals. Lister spoke both locally and regionally to various organizations such as the British Medical Association (BMA), and International Medical Congresses, eager to spread the word. Lister's antiseptic theory was typically better received in the larger provincial towns where younger men, some recent Lister trainees, tended to gravitate.

When speaking to medical students and physicians Lister employed flasks to illustrate an analogy concerning antisepsis. He placed urine in open, straight-necked flasks and in swan-necked flasks and brought all flasks to a boil. Afterwards, the open-necked flasks quickly became contaminated (cloudy), whereas the capped flasks with straight necks took longer to show bacterial growth. The tortuous-necked flasks remained sterile (clear) for as long as three years, since dust and bacteria could not negotiate the curves into the flasks. In other words, there truly was "something in the air" that was infectious. If one could avoid the ingress of air, one could maintain a normal, antiseptic environment.

However, not all surgeons were receptive to Lister's clinical scheme. Mr. Nunneley, from Leeds, epitomized the type of resistance that Lister came to expect — men with preconceived notions, coupling unscientific analysis with ineffective technique. In an 1869 *British Medical Journal* (*BMJ*) article Nunneley strongly condemned any program that was based upon germ theory. Although Nunneley admitted to no personal experience with the scheme, it did not prevent him from commenting on its uselessness. Several of his colleagues had pursued the antiseptic method over a three-year period. Their results were no better than other surgeons. In England, most of the resistance came from the older surgeons who, having been apprentice-trained, were not as well educated or grounded in science as were the younger men. Many, still believing in spontaneous generation, rejected the system outright. Others never exerted the effort necessary to understand the system of antisepsis. They neither studied it thoroughly enough to make an informed decision, nor did they visit Lister to observe him directly. They merely began applying the paraphernalia of antisepsis, not fully understanding what they were doing. When the results were less than satisfying, they denounced the method as useless. Even the esteemed physiologist and pathologist Sir James Paget, a reportedly fair and open-minded man, had difficulty accepting this new way of thinking about wound care. He denounced it after treating a single case of compound leg fracture, stating, "But, at any rate, carbolic acid, applied here with a considerable amount of care and skill, failed altogether to attain its end."[9] When Paget's lecture was published in the *BMJ*, Lister felt compelled to refute his charges, lest such unscientific opinions spread. As the tides of confusion and contention rose, the editors of *Lancet*, a competing medical journal, inquired in 1873:

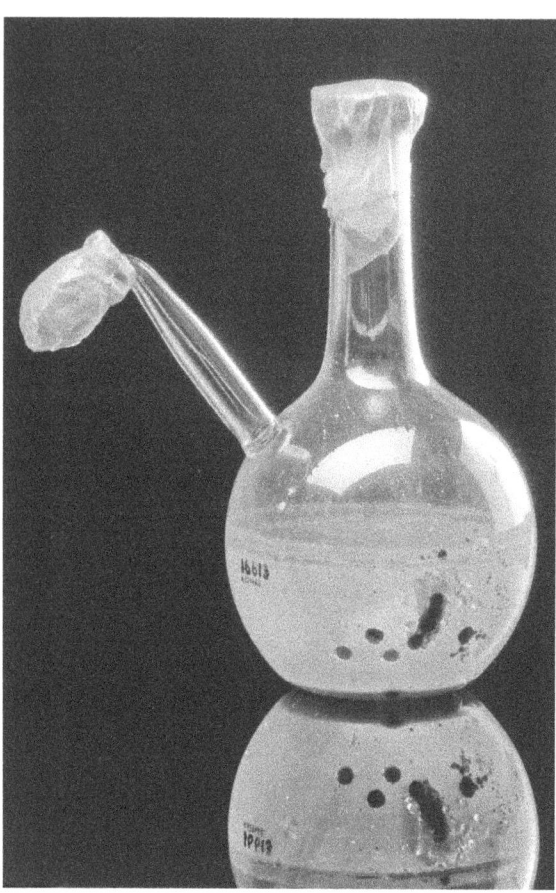

One of Lister's flasks of urine that he used to illustrate the analogous relationship with humans — sterile urine/blood inside a protective cover of glass/skin. As illustrated, straight-necked flasks slowly became contaminated while tortuous-necked ones did not. With any disruption of the protective cover (glass/skin) an infection (sepsis) of the urine/blood ensued. "Something in the air" had to cause the infections. (Reproduced by permission of the Wellcome Library, London.)

Can we not have this treatment fairly and crucially tried in London? There are unfortunately, London hospitals which afford only too good a field for testing the system.... It has taken Professor Lister five or six years to bring his own antiseptic treatment to its present degree of perfection; and we have no reports of anything like similar pains being taken in any of our London hospitals.[10]

But London remained notoriously indifferent to Lister and his theory.

Despite Lister's own successes, employing the antiseptic treatment regimen was slow and awkward in the beginning. To someone already suspicious of its merits, using an awkward scheme proved a strong detraction. But Lister persevered, experimenting as he progressed, unafraid to make changes in any aspect of the scheme if he considered it warranted. If the patient's skin was burned by too strong a concentration of carbolic acid, he diluted it for the next patient. He employed various permutations of dressings, some as thick as seven layers, some designed to filter air, some to be impervious to it. Placing a great deal of faith in Pasteur's claim about airborne bacteria, Lister developed a carbolic acid nebulizer in 1870. This device engulfed the patient and Lister's treatment team in a cumulus cloud of carbolic acid, a preemptive killing of airborne organisms. He employed this scheme both on the ward and in the operating room until 1884 when he no longer considered it useful. Over the years these treatment modifications sometimes frustrated his newer disciples and his detractors. It was more difficult to follow and criticized a target that was continuously undergoing modification.

As he improved his system, his successes mounted over the ensuing years. Once he proved that he could operate with much less chance of infection, he expanded his operative repertoire to include all general surgical procedures from draining tuberculous abscesses to mastectomies and abdominal operations. He could even open knee joints electively for internal repair, although not without rebuke from those colleagues unconvinced of his methods.

## Ovariotomy

Frances Cobbe followed Lister's developments closely. With her attitude towards his antiseptic method varying from dismissive to contemptuous, she could hardly be included among his converts. In the *Zoophilist*, she confessed, incorrectly, that she did not consider animal experimentation to have played any role in the development of Lister's scheme. Furthermore, his method was both useless and ineffective. "Germs flourish in the carbolic spray while human beings are poisoned." She doubted that Lister would ever give up his spray when he has, "for so long a time accommodated facts to fit his theory."[11]

Someone even more critical of Lister was Cobbe's friend and medical advisor, Lawson Tait, the antivivisectionist Professor of Surgery in Birmingham. Tait was an expert in the performance of ovariotomies, procedures in which ovarian cysts or tumors were treated by surgically opening the abdomen. Prior to the 1870s, surgeons performed the operation only reluctantly. The mortality rate from infection was just too high. In the 1870s, several surgeons, including Tait and Spencer Wells, made ovariotomy safer by simply applying principles of cleanliness. Through skill and meticulous work, Tait, in particular, gave the procedure respect and credibility. As operative results improved, ovariotomy evolved into the modern-day laparotomy, an open operation performed to treat numerous abdominal conditions.

To staunch antivivisectionists and feminists such as Cobbe, ovariotomy was immoral. It symbolized a violation of women. Many equated the operation with spaying, removing the female essence, or even as a form of vivisection.[12] As Cobbe stated, "Not rudely and irreverently can these mysteries be explored without injury to the finer susceptibilities and modesties of humanity, least of all the young."[13] Even though a physician had the best of intentions when attempting to solve a woman's ovarian problem, to Cobbe, such treatment represented male doctors physically attacking innocent females. With an antivivisectionist press promoting this attitude concerning medical science and women, one had only to connect a few more dots to complete the obvious metaphor; ovariotomy was rape. Women, like vivisected animals, were the victims of scientific aggression.[14]

Ironically, Cobbe and Tait, the champion of ovariotomy, were steadfast friends connected by their mutual disdain for vivisection. Their friendship endured as Tait walked a narrow line, keeping one foot well placed in each of the antivivisection and ovariotomy camps. Both strongly agreed that Lister's antiseptic system was useless. In an article, "Listerism and the Germ Theory," Tait, still clinging to the theory of spontaneous generation, praised Pouchet, who "kept me out of the errors of the school of Pasteur and freed me from the dreams of Lister into which so many have fallen."[15] To Tait, germ theory gave no final answers. Applying it recklessly was both "malicious and misleading."[16]

In the early 1870s, Cobbe's period of antivivisectional dormancy was coming to a close. With a power base expanded by feminists from the upper social strata, dissident groups set against vaccination, anti-contagionists and other followers of unorthodox regimes, the humane movement had coalesced into a relatively well organized faction. In contrast to antivivisectionists, physiologists remained disorganized and apolitical. Up until now, no public relations skills or need to organize politically had been necessary. Their right to exist, to experiment and to expand had not been seriously questioned. But as

Cobbe and others saw the threat of vivisection looming ever larger, they waited for some opportunity to strike a blow for animal welfare. It came from an unexpected event. Physiologists soon faced a challenge when the British Medical Association (BMA) held its annual meeting at Norwich in 1874, maladroitly conducting a public experiment.

# IV

# HER MAJESTY'S ROYAL COMMISSION

"The queen has been dreadfully shocked at the details of some of these [vivisectional] practices, and is most anxious to put a stop to them."
— Letter to Lister from Queen Victoria, 15 June 1875[1]

CHAPTER 7

# Frances Power Cobbe's Petition

Absinthe is an aperitif much enjoyed during Victorian times, despite its known dangers. A yellow-green distilled liquor which turns opalescent-white when mixed with water, it is highly aromatic due to a mixture of wormwood, licorice, fennel, hyssop and other ingredients — with the licorice aroma prevailing. Since absinthe evoked thoughts of "narcotic intrigue, euphoria, eroticism, and decadent sensuality," it was regarded as the cocaine of the 19th century.[1] Absinthe use was especially rampant in France where, at dusk, "whole boulevards in Marseille and Paris were redolent with the perfume of absinthe."[2] An alcohol content of eighty percent certainly did not detract from to its popularity.

Artists loved what it did to them — rendering them euphoric without drunkenness, heightening their senses, sharpening artistic vision, sometimes to the point of auditory and visual hallucinations. Some claim that van Gogh, a heavy user, owed his unique artistic "shimmering" visual effect to its use.[3] When Oscar Wilde walked out of Reading Gaol in 1897, financially and artistically ruined, he consumed increasing quantities of absinthe, so depressed was he over his dwindling fortunes. As he explained to a friend, "After the first glass you see things as you wish they were. After the second, you see things as they are not. Finally, you see things as they really are, and that is the most horrible thing in the world." Wilde sadly succumbed prematurely to absinthe addiction and syphilis, the latter acquired in a liaison somewhere along the way.[4]

With the widespread use of the drink, its toxic effects soon became evident, earning it the monikers "madness in a bottle," the "green peril," the "scourge," and the "plague." To abuse absinthe was to head "straight to the madhouse or the courthouse."[5] Overindulgence led not infrequently to rapid mental and physical deterioration and even death.[6] Many countries banned the use of absinthe in the early 20th century, once its hazards were fully recognized. Safer modern-day derivatives, however, such as anisette and ouzo, are still available today. Not surprisingly, the 19th century medical profession became interested in the effects of absinthe on the human body.

A Parisian physician, Valantin Magnan, director of the Paris Asylum at Sainte-Anne, carried out absinthe research in both dogs and humans. He found that the essences of absinthe, especially *thujone*, a component of wormwood, affected the nervous system. Habitual use could cause convulsions, hallucinations and a "particularly violent form of insanity."[7] As a recognized authority on the toxicity of absinthe, Magnan lectured and wrote about it extensively.

The British Medical Association (BMA) held its annual meeting in Norwich on August 13, 1874. Local BMA representatives Haynes Robinson, John Pitt, Richard White and Horace Turner invited Magnan to lecture on the physiological effects of both alcohol and absinthe. On meeting day, a large crowd of physicians and lay people gathered in the smoking room of the Freemason's Hall where absinthe was to be injected into dogs to illustrate its convulsive effects. Upon the conclusion of Magnan's lecture, assistants brought two dogs into the room, a white one appearing healthy and a second red one, frail and undernourished. Each dog had already been tied to a board, belly up with all four legs secured. Their mouths were taped shut to prevent biting. The white dog, salivating, struggling mightily, crying as though in pain, was selected first. Apparently it was Magnan who made an incision in the dog's upper leg and inserted a catheter into a major vein. Upon injection of alcohol, the dog was said to be rendered immediately "dead drunk."

A man identifying himself as Dr. Tufnell, president of the Irish Royal College of Surgeons, appeared out of the crowd to protest, causing a great scene with the audience. As Tufnel cut away one or two of the restraints, he charged Magnan and his group with performing unnecessary experiments that were downright cruel. Soon Tufnell was joined in the protest by Dr. Haughton of Trinity College, Dublin. After much shouting, confrontation, and trading of epithets about being cruel and a busybody, the crowd finally cooled down. Order was restored enough to enable someone in charge to take a poll among the audience. The decision: Continue with the experiments. However, by this time, Tufnell had disappeared. He returned later with a magistrate who terminated the proceedings. Sadly for the animals, his action was too late. Magnan, or his assistant, had already injected the red dog with absinthe, causing it to convulse for one hour. While the frail dog died later at the scene, the "dead drunk" dog had fully recovered by the next morning.

By September, word of the confrontation had reached John Colam, secretary of the RSPCA. Realizing he could make some political hay, Colam decided to prosecute Magnan, Pitt, Robinson, White and Turner for violating the Martin Act of 1822. Magnan had conveniently slipped back across the Channel, leaving the remaining four to face the charges.

The Norwich court convened in December, crowded by members of the medical profession and influential citizens of the city. Mr. Colam appeared for the prosecution while Mr. Chittock represented the defense. According to Colam, who led off, the five defendants "on the 13th August, last, in the smoking room ... in the said city and county of Norwich, did unlawfully ill-treat, abuse and torture certain animals — to wit, two dogs — contrary to the statute." During the trial, multiple witnesses for each side were called, including Tufnell, Haughton and Sir William Fergusson, one of the most influential surgeons in England and no friend of vivisection. Fergusson attested that securing an animal to a frame and injecting absinthe did constitute cruelty. The nature of the experiments had not permitted the use of anesthetics, which was equally cruel. Furthermore, why hadn't Magnan merely injected the agents, via a tube, into the stomach? That would have been less cruel and more comparable to the human manner of use, anyway. Cruelty was committed with the restraining, the incising and the injecting.

The four defendants, Pitt, Robinson, White and Turner, admitted to being present at the demonstration but they denied taking part in the experiments. Magnan, after all, was the one bending over the animals, working on their legs and wearing the bloody apron. Predictably, witnesses for the defense testified that the experiments had been justified. They claimed to have been unaware of the seizure-causing potential of absinthe before Magnan's demonstration. A Mr. Allen attested that the operations were "beautifully performed." Dr. Copeman, president of the BMA, felt that the experiments had been warranted. He did admit that, at the scene, he had agreed with terminating them since lay people in the audience would not have understood what was taking place. Several other physicians testified that the experiments had been appropriately performed without cruelty.

## Petition

On 9 December, after several days of testimony, the nine magistrates rendered their opinion — in favor of the defense. The plaintiffs had failed to prove that the four defendants had participated in the actual experiments.[8] With the general English press devoting a great deal of attention to the confrontation, it soon became clear that, in spite of the medical establishment's win, the moral and public relations victory belonged to the RSPCA. One editorial in the *Liverpool Daily Post* declared that "we are not ourselves disposed

... of saying that vivisection ought in no case be allowed. But we emphatically declare that we do not trust the physiological conscience in this matter." In December 1874, Frances Cobbe, sensing a wonderful opportunity to move against experimental medicine, produced two pamphlets in London, *Need of a Bill* and *Reasons for Interference*.[9] In an *Echo* article she urged the RSPCA to consider legislative action to restrict vivisection. In January 1875, she changed her points of argumentation into a petition which she deliberately made "studiedly moderate," hoping that even scientists might sign it.[10]

In her tract, Cobbe concluded that the Martin Act was not strong enough to deal with the evils of vivisection. There was only one organization influential enough to combat the practice effectively and that was the RSPCA. In addition to the inadequacy of anesthesia and newer forms of experimentation such as that of Magnan's, Cobbe lamented the one-sided prosecution of "brutal carters and ignorant costermongers," while the "learned and refined gentlemen should be left unquestioned to inflict far more exquisite pain upon still more sensitive creatures; as if the mere allegation of a scientific purpose removed them above all legal or moral responsibility."[11]

Her requests were four. First, the RSPCA, through the activities of a subcommittee, should place restrictions on this increasing evil. Second, Mr. Colam should prosecute as many cases as possible through the Martin Act. Third, if that were unsuccessful, a bill should be introduced into Parliament prosecuting the publisher of any cruel experiments. Finally, if a bill were to be introduced, it should prohibit painful experiments, require compulsory licensing of scientists, and increase the length of time in which to prosecute a case. Cobbe and others ultimately gathered over 600 signatures in six weeks in support of the memorial. With dignitaries such as the Archbishops of York and Westminster, the Lord Chief Justice Coleridge, Tennyson, Browning, Carlyle, Martineau, Ruskin and many others included, her list was imposing.[12]

To give her petition sufficient gravitas Cobbe wanted very badly to acquire one supportive signature — that of Charles Darwin. The two had been acquainted for over a decade and she was aware of his love for animals. If English culture could produce a "Richard the Lion-Hearted," there should have been a "Darwin the Tender-Hearted." He could not stand suffering of any sort. Coming from a family of physicians, he enrolled in medical school in Edinburgh with the expectation of carrying on the family tradition. One unanticipated problem arose — his sensitivity got in the way. Darwin discovered that he could not stand the putrid smells of anatomy, nor, in the days before anesthesia, the cries of agony in surgery. Invited to observe two different operations on children during his medical school year, he was so sickened and repulsed with their writhing and screaming and the blood dripping into buckets beneath the operating table that he quit medical school. He was more comfortable in a less structured environment, roaming the sea shore, examining crustaceans, following his own interests.

Darwin had always had a special rapport with dogs, claiming to friends that he could spot an abused dog just by observing its nuanced moves in response to its master's movements. He could steal the affections of his sister's dog within minutes of entering her house. His own white terrier, Polly, accompanied him wherever he went. Cobbe, meeting him casually on walks, dinners and at church, even exchanged literary compositions with him. She was disturbed by his theory on the origin and nature of conscience, writing critically of it in *Theological Review* in 1871. Darwin, a year later, complimented Cobbe on her *Consciousness of Dogs*, stating that it was the best analysis of the mind of an animal that he had ever read.[13]

Given his scientific reputation, it was inevitable that he would be dragged into the vivisection controversy. As much as he hated to see any being suffer, he viewed experimental medicine as the ultimate hope for mankind. In a conversation with noted civil servant, Sir Thomas Farrer, Darwin admitted to a deep interest in the vivisection question, probably because of personal as well as scientific reasons. Darwin had lost his beloved 10-year-old daughter, Annie, to a galloping form of tuberculosis in 1851, breaking his heart and shaking his faith in God a full eight years before he published *Origin of Species*.[14]

Darwin himself had been plagued by an undiagnosed illness that nearly dominated his entire adult life. In fact, both he and Annie left a very pregnant Mrs. Darwin in their village of Down, traveling to Malvern for each to pursue Dr. Gully's Water Cure. There he chronicled Annie's deterioration and death seven days later, writing back to wife Emma, "She went to her final sleep most tranquilly, most sweetly at twelve o'clock today.... She expired without a sigh. How desolate it makes one to think of her frank cordial manners."[15] Darwin brought a perspective to the debate not available to many — the intense pain of a grieving parent tempered by the knowledge and objectivity of a scientist. If one were to prohibit experiments on living animals, he would be putting a stop to the knowledge of and the remedies for pain and disease. In a letter to Professor Ray Lenkester in March 1871, he wrote,

> You ask my opinion on vivisection. I quite agree that it is justifiable for real investigations on physiology; but not for mere damnable and detestable curiosity. It is a subject that makes me sick with horror, so I will not say another word about it, else I will not sleep to-night."[16]

In early 1875, Cobbe finally put the question to him. Would he sign her memorial to the RSPCA along with other dignitaries? Not surprisingly, he demurred. In her differing and acerbic account of his reasoning, Cobbe stated,

> This pleasant intercourse with an illustrious man was ... brought to a close for me in 1875 by the beginning of the anti-vivisection crusade. Mr. Darwin eventually became the centre of an adoring *clique* of vivisectors ... who plied him incessantly with encouragement to uphold their practice, till the deplorable spectacle was exhibited of a man who would not allow a fly to bite a pony's neck, standing forth before all Europe ... as the advocate of vivisection.[17]

Although Cobbe could not enlist Darwin himself she did manage to get the signature of his daughter, Henrietta Litchfield.[18] Darwin genes might adorn Cobbe's list, but the name would not.

Since the RSPCA was crucial to the fate of Cobbe's memorial, she waited for decisive action from the group. Sadly, it did nothing. The organization was too large, with too diverse a membership. If the group moved too aggressively it would alienate the scientific members, too slowly and Cobbe and her allies would be aggrieved. Finally, Richard Hutton, writing in the *Spectator*, charged the members with indecision, warning that the movement might bypass them.[19] Cobbe had been invited to attend a subcommittee meeting of the RSPCA. But when she entered the room, "my spirits sank, for I saw round the table a number of worthy gentlemen, mostly elderly, but not one of the more distinguished members of their committee or (I think) a single peer or member of Parliament."[20] Not one man possessed sufficient stature to take on experimental science. Instead of outlining some bold plan of action to Cobbe, the chairman asked her if she could get a bill introduced into Parliament to accomplish their needs. Disgusted with their fecklessness, feeling that her efforts had been wasted, she excused herself from the meeting. The RSPCA's president, Lord Harrowby, soon wrote a letter to the *Times* dissociating their society from Cobbe's strong statements in the memorial. Obviously, she could not rely on the RSPCA for any meaningful action.

Then, as Cobbe pondered her options, manna fell from heaven in the form of an obscure, retired naval surgeon. Dr. George Hoggan published an unsolicited letter in the *Morning Post*, 2 February 1875, which stirred public opinion and the antivivisectionists to new heights. Because of its simple eloquence and credibility, Hoggan's article would prove to have more impact on the movement than any other polemic. Hoggan had spent four months working in Claude Bernard's laboratory and the details revealed in the *Morning Post* were a stinging indictment of vivisection, from a man of medicine, no less. He related:

> I think the saddest sight I ever witnessed was when the dogs were brought up from the cellar to the laboratory for sacrifice. Instead of appearing pleased with the change from darkness to light, they seemed seized with horror as soon as they smelt the air of the place, divining apparently their approaching fate. They would make friendly advances to catch the three or four persons present, and as

far as eyes, ears and tail could make a mute appeal for mercy eloquent, they tried it in vain. Even when roughly grasped and thrown on the torture trough a low complaining whine at such treatment would be all the protest made, and they would continue to lick the hand which bound them till their mouths were fixed in the gag, and they could only flap their tail in the trough as their last means of exciting compassion. Often when convulsed by the pain of their torture this would be renewed, and they would be soothed instantly on receiving a few gentle pats. It was all the aid or comfort I could give them, and I gave it often.[21]

Hoggan continued: While writhing in pain during a dissection, some animals, instead of being soothed, might receive a slap and an angry order to be quiet. If one were well behaved enough to endure pain for hours, he could earn a quick death by pithing — achieved by inserting a needle into the animal's medulla.[22]

Hoggan strongly urged support for the RSPCA in its efforts to restrict vivisection. Most physicians held views similar to his, he argued. They wanted curtailment of unrestricted vivisection but not its total prohibition. Hoggan called for banning the use of curare and for complete suppression of private or secret vivisection. That was where the true horrors took place. Countering the claims of some physiologists, he pointed out many instances in handbooks of physiology, where cruelty had taken place, if only in the use of curare. He concluded by recommending the licensing of both physiologists and their laboratories.[23]

Cobbe quickly re-acquainted herself with Hoggan — whom she had met at a dinner party years before. Hoggan's article had stoked the heat of public opinion as high as it had ever reached, diminishing Cobbe's dependence on the RSPCA. Now with the embers of public conscience fully stoked, Cobbe could exploit her political connections. She drafted a proposal, "Regulating the Practice of Vivisection," getting it quickly approved by many dignitaries including parliamentarian Lord Chief Justice Coleridge. Lord Henniker presented it to the House of Lords on 4 May 1875.[24]

Cobbe's actions did not go completely unnoticed by the other side. At the time that she had approached Darwin for his signature he had become alarmed, seeing the many influential signatories that she had recruited in support of her proposal. Her list had gravitas. Darwin alerted Thomas Henry Huxley to the need for action in the House of Commons. In a letter to Huxley, Darwin stated that, unless a bill countering Cobbe's was introduced into the House of Commons, a thoroughly unscientific and impressionable group in Darwin's eyes, scientists could be facing some severe restrictions in their activities. Huxley replied,

> MY DEAR DARWIN — I quite agree with your letter about vivisection as a matter of right and justice in the first place, and secondly as the best method of

taking the wind out of the enemy's sails. I will communicate with Burdon Sanderson [physiologist] and see what can be done.

My reliance as against [Cobbe] and her fanatical following is not in the wisdom and justice of the House of Commons, but in the large number of foxhunters therein. If physiological experimentation is put down by law, hunting, fishing and shooting, against which a much better case can be made out, will soon follow.— Ever yours, very faithfully, T.H. Huxley[25]

Thomas Henry Huxley was a prominent zoologist, known as "Darwin's bulldog." Darwin detested open confrontation while Huxley eagerly defended him in both print and debate. Darwin's unspoken motto was "peace at any price," while Huxley's was "war, whatever the cost."[26] Best known for his famous put-down of Bishop Wilberforce in the great Oxford debate on evolution, Huxley rose to the heights of Victorian science with a mere two years of university education. Originator of the term "agnostic" to describe his own views on religion, he fought to rid science of its religious influences. Still, ever true to his principles as an educator, he supported Bible study for children. He claimed that the "teachings of Christ provided the best code of conduct that the world had ever known." After his death, his intellectual legacy lived on in the form of his grandsons, Julian and Aldous.[27]

Darwin and Huxley conferred with Burdon Sanderson, who in the early months of 1875 organized scientists and physicians in London, Oxford, Cambridge and Edinburgh into a nascent organization. R.B. Litchfield, Darwin's son-in-law, drafted a physiologists' bill and presented it to Lyon Playfair, parliamentarian, who would present it in the Commons. Lord Cardwell would do the same in the Lords. Playfair tried to convince Henniker to withdraw his bill — which he would not. In fact, for two sides so opposed to each other, both bills were surprisingly similar. Both banned painful experiments except under anesthesia but they differed in manner of enforcement. Henniker's bill required all experiments to take place in registered premises, subject to inspection, while Playfair's bill only regulated painful experiments.

Hutton and Cobbe refused to budge on this last point as they felt the definition of "painful experiments" was too open to deceit. The press, both scientific and lay, was of mixed opinion. Debates within the press yielded a great deal of heat but little light. Despite being an ardent antivivisectionist, Queen Victoria had to present a neutral public presence consistent with her position. Within her court she had stated, "Nothing brutalizes human beings more than cruelty to poor dumb animals whose plaintive looks for help ought to melt the hardest heart."[28] She would not even allow docking of her horses' tails. Her court continued putting pressure on Richard Cross, Home Secretary, to get the problem resolved. Still, he refused to act on either bill. After much editorializing, gesticulating and pontificating on the part of the public, Cross finally, on 24 May 1875, decided to appoint a Royal Commission of Enquiry "on the practice of subjecting live animals to experiment for scientific purposes."[29] Now, no more chances for gentlemanly compromises between the two parties — each could only glare at the other across that legislative chasm.

Richard Cross charged the commission with three tasks: to determine the extent of vivisection in England, to establish whether any cruelty in experimentation does or does not exist, and, if cruelty does exist, to assess what would be the best means for preventing it.

The selected commission members represented a good balance between the opposing interests. It was chaired by Lord Cardwell. Thomas Huxley, dean of British science, and John Erichson, Professor of Surgery, University of London, were both pro-vivisection, while the Quaker, W.E. Forster of the RSPCA and editor R.H. Hutton both represented the antivivisection side. Sir John Karslake and Lord Winmarleigh were two "uncommitteds," whose vivisectional opinions were unknown.

The choices proved wise. All members functioned well within the committee framework. Meeting between 5 August and 15 December 1875, they interviewed 53 deponents with 3,764 questions.[30] The witnesses consisted of veterinarians, physicians both for and against vivisection, 12 practicing physiologists and several private citizens. Frances Cobbe was not included in the list, despite her prominence in the debate. Appearing early, Burdon Sanderson gave a good picture of the amount of physiological activity extant in England and the state of research and teaching there. He testified that England should have full-time physiologists practicing without restriction, just as they do in Europe, if English physiology is to keep up with work on the Continent — whether the experiments were painful or not.

Pointed queries indicated the ideological leanings of the questioner attempting to make points for his side. Hutton pressed physiologist Michael Foster:

> 2411. [Hutton] ... it is the intention, is it not, ... to introduce the general system of study abroad very much more generally into England than it has hitherto been introduced?—[Foster] *I think our study is a study entirely of our own; I mean; I think we teach physiology in a way that is not taught on the continent at all.*
>
> 2412. The experimental method is derived very much from the continent, is it not?—*The experimental method is coeval with physiology.*
>
> 2414. Still your object is to extend the experimental method in England, is it not?—*My object is undoubtedly to advance physiological science, for which the experimental method is one good means.*[31]

When commission members questioned RSPCA president John Colam he had to admit that, even after detailed study, he knew of no instances of physiological cruelty in England, even though vivisection was frequently practiced. Nevertheless, Colam pleaded for a law that provided three forms of protection: First, he wanted prohibition of painful experiments on animals, along with licensing of both physiologists and their place of work. Finally, he hoped for the implementation of reliable methods of laboratory inspections.

Next up before the commission was Joseph Lister, implacably set against any governmental interference in physiology.

CHAPTER 8

# "This legislation is wholly uncalled for"

Joseph Lister, now eight years into his antiseptic regimen, appeared before the Commission in November 1875. Just four years earlier, Lister had earned Queen Victoria's favor by employing his antiseptic system to drain a painful abscess from her armpit, an experience reported by the queen to have been a "most disagreeable duty most pleasantly performed."[1] Just prior to his testimony before the commission, Lister received a letter from the queen, an ardent antivivisectionist, through her secretary, Lord Ponsonby. He related that the queen had been "dreadfully shocked at the details of some of these [vivisectional] practices and is most anxious to put a stop to them."[2] She requested that Lister and other leading men of science condemn these horrible practices when they appeared before the Royal Commission. The forthright Lister wrote a long and detailed reply to the queen, asserting that, regrettably, he could not comply with her request. He admitted to having often performed experiments on lower animals — studies designed for the benefit of humanity. Furthermore, "an act is cruel or otherwise, not according to the pain which it involves, but according to the mind and object of the actor.... I am therefore clearly of opinion that legislation on this subject is wholly uncalled for; while any attempts of that kind might prove very injurious by checking enquiries calculated to promote the best interests of Her Majesty's subjects."[3]

When Lister appeared before the committee in November he testified that, had it not been for his early animal experiments, "I believe I could not by possibility have made my way in the subject of antiseptics."[4] With regards to Lister's earlier development of the catgut ligature, one Commissioner, John Erichsen, author of the book on hospitalism, posed the question to Lister:

> [Erichsen] Am I right in thinking that it was necessary that you should discover some substance, to use as a ligature, which did not produce the irritation which is occasioned by an ordinary ligature?

[Lister] *Yes.*

[Erichsen] And that it could only be ascertained by experiments on living animals?

[Lister] *Yes, certainly.*

[Erichsen] Had you not made experiments on brutes, you would have had to experiment on man; there was no alternative, was there?

[Lister] *There was no alternative.*

Lister took the opportunity to repeat his opinion before the commission that this "anti-cruelty" legislation was uncalled for. The commissioners sensed among "some minds" strong opinion against any legislation that "appears to be connected, as in the case of Mr. Lister, with a notion that such interference implies an imputation of cruelty upon those who are engaged in these investigations."[5]

As testimonies before the commission continued, proceedings were going very well for the scientific side until Emmanuel Klein, an Austrian histologist (the microscopic study of tissue), and one of the authors of the *Physiological Handbook* took the stand. His testimony proved so damning that it jeopardized any chances of the physiologists escaping unscathed. Under questioning, Klein admitted that, when he worked, he did not care if the animal suffered pain or not. He bothered with anesthetics only for his own convenience — if he wanted to avoid bites and scratches from recalcitrant cats and dogs:

> or [as] a cook putting a lobster into boiling water ... just as little can the physiologist ... be expected to devote time and thought to inquiring what this animal may feel while he is doing the experiment. His whole attention is only directed to the making [of] the experiment, how to do it quickly, and to learn the most that he can from it.[6]

Given multiple opportunities to correct himself or modify his views, Klein blithely pressed on, leaving the commission members perplexed. Huxley had been out of town during Klein's appearance before the commission. When he discovered the content of Klein's testimony he felt that the ground was "cut away from beneath my feet; the advocates of legislation and restriction are furnished with all the arguments they want."[7] Klein's callous, incautious rhetoric did more damage to the cause of science than all the efforts of the antivivisectionists combined. Huxley was now ready to settle for any law that would render this kind of man impotent. Making matters worse, when Klein was given his proofs to check for accuracy, he tried to alter them in favor of the vivisectionist side, resulting in the commission's printing both the initial and corrected versions for all interested to see.

Cobbe saw an opportunity. She wrote *Public Money: An Enquiry Concerning an Item of Its Expenditure* in which she reproduced, in juxtaposed columns, Klein's original testimony and that which he had altered. Readers could compare his statements side by side in a very damning fashion. This essay persisted in print as late as 1892. His testimony would be cited again and again in antivivisectionist literature.[8] Just as the antivivisectionists fueled their current movement by fanning the fading embers of Magendie's atrocities 30 years after his retirement, Klein's cruelty and disingenuousness were similarly exploited.

Finally, in January 1876, the Royal Commission issued its report in the form of the famous Blue Book. The members formally recognized that it was impossible to prevent the practice of vivisection. Total prohibition would not be a reasonable position. They did acknowledge a great need for the regulation of vivisection as the opportunity for abuse was so great. There was no doubt that inhumanity can be found even by people in very high position, citing Magendie as an example. Then there was the question as to whether or not cruelty in English vivisection had ever existed. Most of the press claimed that British physiologists had been exonerated from the false stories of cruelty circulated about them. Cobbe, however, asserted that the committee members deliberately avoided any such conclusion.[9] Nevertheless, it was clear at this point that legislation was inevitable. That was still the public's desire.

## Animal Protection Society

In the autumn of 1875, while the Royal Commission had been forming, Hoggan suggested to Cobbe the need for a new organization, one that could take on the recently organized scientists. Cobbe reluctantly agreed, realizing that she might be charged with the onerous work load of such a group. She, Hoggan and Hutton represented a good nucleus, but a first rate organization required influential people from disparate backgrounds, such as clergymen, the literati, and people from within Parliament.[10] Politicians from the humanitarian side could embrace her society and, at the same time, move effectively in and out of Parliament. Recruitment, particularly by Cobbe and Hutton proved effective.

The organization was up and running with their first committee meeting on 2 December 1875 at the home of George Hoggan.[11] As a result of Cobbe's ministrations, this group shortly became the most influential antivivisection society then in existence. She enticed the Archbishop of York and the renowned Parliamentarian and reformer Lord Shaftesbury to join as the titular leaders of the society. Shaftesbury functioned as the interface with Parliament while serving as executive of the newly formed Society for the Protection of Animals Liable to Vivisection (SPALV), later known as the Victoria Street

Society (VSS). Anthony Ashley Cooper, the Earl of Shaftesbury and eminent Evangelical statesman, had spent most of his life fighting diverse social evils extending from the poor treatment of "lunatics" to the sad state of ragged schools.[12] Antivivisection agitation was another thankless humanitarian cause for which Shaftesbury freely gave of his time. Adored by Cobbe, Huxley dismissed Shaftesbury as "that pietistic old malefactor."[13] Cobbe assumed the position of honorary secretary of VSS from its inception, resolving at that time "never to go to bed at night leaving a stone unturned which might help to stop vivisection."[14] From 1875 to 1884 she emerged as the face of the antivivisection movement. She then wielded dwindling power from behind the scenes until 1889. Hoggan held a comparable position until 1878 when he left the society over the board's policy shift to total prohibition of vivisection.

Other antivivisection groups existed in England, some joining forces with VSS over time, while some remained independent. By the end of the decade, similar societies had formed in Germany, Sweden, Denmark, Italy, Switzerland and America. No other organization, however, ever matched the power and influence of Cobbe's Victoria Street Society.

In 1881, the VSS made one more move to improve its level of effectiveness. It published its first edition of the *Zoophilist*, which replaced the *Home Chronicler* as the literary arm of the society. This monthly carried a potpourri of antivivisection news, such as articles on animal cruelty, failures of vivisection or major differences of scientific opinion between physiologists. Another recurring column was devoted to "Physiological Fallacies," in which the editors openly disagreed with vivisectors on a variety of scientific points. In short, among other functions, the *Zoophilist* served as a propaganda wing for the VSS. Here Cobbe carried on a steady stream of rhetorical attacks against vivisectors for nearly 20 years.

## The Bill

In early 1876, advocates for each side of the vivisection legislation began a year of lobbying and maneuvering, with confrontations, deputations, subdeputations, readings and just plain argument. The government claimed that the bill, in its final form, would reflect the Royal Commission's conclusions, but neither side was fully mollified by that assertion. Richard Cross, Home Secretary, delegated to be the disinterested usher of the legislation through Parliament, asked both sides for suggestions regarding content of the bill. Lord Carnarvon, antivivisectionist, seemed objective when he proclaimed that the bill should reconcile the high laws of medical science with the still higher laws of morality and religion.[15] While such a proclamation sounded innocent

enough, it did suggest a hierarchy of morality over science. The scientists, who were periodically updated by a Lord Cardwell as the legislation moved through Parliament, should have been duly warned, but they were not. Carnarvon then crafted into the bill a statement allowing vivisection "with a view only to the advancement by new discovery of knowledge which will be useful in saving or prolonging human life or alleviating human suffering." One might as well require another to guarantee his results before embarking on any journey of discovery. Carnarvon also completely exempted dogs and cats from vivisection. Hutton had tried to slip that same clause into the Royal Commission's recommendations, only to have it unanimously rejected. There were lesser stipulations but these were the two most contentious. The medical side, apparently sleeping, offered no counter proposals to these blatant violations of the spirit of the Commission.

Lord Carnarvon planned to introduce the bill into Commons on 15 and 22 May 1876. While the medical side had not even examined the bill, Shaftesbury had the temerity to state that the bill did not go far enough. He claimed that the country was in favor of total abolition and the bill should reflect that sentiment.[16] Cobbe at this point was both "pleased with the bill and optimistic about its fate."[17] Apparently emboldened by medicine's lack of resistance, the RSPCA wanted equine species included in the ban as well. They also recommended that experimenters acquire a character reference from a "layman of eminence or position" before performing a painful experiment.[18]

The medical press, more alert than the scientists, was appalled by the bill, stating that it would mean the end of all research. When the proposal was read before the Lords on 15 May 1876, the scientists were reportedly dumbstruck by the extremes of Carnarvon's proposal. Huxley was infuriated by Cardwell's lack of action. He was supposed to keep the physiologists alert to legislative developments. Several weeks of frenetic activity took place on the scientists' side. Then, with the unexpected death of Carnarvon's mother, the physiologists gained some additional time.

With Carnarvon out of town, the scientists organized with the General Medical Counsel (GMC), a body statutorially charged with establishing medical training and maintaining standards throughout England. Lister, the newly appointed head of the GMC's commissioners, argued strongly that any legislation regulating vivisection was unwarranted. Cruelty might exist on the Continent, but that was not the case in Britain.[19] But Lister could not muster sufficient support within the council to stop the legislation. The GMC, along with the BMA, joined with Ernest Hart, editor of the *British Medical Journal*, in acquiescing to the legislation. However, they insisted to both Carnarvon and Cross that cats and dogs must be kept available for research. Seeing now the burgeoning power of the medical establishment, antivivisectionists realized that some concessions had to be made. Feeling that he had no alternative, Carnarvon reluctantly agreed to a clause that permitted experiments on cats and dogs. While Hutton was heavy with disappointment, Shaftesbury quietly agreed to the concessions.[20]

Ernest Hart, however, was not satisfied. The antivivisectionists had not surrendered enough. On 10 July, he, along with a deputation exceeding 100 men, met with Cross, who was now fully in charge of the bill. Hart expressed medicine's indignation over the entire affair and presented other lesser amendments. With this show of force, Cross, the VSS and RSPCA all reassessed their positions. The points in the bill that favored their side were probably all that they were going to get. Furthermore Cross, kept busy communicating back and forth with both groups, indicated that timing was optimal. If no bill materialized from all of this time and activity, there would likely never be a bill at all. While Hart represented an intransigent group that was willing to let the whole process die, the larger group, led by Huxley and Burdon Sanderson, preferred getting the bill passed with the newly favorable terms included.[21]

Finally, on 18 July 1876, Cross wrote to Carnarvon, "I am afraid that these Medical men are determined to stop legislation but I am told privately that if you and I were to see one or two of the best of them *without* E. Hart that something might be done. What say you?"[22] That meeting, held 22 July with Joseph Hooker, Sir James Paget, Michael Foster and Burdon Sanderson, resulted in the granting of modifications sought by the scientists. Cats and dogs could be experimented upon. The prohibition against dissecting "cold blooded animals" was changed to "invertebrates." Frogs were still fair game to the physiologists. With these modifications the bill received the Royal assent, becoming law on 15 August 1876.

## The Act

In its final form the Cruelty to Animals Act of 1876 contained multiple requirements. Anyone aspiring to experiment on living vertebrates must receive certification from the Home Secretary. His place of work must not only be licensed but subject to inspection as well. Licenses must to be renewed annually. Experiments shall only be performed with a view to the advancement, by new discovery, of physiological knowledge or knowledge that might be useful in saving or prolonging a life. No experiments may be performed before the public or for purposes of gaining manual dexterity. Experiments on cats, dogs, horses, mules and asses without anesthesia must bear certification that the objectives would be frustrated if these animals were not used. Curare was not to be considered an anesthetic. Fines would vary from 50 pounds for first offense to 100 pounds for subsequent infractions.

With so many strong personalities representing the extremes of both sides of such a contentious issue, it is not surprising that many people were left unsatisfied. Anguished cries of betrayal, deceit and favoritism arose from both sides. Claims of "this is worse than no bill" and "physiologists protection bill" filled the air and the press. While physiologists were not happy with this new governmental scrutiny they were destined to endure, they were resigned to the fact that legislation was preferable to the incessant harassment by the antivivisectionist zealots that they had been forced to face in the past.[23]

In a September *Contemporary Review* essay, pro-vivisectionist and liberal MP Robert Lowe, lamented that the entire Vivisection Act had been ill-conceived. Legislation based upon "mere compassion" has never resulted in good laws. Medical professionals within the United Kingdom have been slighted by the manner in which the Commission has treated them. More specifically, the physiologists, as the accused, were first acquitted of the charge of cruelty, then they were sentenced to be under surveillance of the police for the rest of their careers.[24] No other group in Britain, professional or otherwise, had ever been treated in such a manner. By simple decree, contemporary scientists with the most beneficent of aims, may not now inflict even the least amount of pain on any creature, while other members of society are free to subject animals to the most exquisite types of pain, without any chance of punishment at all. So long as the common man can demonstrate that he tortures in the name of cruelty, gluttony, money, or amusement, that is, for any reason except for the benefit of mankind, he can proceed with impunity; "but woe to him if in his infliction of pain there is any alloy of science or philanthropy."[25] In short, Parliament could have produced the best legislation merely by making two simple changes to the current law. First, increase the penalty for illegal dissections from 50 to 100 pounds. Second, purge the word "domestic" from the current statute, thereby placing all animals under the protection of that law against cruelty.[26]

In the October issue, Cobbe answered Lowe's charges, writing "Mr. Lowe and the Vivisection Act." She claimed that, in their efforts at legislation, the antivivisectionists were merely attempting to stop the worst form of cruelty from spreading into English schools from foreign laboratories.[27] Vivisection in its current form must be restricted or abolished since it involves "protracted and hideous *tortures*."[28] Cobbe reminded her readers that, no more than a generation ago, students of anatomy, too zealous in their pursuit of dissection, used the likes of murderers such as Burke and Hare to obtain their dead subjects for study. Such bad behavior resulted in the Anatomy Act with its system of state inspections, enacted with the full cooperation of the medical profession. It was the same with vivisection. If inspections were needed where only dead matter is concerned, certainly "it is called for where the quivering flesh of living animals is subjected to the scalpel."[29]

With each side dissatisfied, one might make the claim that the legislation was a fair compromise. Lister complained that "the faddists have had their way."[30] He was so disappointed with the enactment of the bill in August that he never applied for a license, choosing instead to experiment mainly with Professor Tuissaint at the veterinary school in Toulouse, France. Of course Cobbe considered the Act a disaster for her side as well. From that point onward she was never quite the same, feeling that Carnarvon had failed. "We asked for an Act to protect animals from vivisection. The Home Secretary has given us an Act to protect Vivisectors from prosecution." Over the next 20 years she repeatedly second-guessed herself. Had she done the right thing by getting the RSPCA and Parliament involved? The movement might have been more successful by just prosecuting individual cases of cruelty as they arose. "Justice and mercy seemed to have gone from the earth," she lamented.[31]

According to Sally Mitchell, one of Cobbe's biographers, her stubborn and irrational moves took origin from this event. Cobbe placed much of the blame for the bill's passage on her adversary Huxley, who she felt "connived" to substitute a measure different from the Commission's intent. A simmering hatred — for the process but especially for physiologists — set in. She could always tolerate the presence of people representing the other side of suffrage or religious debates — but never someone sympathetic to vivisection.

With her hopes shattered, her sunny, witty disposition changed; Cobbe considered more extreme acts against her opponents. At this time in 1876, the *Home Chronicler*, under the editorship of former VSS secretary A.P. Childs, still served as the literary outlet for Cobbe's antivivisection polemics. In one article, "The Policy of the Future," she vowed to make vivisection infamous since antivivisectionists' efforts to make it illegal had failed. She suggested publishing names and addresses of vivisectors, holding open air meetings in Hyde Park which would hopefully result in rioting. She entertained the strategy of boycotting hospitals that allowed experimentation in their medical schools.[32] Shaftesbury, aghast at her suggestions, tried to be a voice of reason and moderation. He began checking her activities more closely so that he might preempt her from putting her more radical ideas into action.

## Efforts at Total Prohibition

For months Cobbe had been mulling the pros and cons of changing VSS policy — from mere restriction of vivisection to total prohibition. Then in the

November 1876 VSS meeting she carried out a power play, issuing an ultimatum to the society. The board must adopt a policy of total prohibition or she would resign. After a contentious debate, Cobbe finally agreed to a compromise compatible with the sentiments of Hoggan, who wanted prohibition of all painful experiments.[33] That policy lasted a mere two years at which time Cobbe and the VSS board formally changed their platform to one of total prohibition of vivisection. With prohibition being too extreme a position for Hoggan, he submitted his resignation.

However, the new policy made little practical difference since the likelihood of VSS pushing any significant antivivisection legislation through Parliament was slight at this time. With the Act of 1876, the public's thirst for legislation had been satiated and most legislators did not want to deal with such a contentious topic again. In response to public sentiment, the VSS changed tactics, striving for greater public education in the form of meetings, lectures, sermons, placards and the like. Still, Cobbe kept the interpersonal battles going. She informed long-time friend, Louisa Carpenter, wife of William, the antivivisectionist physiologist, that she must regrettably end "all personal intercourse" with them. William was the brother of Mary Carpenter from the old ragged school days — Cobbe was cutting off dear old friends, people still somewhat sympathetic to her cause.

Cobbe was not yet through with her campaign. Under her direction, the VSS pasted the walls and fences of London with 1700 handbills, 300 sensational photographs, and illustrations from physiological textbooks that vividly revealed, some even exaggerating, the horrors of vivisection.[34] Both friends and allies felt that she had gone too far. The level-headed Shaftesbury counseled her again, "Public Opinion is, with God, our only Hope."[35] He began editing her leaflets. Her language was often too strong, the information sometimes inaccurate.[36]

As if her exposé of photographs and handbills had been insufficient, Cobbe later saw an opportunity to strike a similar blow against Claude Bernard. In 1879, he produced one of his best known works, *Physiologie Operatoire*, for fellow physiologists. Since the book presented his experiments in great detail, along with illustrations, Cobbe decided to provide the public with "an ocular illustration of the meaning of the much disputed word, *vivisection*."[37] In her essay, *Light in Dark Places*, she provided excerpts from *Physiologie Operatoire* plus a similar vivisection manual produced by Russian physiologist Elie de Cyon, as illustrated. "Thus every illustration in this pamphlet may be taken with certainty to be *a Vivisector's own picture of his own work*, such as he himself has chosen to publish it."[38]

Through the prolonged legislative fight, physiologists had been forced into a reactionary position by antivivisectionists — frequently a little late to the trough. In 1882, they formed the Association for the Advancement of Medical Research (AAMR), an organization through which physiologists hoped to improve their public image in two different ways. First, through placards and medical associations, they softened their profile by associating with the British general practitioner — a group still venerated by the public at large. These men were still viewed by the public as the kindly family doctors, "the warriors against pain, comforters of the afflicted."[39]

The scientists' second strategy, however, would prove a taller order. The public needed some gentle nudging. If physiology was to survive, the public needed to either get over their sensitivity to the pain associated with vivisection or at least learn to come to terms with it. On the consideration of public good versus experimentation, the public was slowly beginning to side more with physiologists than with Cobbe and her allies. To her, any infliction of pain on a lesser being corrupted a man's soul. Any knowledge gained through painful experimentation was information purchased at too high a price. If the antivivisectionists could not see beyond the infliction of pain on a few, for the potential benefit of the "sufferings of thousands and thousands of human

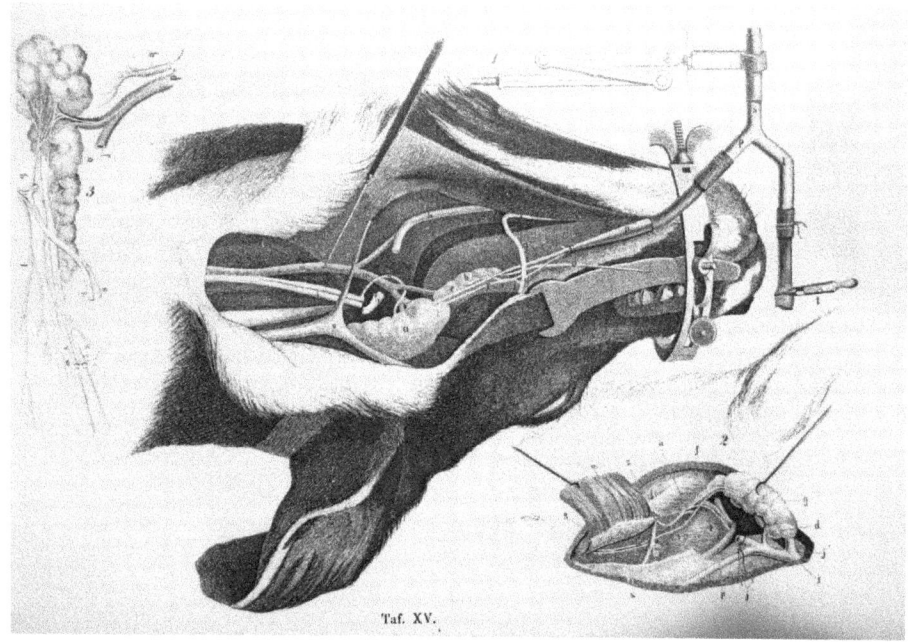

Dog in "nosegay." Cobbe derisively used the word for the animal holder. He hoped that the sharp points holding the dog's snout securely in the device and the open neck wound would repulse readers. (From Elie de Cyon's 1876 *Methodik der Physiologischen Experimente und Vivisectionen: Mit Atlas*.)

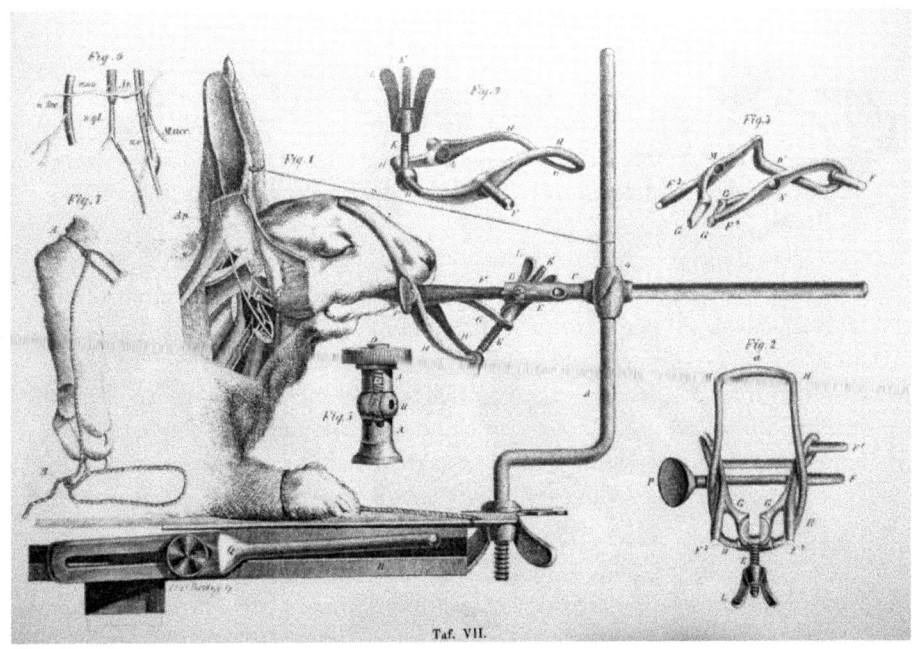

Rabbit in holder. This device holds a rabbit, typically less contentious than a dog to the experimental conditions. Note clamps encompassing the face for dissection in the neck. (From Cyon's *Atlas*).

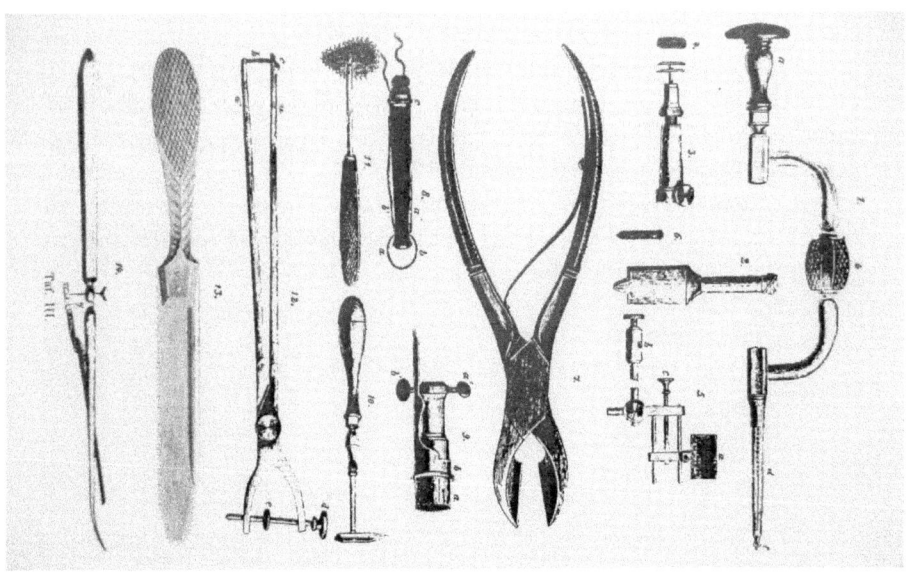

Physiological tools. Here is a sampling of physiological surgical instruments that Cobbe found so shocking. While stark in appearance, these tools of 1876 are little different from some used today. (From Cyon's *Atlas*).

beings of the present and future generations," one could then argue that the antivivisectionists had really ceded that higher ethical ground of pain relief to the vivisectors.[40] Making an immediate, small sacrifice for a later potential benefit of many was beginning to make too much sense for the prudent person to dismiss.

Even if physiologists could prove convincingly that they cared as much about pain relief as did their adversaries, that did not let them entirely off the hook. They had to prove, through tangible achievements, that they were ridding society of suffering and disease. Even Claude Bernard, early in his career, admitted that, despite all of the knowledge experimental scientists had accumulated up to that time, none of it had directly resulted in a single practical remedy for human suffering. In spite of that, Bernard was unyielding in his belief in vivisection. When asked later about the utility of vivisection, he stated:

> You ask me which are the main discoveries we owe to vivisection in order to emphasize them in arguments defending these kinds of study. When it comes to that, one can only cite all of the accomplishments of experimental physiology; there is not a single fact that was not the direct and necessary result of vivisection."[41]

It is true that working physiologists the world over were accumulating bits of knowledge in a disparate and disorganized fashion. Separately, these bits may have been mere dots on a blank canvas. With time, when scientifically juxtaposed, those points might amount to nothing — or they might fall together creating some beautiful mosaic of scientific achievement. Most scientists, through their life's work, create only a small piece of that image, merely expanding one small aspect of a puzzle. Now, in 1880, one other scientist, Pasteur's junior by 20 years, necessarily entered the scene late. His contributions would prove so great that he is today considered the other co-founder of modern bacteriology.

# V

# GERM THEORY EXPANDED

His [Koch's] decision to experiment "not with humans but with the parasite in pure culture," was more than a move from the hospital ward to the laboratory, for it changed the very object of the investigation. New knowledge about diseases was now based not so much on the observation of sick humans as on the reproduction of pathological processes in experimental animals.[1]

CHAPTER 9

# Robert Koch: Templates of Hospitalism

August 1880 found Lister in Cambridge at the British Medical Association, delivering a speech, a summary of notable contributors to the field of pathogenic microorganisms. Lister reported on a rising luminary, Robert Koch, a young German bacteriologist who possessed unmatched methods for demonstrating the presence of diverse microorganisms. Remarkably, Koch accomplished these feats through meticulously planned animal experiments combined with ingenious techniques for staining bacteria, all while intellectually isolated as a country doctor.[1] Although new to the scientific scene around 1875, Koch's successes, when viewed over the entire spectrum of his career, matched those of Louis Pasteur.

His path to prominence was an unusual one. Two childhood talents which he developed under the guidance of his maternal uncle in Clausthal Germany would serve him well in his later career. The first, a gift for photography, arose at a time when producing high-quality daguerreotypes was no small feat. Secondly, he learned taxonomy, the scientific classification of plants and animals, providing him with precocious insights about biologic organization. After high school Robert attended the prestigious University of Gottingen, with plans to become a natural scientist. After coming under the influence of such noted scientists as anatomist Jacob Henle, an early proponent of germ theory, and Professor Wohlers, synthesizer of urea, he changed his major to medicine. However, it was a physiologist, Georg Meissner, expert in animal experimentation, who most influenced the young student, instilling in him a love for experimentation. Under Meissner, Robert won a coveted scientific prize for his work on "The Presence of Ganglion Cells in the Uterus." Robert received his medical degree, in 1866, after passing his "Facultates-Examen" at age 23. Uncertain about his future plans, Koch traveled to Berlin for a three-month lecture course from the famed pathologist Rudolf Virchow.[2]

He had no inkling of how their paths would clash less than a decade later. Suppressing a strong desire for worldwide travel, Koch decided to settle down instead, marrying his childhood sweetheart, Emmy Kraatz, in 1867. The couple then moved to a series of small provincial towns, each anxious for its own physician. He was immediately loved and sought after for his kind manner and obvious competence, but making a living in these poor mountain towns was difficult. Even in these bleak, non-academic surroundings, a definite bacteriological bent was becoming evident. In Rakwitz — now part of Poland — he visited nearby marshes, collecting swamp water to examine protozoa and algae under his microscope. Life was starting to fall into place for the young family until 1870 when the war with France erupted. With his severe near-sightedness, Koch could have avoided military service but he volunteered instead, causing a two-year hiatus with his family. Koch, assigned to a field hospital of the 10th Army Corps at Mainz, later recalled that his experience there caring for the war wounded was worth "more than six months in a surgical clinic."[3]

For a major conflict, the Franco-Prussian War was incredibly brief. The military campaign lasted a mere four months, from July into October 1870. France suffered crushing defeats at Sedan in September and at Metz in October. In a second phase of the war, both countries languished through much of the winter with Prussia enforcing a tight military blockade around Paris, known as the Iron Ring. The French could do little but writhe in their constraints. With a routed army and no central control, anarchy prevailed, especially in Paris. Finally, in May 1871, a fragmented French army managed to end the chaos by gaining control of the city, and acceding to the enemy's demands. Prussia's domination of France was as complete as it was humiliating. The war was formally over.[4]

Historians have called the Franco-Prussian confrontation the most important international conflict from the time of Napoleon I to the first World War. Its conclusion ushered in the modern European era with Germany replacing France as the world's most powerful nation. In the settlement, the Prussians extracted five billion francs in war reparations from the French. For the proud and patriotic French, the defeat was not easily forgotten. Resentment of the Prussians lived on through generations. Adding to Pasteur's angst, France was forced to cede his beloved city of Strasbourg, all of Alsace and much of the territory of Lorraine to Germany.

Understandably, a rivalry developed between Pasteur and Koch related both to their nationalism and their experiences in the war. But something positive developed as a consequence. The two scientists not only placed germ theory on sound footing, but they established the discipline of bacteriology as well. Just as with Pasteur, the war served to sharpen Koch's nationalism and to intensify his feelings against the other country. That tension, held in common, colored the scientists' already competitive relationship. Koch's work with the war wounded not only helped his country, but also gave him valuable experience in evaluating and treating wound infections. He exploited this experience a mere eight years later in his pioneering bacteriological work.

## Country Doctor

With the resolution of the war, Koch and his family settled in Wollstein, Prussia, later known as Wolsztyn, Poland. Here he spent eight productive years, moving from obscurity to near worldwide fame as a result of his investigative work. He and Emmy rented a large house which also served as his clinic. The young investigator devoted part of one examination room to his ever increasing laboratory interest. Influenced by his Gottingen days, Koch housed a collection of animals including guinea pigs, dogs, rabbits, mice and even two monkeys, all of whom became part of his experiments at one time or another. His practice thrived. One former Wollsteiner recalled, "What a doctor! There was something special about him. How often did I hear my mother say, 'If Dr. Koch came into your sick room, you immediately felt calm and secure.'"[5]

But being a country doctor was the last thing Koch wanted to be.[6] His career interests turned more towards the academic when, in 1866, he attended lecture courses by the famous Rudolf Virchow. By the time Koch entered the microbiological scene, Pasteur's ideas concerning microorganisms, putrefaction and fermentation were becoming more widely known and Lister's antiseptic work was well under way. Both men were undeniably pioneers in the study of microbes but Koch brought a different approach to it than did Pasteur. Koch was more the morphologist, interested in the discovery of bacteria, their various physical and behavioral characteristics and how organisms related to morbidity. His idea of controlling disease related more to preventive measures such as diminishing overcrowding, improving water supplies or cleaning up vermin-infested sections of a city based upon scientific information. Pasteur disliked the term "applied scientist," but after his great contributions of putting spontaneous generation to rest and gaining acceptance of germ theory, that was arguably what he became. Pasteur manipulated bacteriological phenomena to achieve an effect — an immunized subject. With their work, both Koch and Pasteur ushered in an entirely new paradigm, completely changing how one classified and investigated diseases.

Earlier, Thomas Sydenham, the famous 17th-century London physician, taught students how to identify diseases based upon symptoms — a purely empirical approach. Just as one could recognize friends by their height, shape, bodily habitus and actions, enemy diseases were similarly identified by their silhouette of symptoms. Since most physicians still believed that an imbalance of humors produced disease, the idea of a specific agent causing a particular disease was a completely foreign notion. They could not have imagined using etiology (disease causation), as a criterion for classifying diseases.

Pasteur and Koch were not the first to incorporate this new theory about germs into their reckoning about how infectious diseases developed. Pioneering 19th-century French physician Bretonneau presciently stated that specificity of disease was due to specificity of cause. Each disease "developed under the influence of a contagious principle capable of reproduction."[7] Jacob Henle, Koch's old Gottingen teacher, had similarly written about contagion as a concept but he had never demonstrated it through any sort of experimentation. It was just a theory. The first person to conflate causation, infection and disease as such was Agostino Bassi. He published a book about muscardine or "silk worm rot" in 1836 in which he recognized that a "fungus" parasitized the silkworm — an entirely new theory.[8] Pasteur, in his early work with silkworms, gave Bassi full credit since Bassi's work was decades earlier than his own. Contagion meant the spread of disease by contact between a diseased and a healthy being. But many scientists, especially physicians, still remained very skeptical of both infection and contagion. The older, more firmly entrenched icons of science, such as Virchow and Theodor Billroth of Vienna, even at mid-century, still denied that microorganisms played any significant role in infectious disease.

In the early 1870s, an acute epidemic occurred among the sheep and cattle of Europe. Anthrax, a disease as highly infectious as it is lethal, caused great concern among farmers. But the farmers' misfortune provided Koch with a golden opportunity. As the local health official in Wollstein, it was his job to examine sheep that died in the epidemic. Anthrax was a truly fearsome disease. The French called it *charbon* (coal) because it turned red blood to black. Early in the disease only subtle manifestations such as a lamb or cow listlessly holding its head low gave any clue that something was wrong. A disease more of cattle than humans, anthrax was so virulent that it could decimate a herd virtually overnight, leaving lifeless, anthracitic bodies scattered throughout the field. Animals that ingested the organisms became septic with high fevers within hours. As the disease advanced, the animals bled from all orifices, due to incompetence of their blood-clotting systems. Rapid decline ensued, with the animal passing into delirium, then coma, followed by death. At autopsy, a turgid, massive, black spleen was the pathognomonic finding. Scientists already knew that the blood of animals dying of this virulent disease contained rod-shaped bacteria at postmortem, but they did not understand its significance. Koch too noted microscopic organisms in the blood. In fact, he later proved that the disease was contagious by transmitting anthrax from one animal to another. To Koch the infectiousness of the bacillus was no longer in question, but in the real world, direct infection did not always occur in a predictable manner consistent with a contagious disease. For example, a solitary animal could contract anthrax from merely grazing solo in a pasture. If contagion meant the passing of disease from one living being to another, how could a solitary animal contract the disease? Anthrax, it appeared, did not always follow the rules. Was there something in the soil or was some other unrecognized infectious mechanism in play? Koch soon found the answer. In April 1874, while examining infected sheep blood, he observed changes suggesting that anthrax bacteria could become virtually inert. "The bacteria swell up, become shinier, thicker and much longer. Slight bends develop. Gradually a thick felt develops. Within the long cells, cross walls appear and small transparent points develop at regular intervals."[9]

Koch had just discovered endospores, a virtually indestructible form of the anthrax organism. Like a turtle contracting into the safety of its shell, protected, if the environment turns temporarily unfriendly, the spore is able to withstand external assaults. With the return of a more friendly environment, the spore can reemerge. Farmers around Wollstein, by tradition, had been in the habit of burying the carcasses of animals dying of anthrax in the pasture essentially where they fell. Later Koch solved this puzzle by demonstrating that earthworms consumed those spores which had been lying inert in the soil since the time of burial. The sheep or cow in turn became infected by ingesting the worm as they grazed on grass. In the friendly environment of the ruminant's bowel, the spores then evolved back into the infectious anthrax bacilli. That missing link of contagion had finally been resolved.

Beginning in December 1875, Koch singlehandedly elucidated the entire life cycle of *Bacillus anthracis* in a matter of months, first by inoculating a rabbit with the organism. Within 24 hours, he found the rabbit on its back, legs in the air, color now blue-black. On postmortem its spleen was huge, oozing black, slimy fluid. All of the rabbit's tissues teemed with the anthrax organism. Through a small slit in the cornea of another living rabbit, Koch inserted splenic tissue from the dead rabbit. After this second rabbit died, autopsy revealed widespread dissemination of bacteria, from eye to blood and spleen. After repeating this manipulation many times, Koch was confident that he had not only demonstrated the full life cycle of the anthrax bacillus, but also proved its infectious nature. In the process he had developed a new culture medium, the anterior chamber of the eye, that is, the liquid area immediately behind the cornea. The eyeball represented a perfect culture medium for bacteria with its sterile interior and ample supply of nutritious proteins and minerals. Koch began visiting the local abattoir to acquire cows' eyes for his new culture method. With such a convenient, new repository he could reap and sow bacteria as he wished.

## Appointment in Breslau

Excited by these new developments Koch considered publishing his results immediately. But working by himself in a small town away from scientific centers, he began having self-doubts. Had he done everything correctly? Rather than possibly making a fool of himself, he decided on a more prudent course. He would present his work to an authority in the field — consider that expert's criticisms privately, then make the necessary corrections in the protective shadow of anonymity. Koch therefore arranged an audition with Ferdinand Cohn, Professor of Botany in Breslau. Cohn was similarly involved in pioneering studies with microorganisms, except his subjects were plants rather than animals. As Koch boarded an overnight train in Wollstein, he must have been a strange sight, accompanied by his apparatus, flasks, reagents, living mice, rabbits and frogs — all en route to Breslau.[10] Arriving at the institute the next day, he set up fresh cultures so that Professor Cohn might see the process starting at step one. In his three-day stay, Koch produced pure cultures of anthrax, elucidated the organisms' transformation from spores — residing in the anterior chamber of the ox's eye — to chains of bacilli, through which he then infected subsequent generations of mice. To transmit the disease to other mice, he impaled each with a sliver of wood coated with anthrax.[11] The next day all cultures from these mice were swarming with new growth. Cohn was fascinated. Here was this solo practitioner, isolated in the outlands, showing new tricks to the experts. By Koch's third day in Breslau, the entire university was aware of this unusual visitor. Even the famous botanist Julius Cohnheim, Director of the Institute of Plant Physiology, came to observe. Returning to his institute, he told his assistants:

> Now leave everything as it is and go to Koch. This man has made a magnificent discovery, which, for simplicity and the precision of the methods employed, is all the more deserving of admiration, as Koch has been shut off completely from all scientific associations. He has done everything himself and with absolute completeness. There is nothing more to be done. I regard this as the greatest discovery in the field of pathology, and believe that Koch will again surprise us and put us all to shame by further discoveries.[12]

Cohn was so impressed that he arranged to publish Koch's results in his own prestigious journal.[13] It was a different Koch that boarded the train back to Wollstein, buoyant, energized — his pioneering work fully authenticated.

Two publications resulted from these early efforts: One paper dealt with the etiology of anthrax and a second with photographic microscopy. Making use of his old childhood photographic skills, Koch worked diligently on capturing bacterial images using only sunlight. Since microscopes were not yet electrified, the luxury of artificial light was unavailable. This was also the era of preparing your own cassette, positioning the microscope optimally in relation to the window, using silver iodide emulsion, and waiting on exposure times of minutes just to capture that image. Even keeping the microscope in focus could be difficult. Amazingly, Koch carried out this meticulous work by stealing time in between patient visits. Getting three to four acceptable photographs with four hours of effort was typical. Still, the effort was worthwhile since the photos brought instant credibility both to skeptics and new viewers. Even the most meticulous drawings of bacteria could not compare with the impact of seeing the actual images. The persuasive power of a photomicrograph to any agnostic of germ theory could hardly be overestimated. Koch produced the world's first photomicrographs of bacteria and his was the first such publication ever.

He made other technical improvements, in collaboration with workers from Zeiss, the microscope company, such as immersing the top of the glass slide with mineral oil, which allowed the oil to touch the microscope lens. By replacing air with oil in this limited space, he minimized distortion of the light beam, thereby improving image detail.[14] Koch collaborated with Carl Weigert and Paul Ehrlch of Breslau, both experts in the chemistry of organic dyes. If the correct dye could be matched to the appropriate bacteria, the dye would be taken up in the capsule of the bacteria, giving it a color. Now the viewer could more readily differentiate the organisms from debris and other objects. Methyl violet generally worked best, staining the bacteria blue.

Koch next returned to the study of his old military interest — wound infections. In doing so, however, he first became embroiled in a heated, ongoing dispute between two schools of thought — a debate requiring resolution before he could focus on infections, *per se*. As described by Koch biographer Thomas Brock, some scientists felt that each specific bacteria had its own unique origin while others believed one bacteria could branch into many different cell lines — a sort of microcosm of the evolutionary debate. Koch sided with Ferdinand Cohn, who claimed that each bacterial strain descended from a specific origin or a specific reproductive lineage.

In the other corner was the influential Swiss botanist Carl von Nageli who argued in favor of a primordial organism, much like a stem cell — a cell of pluripotential power — that could develop along one of several lines, in response to the environmental conditions in which it was placed. Von Nageli even boldly stated that in 10 years' work, he had never seen two distinct species. If von Nageli's theory were true, it weakened the base upon which germ theory tenuously rested, since the scheme of one specific organism for one specific disease would no longer apply. Instead, it would be one vague organism causing a panoply of diseases. Further supporting von Nageli's theory was German Edwin Klebs. During the Franco-German war he had performed a microscopic study of gunshot wounds in 100 autopsied soldiers. In nearly every infection he found bacteria of differing types — an observation that should have supported Koch's side. However, since prevailing medical opinion at that time supported the pluripotential theory, Klebs merely went along with the majority, naming the supposed bacteria *microsporon septicum*.[15]

After studying the methods of his two predecessors, Klebs and von Nageli, Koch discovered that both had been insufficiently stringent in their work. From direct observation he recognized that the bacteria of wound infections were not only smaller than the anthrax organism, but were also more difficult to see in blood. Klebs and von Naegli had probably not even seen the important organisms. Koch discovered that one had to stain the specimens with aniline dyes (chemical derivatives of benzene) and view them through the oil immersion lens which

> completely altered the pictures. In the same slides which had previously shown nothing, the smallest bacteria are now visible with such clarity and definition that they are very easy to see and to distinguish from other colored objects.... Now we can see bacteria which can be distinguished by size and shape.[16]

Next, using mice as his model, Koch produced an experimental infection in blood that would serve as one archetype of infection. Injecting bacteria in low doses, he made multiple, successive passages in mice, injecting blood from mouse one into mouse two, then to mouse three and so on. He produced 17 successive generations of bacteria and infection in that manner. Each mouse died of uniform symptoms in about 50 hours, suggesting a uniform pathology, a uniform disease.

## Templates of Infection

In his next experiment, rather than simply concentrating on blood infection (sepsis), he studied different forms of infection: gangrene (death and decay of soft tissue), anthrax, abscess, pyemia (another kind of blood infection) and erysipelas (a spreading infection in the skin and subcutaneous tissue).

From this experience, Koch recognized the value of pure bacterial cultures, that is, cultures in which all extraneous organisms had been eliminated. Then when he inoculated with a specific bacterial type, purified through gen-

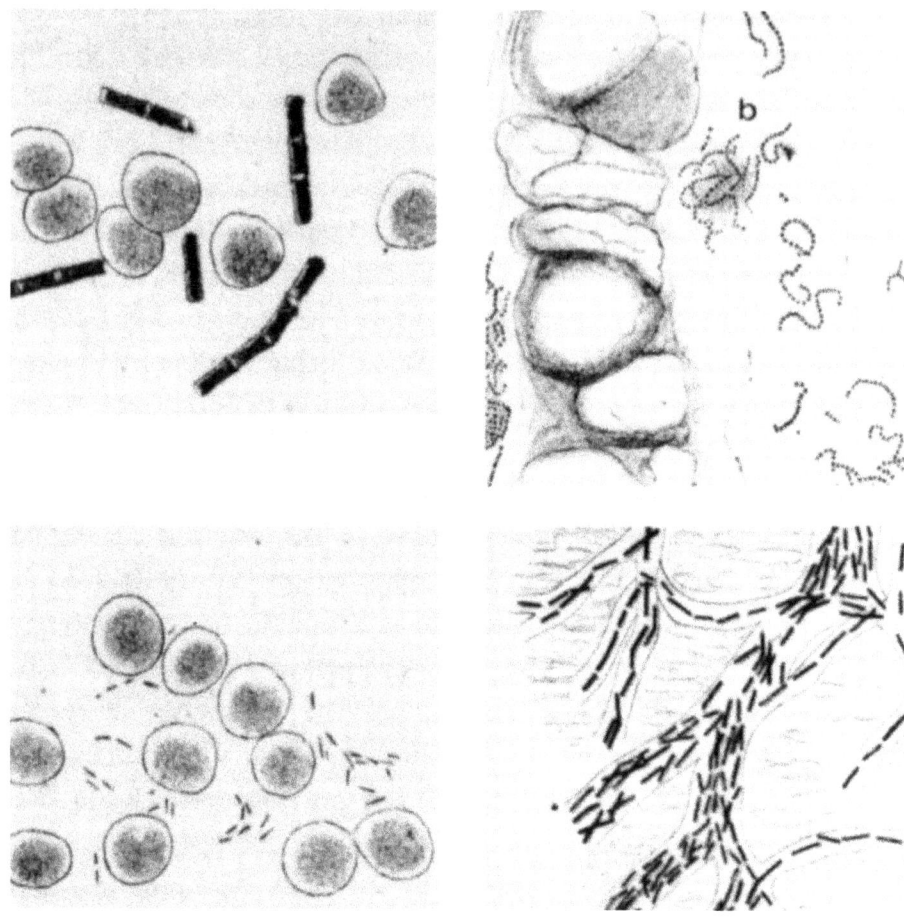

Koch's own drawings illustrating differing aspects of sepsis. *Clockwise from upper left:* (1) Cylindrical anthrax organisms in the blood of a mouse. (2) Micrococci in chains appearing next to cartilage of a mouse's ear. (3) Capillaries filled with chains of bacilli. (4) Septicemia: Small cocci in mouse's blood. (Courtesy of ASM Press and Thos. D. Brock, p. 78).

erations of animals, he could then have confidence that the subsequent phenomena observed in the animal were the result of that particular bacterial strain. If the inocula were of mixed strains, the changes in the animal would more likely be mixed and unpredictable. Still, how does one go about getting a pure culture? Pasteur claimed to acquire them merely by taking a small liquid portion from the culture broth, a virtual alphabet soup of organisms. Under such conditions, extracting the desired bacterial strain relied too much on faith and too little on technique. Koch would later solve this problem of purity by perfecting a plating technique in which bacteria were spread on a surface, like butter on bread.

Unfortunately, with his limited resources in Wollstein, Koch had to rely, for the time being, on the next best cultivation apparatus — the animal itself. Inject the first generation of animals with bacteria, then inoculate the second generation with bacteria grown from the first generation and keep that pattern going for as many generations as one wished. With this method each culture successively purified the stronger strains of bacteria in mice. Since some of the weaker strains died off, the next generation was comprised of newer, hardier bacteria, resulting in a purer form than the last — Koch's so-called "enrichment culture."[17] He documented these experiments in his book, *Investigations into the Etiology of Traumatic Infective Diseases*. Those images presented by Koch's animals served as analogues to the various forms of infections presented in his book — septicemia, abscesses and soft tissue infections. They were templates of infectious disease — patterns of animal illness analogous to what clinicians had been seeing in humans for years. Koch had produced his own laboratory form of hospitalism in animals, independent of both Pasteur's and Lister's similar work.

Once he completed his book, Koch took a tour, visiting Cohn in Breslau and Cohnheim in Leipzig. It was Cohnheim who convinced Koch to meet with the influential Virchow in Berlin in the hopes that he might be impressed with Koch's new findings. But Koch, a minnow in Virchow's ocean, proved no match for the great agnostic of germ theory. Virchow's reception of Koch was icy. Of Koch's work on anthrax, he commented, "The whole thing to me seems highly improbable." Virchow was even less impressed with the younger man's microscopic photography. Koch later told a friend, "What Virchow couldn't see

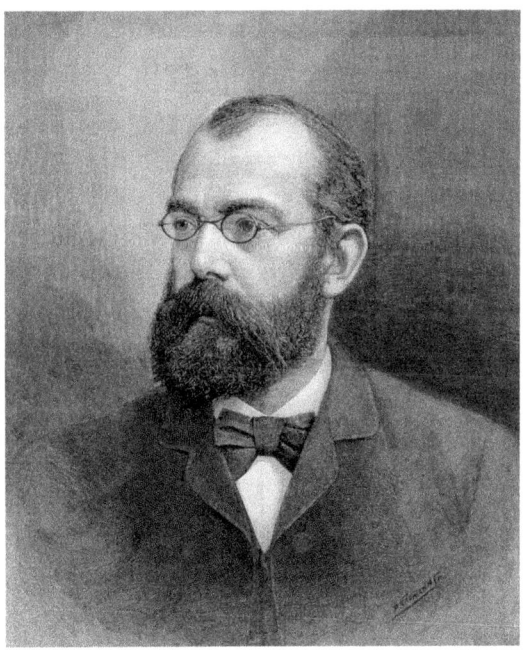

Wood engraving of Robert Koch by P. Naumann. Aged 40, he was already established as a bacteriological savant and was launching his work on cholera in Egypt. (Reproduced by permission of the Wellcome Library, London.)

through his spectacles, he did not want to know about."[18] Dismayed, Koch bid him farewell. In four short years he would have a great pronouncement concerning tuberculosis that would finally make a believer out of Virchow.

Despite Virchow's doubts, Koch's reputation spread. He became increasingly dissatisfied living in Wollstein — he needed to work in a large, active city among fellow researchers. Finally, with intercessions from Cohn and Cohnheim, Koch arranged a position in the Imperial Health Office in Berlin. Arriving at 57 Luisenstrasse in July 1880, he was entering a new and productive era. His only responsibility would be full-time research. In addition, he had two assistants with whom he could exchange ideas, Georg Gaffky and Friedrich Loeffler.[19] Both became prominent bacteriological figures in their own right. The volume of work originating from 57 Luisenstrasse over the next decade would be prodigious. Koch, later reflecting on the fecundity of this period, claimed that gold lay everywhere on the ground — "all that was needed was the ability to distinguish what was gold."[20]

## Koch's Pure Culture

With a better work environment and his experiments on wound infection completed, Koch could now pursue something long overdue — a technique for obtaining pure cultures. Most bacteriologists realized that merely reaching into a culture broth, which was no more than a melange of bacteria in a bulbous flask, and extracting the precise strain of bacteria one wished to grow was less than an ideal method. Koch criticized Pasteur's technique of using just such an admixture of bacteria while believing that he was obtaining a pure culture. Furthermore, "it should be heeded by the Pasteur school in its noteworthy but blindly zealous researches, since this renders it doubtful that they have obtained in pure culture the organisms of rabies, sheep pox, tuberculosis and so forth."[21]

While criticizing Pasteur, Koch may have been committing his own transgression by using another man's work without giving full attribution. Stories of the origin of his inspiration differ. One biographer, David Knight, relates that one morning Koch noted a colored material growing on the surface of a boiled potato carelessly left on his lab counter.[22] But Joseph Schroeter, a student of Cohn's, had reported growing pigmented bacteria, some red and some blue, on the surface of incubated potatoes. This bacterial pigment was a constant, surviving from one generation of bacteria to the next. Schroeter noted that each bacterial species had its own physical characteristics when cultured in this manner, allowing one to readily distinguish one bacteria from another merely by looking at them. Koch's biographer, Robert Brock, alleges that it was through Schroeter's work with potatoes that Koch became aware that bacterial colonies could be identified by their external appearance.[23] Nevertheless, the idea of using such a phenomenon to create pure cultures belonged exclusively to Koch. Bacterial growth on a solid surface could provide that critical difference in getting a pure culture. It is more accurate to pick an item off a tabletop than to reach into a churning tub of alphabet soup. In the soup, one might hope to retrieve only one letter but inadvertently pull out six or eight others as well. When Koch exploited this principle of pigmented bacterial growth on potatoes, he adapted the process to a glass environment for easier use. Still, since all existing culture media were liquid, Koch needed some agent to add to the liquid to render it solid at room temperature. By converting the liquid into something solid, he was transforming the stew into that desired tabletop, with organisms now sitting on the surface rather than swirling in fluid. He first settled on gelatin as his medium but later, through the advice of an assistant, changed the agent to agar, a seaweed product solid at room temperature. Koch's initial glassware was later changed to the Petri dish, a round, flat-bottomed bowl with glass cover, still in use today. Koch could now sterilize the glass and agar separately, before allowing the latter to solidify at the bottom of the glass container. This surface was the slice of bread to be buttered. Using a sterile platinum wand, subsequently coated with the bacteria desired from the inoculum or infection, he merely dragged the wand across the surface of the agar, sowing the seeds of bacterial growth.

That was Koch's "plating" technique. As organisms grew on the surface, he could put the enclosed glass under his microscope and more finely select the bacteria he wanted, swabbing them on a new culture plate, guided by their appearance. Each succeeding generation of bacteria produced a purer culture.

As Koch stated it, "The pure culture is the foundation for all research on infectious diseases."[24] It did provide several benefits. First, it provided purity of bacterial strains to a superb level, never before attained. Koch felt that culturing through three or four generations produced a pure culture, for practical purposes. However, with some microbes, such as anthrax, he cultured strains out to 20 or even 50 generations, in effect eluting any bacterial or metabolic impurities from the culture completely.[25] Purity of culture promoted clarity of experimental results.

## Speciation

One unanticipated dividend of the pure culture: Koch quickly recognized that colonies of bacteria possessed their own distinct physical characteristics, something unappreciated until bacteria could be seen more distinctly on a solid media surface. Some colonies were waxy and smooth, while others might be dark and rough, or light and translucent. With such unique physical and behavioral traits, Koch began applying Linnaean taxonomic principles, classifying them by genus and species just as scientists had been doing for the plant and larger animal kingdom for many years. The solid plating technique therefore brought order to a previously chaotic microscopic world.[26]

Admirers of Koch's new technique began appearing even within the competitive Pasteur camp. Émile Roux admitted that "culture in solid media is very useful because it permits us to observe the form of the colonies and because it readily permits the separation of diverse organisms."[27] The technique was so simple and so reproducible that it was widely adopted, changing the method of bacterial culture for all time. Koch's paper, "Methods for the Study of Pathogenic Organisms," published in 1881, became known as "The Bible of Bacteriology" since it explained in detail all of the necessary steps for culturing and studying microorganisms. Koch's technique both modernized and standardized bacterial methodology.

As fellow scientists became aware of Koch's proficiency and originality of thought, his reputation soared to a level equal to that of Louis Pasteur, a rival 20 years his senior.

CHAPTER 10

# Louis Pasteur: The Infinitely Small Are Infinitely Great

While Koch had been so consumed covering new bacteriological ground, Louis Pasteur had not been resting on his laurels. In 1877, he had begun working on anthrax, like Koch, but with a different aim. Prior investigators had microscopically examined blood from animals dying presumably of anthrax, only to get mixed results; some found organisms in the blood and some did not. Bringing his systematic methods to bear, Pasteur examined the blood of a lamb 16 hours after death and saw anthrax organisms. But the blood of a horse, examined 24 hours after death, revealed two different bacteria — anthrax and another unknown one. In a cow, examined 72 hours after death, Pasteur saw a heavy growth of that unknown organism and only a few anthrax bacilli. It was clear that bacterial populations varied with time of death. When he injected blood from the animals dying at 24 and 72 hours into other animals, their deaths were speedy and differed greatly from the blackened tissues and enlarged spleens typical of anthrax. In contrast, blood from the lamb, dead at 16 hours, caused a death identical to anthrax when inoculated in other animals.

Pasteur was not only able to separate the two organisms, but in the process he discovered the source of putrefaction and how man and animal return to dust. This second organism he called *Vibrion septique*. While anthrax was aerobic, heavily dependent upon ambient oxygen for survival, subsequent studies with the vibrio organism showed that it was not. It was not only anaerobic but it produced carbon dioxide as a byproduct. He discovered that *Vibrion septique* was ubiquitous. Billions normally reside in the intestinal tract of healthy animals, including man. Long and translucent, these organisms could slither, serpentine style, through the intestinal wall of a moribund animal, invading the body immediately after death.[1] In such a manner the process of putrefaction began. Pasteur found that this vibrio slowly deconstructed the body, returning it to the soil and air from whence it came. As the process emits carbon dioxide, one notes massive abdominal bloating, such as cattle lying in the field on their backs, all four extremities protruding like the four fingers of an inflated rubber glove. As the putrefactive organisms break down protein, certain aromatic amines, such as putrescine and cadaverine, are released into the air, accounting for the offensive odors emanating from the dead. The body is thus chemically deconstructed from within, imploding, progressively shrinking in size. Only the skin, slowly oxidized from without, is unaffected by the putrefactive process.

Pasteur fully appreciated the beneficial role played by this vibrio. It completed the circle of life by clearing out the dead, returning the body to dust. As Pasteur gained more information it became clear that there are beneficial germs that work through fermentation, producing products such as wine, beer or cheese; pathogenic germs that cause infectious diseases in both man and animal, and germs like the septic vibrio that clean up the environment. Pasteur became fond of stating that, when it comes to the role of microorganisms in the regulation of nature, the "infinitely small" are "infinitely great."[2] As he became more enlightened with time and further reflection he could have added a corollary: The body itself is a collection of ferments, the deconstruction of disparate organic compounds in the proper stew of enzymes and bacteria. Whether considering the digestion of food, various bodily infections, the putrefaction of advanced gingivitis, even the "natural" aroma of unwashed human skin—all are noxious ferments.

Even though Pasteur was convinced of the prominent natural roles played by bacteria in his ever-expanding research, others were not yet convinced. He occasionally lectured the members of the Academy of Medicine about microorganisms and how physicians might avoid infections or even death from bacterial origin. In one such lecture to surgeons in January 1874, before he had ever communicated with Lister, Pasteur caused some consternation by stating, "If I had the honor of being a surgeon, I would never introduce into the human body an instrument without having passed it through boiling water or, better still, through a flame and rapidly cooled right before the operation." He further warned, "You should only use instruments and bandages, that have been previously exposed to a temperature of no less than 266–302°C."[3] Inexplicably, even in France no one followed the celebrated scientist's advice. When it came to human disease, many in the Academy were plainly indifferent to his views. What would a chemist know about diseases and microorganisms?

Of course Pasteur knew a great deal about disease, approaching it from a different perspective. He had developed his own sophisticated version of sterile technique (asepsis)—born in response to situations arising in his workplace. He realized that mistakes committed in his laboratory, through ignorance or carelessness, would render his experimental results chaotic and useless. He enacted a reliable routine to avoid calamity. Don't stir up dust. Wash your hands both before and after dealing with contaminated matter. Sterilize surfaces and objects with heat before and after use. Keep cultures covered, protected. Pasteur hated to shake hands, which added to his imperious persona. If he could not avoid the ritual, he hastened to a sink as soon as possible afterwards, discreetly washing off those dirty acquired bacteria.

Even though he had not worked regularly in hospitals, Pasteur had occasion to pass through them, sometimes even bringing a team equipped with sterile needles, pipettes and culture plates for acquiring samples from patients. Like Lister, he saw hospitalism first hand. It took him little time to recognize that most French physicians and nurses were indifferent to, if not completely ignorant of, his new theory about germs. He felt repulsed by the hospital odors, the filth of the floors, the beds and the personnel. Paris was no different than London. Pasteur felt pangs of despair about the depth of microbiological ignorance around him.

## Puerperal Fever

Despite such complacency in colleagues, Pasteur did have several opportunities to extend the reach of germ theory. In March 1879, he attended an Academy of Medicine meeting, listening while an obstetrical authority, Dr. Hervieux, lectured on the causes of puerperal fever, the infection so frequent on maternity hospitals. On some wards mortality approached 50 percent. Postpartum women were predisposed to infections, especially in the first week after delivery. The uterine lining where the placenta had been attached was now like an ill-ventilated, large, deep abrasion — combining all of the elements of a perfect bacterial culture bed. On a previous occasion Pasteur had sampled the blood of a woman dying under such circumstances. He found her blood loaded with sausage-like strings of bacteria, later named streptococci. Pasteur knew the scenario well. As Hervieux continued his lecture, he spoke disparagingly about germ theory, attributing the disease instead, to the impure "miasmatic" air.[4] Pasteur became increasingly upset, finally interrupting this man spewing misinformation. Suddenly he found himself on the stage, shouting, "What causes the disease is nothing of the kind; it's the physician and his staff who carry the germ from a sick woman to a healthy one." He heard shouts of "sit down" coming from the audience, but he persevered. Pasteur drew some streptococci on the board. "There — that's what it is like."[5] Disgusted, he limped off the stage, virtually divorcing himself from the Academy of Medicine. But his determination to show them the truth about germs was hardened more than ever. He would show them the truth about germs and the huge part these "infinitely small" organisms played in the production of disease.

## Staphylococci

Around the same time Émile Duclaux, one of Pasteur's assistants, suffered from a series of boils. Pasteur collected pus from them and initiated a series of cultures. He noted in all samples, clusters of cocci (spherical organisms), all bunched together. He named them staphylococci, depicting a "cluster of grapes." Soon after, when invited to visit a young girl at a Paris hospital suffering from osteomyelitis of her tibia, Pasteur readily accepted. As the surgeon exposed the bone, Pasteur took a sample for culture. Later, under the microscope, he recognized this organism to be the same type that had infected Duclaux—it was a staphylococcus infection of bone: A furuncle of bone— it was the same infection—appearing as a different disease (osteomyelitis), because it occurred in a different type of tissue.[6]

Pasteur pressed on in his laboratory, which was now beginning to resemble a menagerie with chickens, rabbits, mice and a few sheep in the pens. He, like Koch, was now sacrificing animals by the hundreds for experimentation. Animals were the capital for experimental medicine. They made it flow. Medical scientists, bacteriologists in particular, dealt in animals by the tens and hundreds. Any series of injections might involve at least 10 animals, with a second generation of 10 inoculated, followed by a third, fourth and fifth generation, up to perhaps 15 or 20 generations. Expending 100 lives to explore or prove a specific point would not have been at all unusual. One could expend many animals in the course of proving some minor physiological principle. Smaller animals such as the mouse or guinea pig were desirable in that they were cheap, small and inexpensive to maintain. Additionally, since mice oozed no personal charm like the dog, they were more easily sacrificed.

Antivivisectionists, while more exercised by open operations on awake animals, were still bothered by this form of bacteriological experimentation. In a *Zoophilist* article, "Experimental Pathology," Cobbe complained that an inordinate level of importance had been given to this method of research. Inflicting disease on animals, then studying the changes in their bodies, was invalid, whether achieved through simple inoculation or, as Koch had done with anthrax, injecting organisms into the eyeball. The suffering such actions caused was extreme. And Pasteur with his attempts at developing a vaccine: "What could be more desirable than to kill the microbe—which Pasteur assures us exists with every disease?" Such remedies have been tried with various diseases and the trial has been attended with an alarming increase in the death rate — "not of *Microbes* but — of *Patients*."⁷

It was 1879 when Cobbe made her references to vaccines, at a time when Pasteur was well along with his anthrax experiments. The disease had been devastating livestock throughout France. With assistants Charles Chamberland and Émile Roux, he had gone through the initial set up for their study, growing the bacillus and infecting large groups of guinea pigs with their injections. His interest in anthrax was different than Koch's since Pasteur was aiming for a vaccine to confer immunity to cattle. First, Pasteur would need to diminish (attenuate) the virulence of the organism to the point of innocuousness before he could consider administering such a vaccine to sheep. His initial attempt at a vaccine involved a simple serial dilution of anthrax cultures, hoping to attenuate them. But this preparation — diluted to a point of seeming innocuousness-was completely ineffective. It still resulted in nothing but dead animals.

## Chicken Cholera

As Pasteur paused to reflect on this dilemma, a new problem arose, diverting his attention. An epidemic of chickens had suddenly erupted, spreading through much of France. Farmers were familiar with its early clues. Their birds become immobile, let their wings fall to their sides, feathers ruffled and heads bowed. It was chicken cholera, a highly contagious infection capable of killing entire flocks overnight. When the French government requested Pasteur's help with this new emergency he had little alternative but to put his anthrax study aside.

It was back to the laboratory to make space for more pens, this time for experimenting on chickens. First, he had to build a ready supply of organisms by culturing the appropriate bacteria. Over the ensuing months Pasteur and his team tried every combination of culture techniques, but experienced nothing but failure. They tried differing nutrients and temperatures, all to no avail. Finally, in a special broth at an incubation temperature between 110 and 115°C, organisms began to sprout. These were truly virulent bacteria — breadcrumbs tainted with them caused death in chickens within hours. Then a wonderful act of serendipity occurred, one which Pasteur would later exploit. He instructed Roux to inoculate some chickens with cultures that were several weeks old. Expecting death within 24 hours, Pasteur was surprised to find the chickens strutting and clucking about the next morning, apparently normal. As Pasteur left the laboratory for several weeks of vacation, he was wondering, "Was that inoculum too old to be effective?" Upon his return he had forgotten about the chickens that refused to die. As he resumed his routine, he inoculated a larger group of chickens. Returning the next day, he expected the entire group to be dead, but pecking about among all of the other dead birds were the two which had been inoculated just before his vacation. They appeared to be immune to the cholera organism. Apparently aging of the virus alone diminished its virulence. By enfeebling (attenuating) the organism he could inoculate the chickens and produce a milder, non-fatal disease. The group had chanced upon a mechanism for producing a vaccine. Despite his inartful stumbling onto the mechanism for producing a vaccine, this was arguably one of Pasteur's most important discoveries.[8] It opened an entirely new vista, a scientific pathway for treating disease through exploitation of the immune system. Pasteur had made an improvement upon the work of Jenner who, in 1796, used a benign disease, cowpox, to provide human immunity to smallpox. With further experience Pasteur became confident that he could make a vaccine by manipulating the microorganisms' environment. Why could he not do the same for other diseases besides chicken cholera? Why rely on some natural phenomenon, like cross immunity — cowpox conferring immunity for smallpox?[9]

Pasteur needed time to work out the specifics. Was it something in the air, such as oxygen, that produces the attenuation? How much time was required to produce a safe inoculum? How many injections would be required, and at what dosage? It took the team three months to obtain the answers. Pasteur set up many cultures, planning to inoculate chickens with specimens of increasing ages. With the first inoculation, using three-day-old cultures, all of the chickens died. The same happened at one week. With cultures one month old, two out of ten chickens survived. Next, cultures six weeks old caused half to die and half to survive. Finally, in early 1880, receiving inoculations that had been incubated for three months, all 10 chickens survived. They also survived an otherwise fatal injection of fresh organisms — fully immunized. Pasteur had a bona fide vaccine. The French government completed a chicken vaccination program throughout the country, once again grateful to the savant for saving an industry.

## Anthrax Revisited

Pasteur could now return to his anthrax project. Could he manage to produce an effective vaccine for this killer of sheep, cattle and man? Applying the principles learned with chicken cholera, his group made many cultures of anthrax and tested it at various ages against animals. As anthrax aged, however, it produced increasing numbers of spores. With the spores, attenuation was impossible — with them in the picture, no vaccine could be produced.

How could they get rid of the spores? This dilemma sent Pasteur into one of his contemplative interludes, pacing back and forth, avoiding conversations, muttering to himself. As with the chicken cholera, the group experimented, varying the nutritive elements in the broth as well as the temperature of the incubator. Finally, they discovered that a neutralized chicken broth at a temperature of 42° to 43°C made the difference. Under these conditions the rods of anthrax were incapable of forming spores. Therefore, aging the rods for varying lengths of time under these same conditions resulted in their attenuation. In the case of anthrax, it only took 12 days for the rods to be sufficiently attenuated that all sheep not only survived the inoculation but also the injection of the fresh and virulent rods. The sheep had been given a benign form of the infection, thereby protecting them from the virulent and deadly type.

The team had their vaccine. Pasteur, impulsive as ever, wanted to tell the world, while Roux and Chamberland were a bit more circumspect. How about cattle? Would a vaccine designed for sheep work with other types of livestock or not? It would have seemed wise to get some real clinical experience before any grand pronouncements? But Pasteur's mind was already made up. In February 1881, he presented his work in detail, to the Academy of Science, claiming that the world would soon be rid of the anthrax scourge. As the news spread, farmers were delighted, but scientists and physicians remained suspicious, even resentful. Veterinarian Monsieur Rossignol, who edited *The Veterinary Press*, sarcastically wrote,

> Will you have some microbe? There is some everywhere. Microbiolatry is the fashion; it reigns undisputed; it is a doctrine which must not even be discussed, especially when its Pontiff, the learned M. Pasteur, has pronounced the sacramental words, "*I have spoken.*" The microbe alone is and shall be the characteristic of disease; that is understood and settled; hence forth the germ theory must have precedence above pure clinics; the microbe alone is true, and Pasteur is its prophet.[10]

In late March 1881, Rossignol and some associates at the Agricultural Society of Melun, who had no faith in Pasteur's vaccine, began musing. How might they give this man his justly deserved rebuke, some prominent form of humiliation? Rossignol owned a farm, Pouilly-le-Fort, near Melun. He, along with Baron de la Rochette, president of the Agricultural Society, formulated a proposition for Pasteur. If Pasteur would be kind enough to give a public demonstration of his methods of vaccination for this dread disease, they would provide all of the animals and the space at Pouilly-le-Fort farm. Their proposition: One group of animals would be inoculated with his vaccine, while a second group would go without vaccination. Then, weeks later, all animals of both groups would receive an injection of deadly anthrax microbes. Two days later all parties would convene to ascertain which animals were alive and which were dead. In a follow-up article, *The Veterinary Press* proclaimed that Pasteur had an opportunity to "demonstrate that he had not been mistaken when he affirmed before the astonished Academy that he had discovered the vaccine for splenic fever, a preventative [sic] of one of the most terrible diseases with which animals and even men could be attacked."[11]

Surely Pasteur would not accept this challenge with a vaccine so new and untried, except for a small laboratory series of 14 sheep. Roux and Chamberland were on vacation when the challenge was made, but during the interlude between challenge and answer, the other laboratory associates inquired of Pasteur why he would even consider this challenge at so early a time. "What succeeded with fourteen sheep at the laboratory," he replied, "would work as well with fifty at Melun."[12] When his assistants heard Pasteur had sent Baron de la Rochette a reply to the affirmative, they sat incredulous, stunned by his brazenness.

# Chapter 11

# Showdown at Melun

One week before the demonstration, Pasteur wrote to Roux and Chamberlain notifying them of the event. Requesting that they interrupt their vacations, he wrote, "The vaccination experiments will begin at Melun on 5 May. I very much wish you to return by 3 or 4 May at the latest. This is a big and important event. We must have a serious talk about it before we begin."[1] Upon their return, Pasteur informed them of the details of the experiment. The first inoculations would take place on 5 May and the second on the 17th. The veterinarian society was making 60 sheep available for the study. Twenty-five sheep would receive the vaccination with an equal number getting no inoculation. The remaining 10 sheep would serve as controls, by occupying the same environment but receiving no inoculations at any time. Later, as an afterthought, Rossignol suggested inoculating 10 cows as well, to which Pasteur agreed. Then, as a concluding step, on 31 May, the third series of inoculations — a virulent strain of anthrax — would be given to all 50 sheep. In other words, 25 sheep would be injected with live anthrax after receiving two protective inoculations, and 25 would be injected without ever receiving the protective inoculations. Two days later, all participants would record the results — how many sheep, both treated and untreated, would be left standing?

A commission of veterinarians would judge the entire affair, ensuring that the rules were followed correctly. At the termination of the experiment, commission members would also render a judgment of the results.

Even though Roux and Chamberland thought the demonstration was premature and ill-advised, they had both already resigned themselves to cooperating with Pasteur. Still, they could not help but worry: Too strong an inoculum and all of the animals would die — too weak and they would all survive, making fools out of the scientists. Resisting at this late a date, of course, would be of little use. Whenever Pasteur discussed the matter, he predicted, with total confidence, that all unvaccinated sheep would die and all of the treated sheep and cows would survive.[2] When Koch learned of Pasteur's latest gambit, he felt that the man's ambition had finally exceed his capabilities.

## Improved Attenuation

Pasteur was not aware that Roux and Chamberland, in his absence, had made a significant change in how they attenuated anthrax. While Pasteur had used oxygen to weaken the organisms, Chamberland had discovered a better method — exposure to potassium bichromate.[3] When Pasteur heard of the change, he eagerly appropriated the newer method for the upcoming demonstration. That improvement in technique at the hands of his assistants possibly saved Pasteur from great embarrassment since it yielded an organism of more consistent attenuation.

On 4 May, with vaccines in hand, Pasteur and his three assistants Roux, Chamberland and Louis Thullier, took the train to Melun, where they spent the night in a hotel. The next morning, they rode through the rolling green pastures, wood and stone outbuildings, hedgerows and prominent stone fences towards the farm, Pouilly-le-Fort. Upon their arrival, they were astounded to see a huge crowd gathered for the occasion. The general medical and veterinary press had played up the event to a point of high theatre. All roads, in and out, were clogged with carriages, coaches and people. Members of the press corps were visible, along with veterinarians, physicians, and politicians. Local farmers arrived dressed in their boots and aprons, as though they were attending the occasion in between chores. A number of people had apparently come out of pure curiosity, just to see the famous scientist up close. Pasteur instinctively felt that the farmers were the only group that might be rooting for him. They were anxious to see the end of this infectious curse, which had cost them dearly both in grief and money. Both Roux and Chamberland, who had made daily trips to the farm in preparation for the experiment, had been made uneasy hearing the idle chatter around the farm. Most of the people around Melun did not believe in Pasteur's methods. Seeing him humiliated would be a wonderful conclusion to the whole affair.

As Pasteur's team approached Rossignol's farm, they spotted him sitting near the entrance sporting a sardonic grin, appearing very self-satisfied. He had reason to be smug; there was no way he could lose. If Pasteur were successful, Rossignol would be recognized as the one who helped expose his greatness. If not, then Rossignol was the man who had forced the pretender's hand.

Pasteur and his entourage had to force their way through the raucous crowd. The atmosphere was more circus-like than scientific, with continual

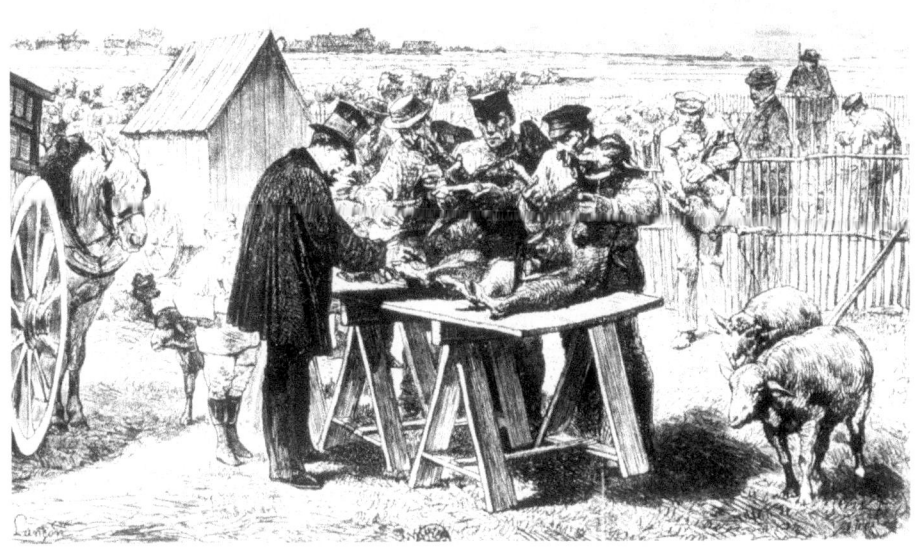

Illustration of Pasteur's showdown at Pouilly-le-Fort, Melun, in 1881. Aides are setting up groups of sheep for Pasteur, in the stove-pipe hat, and his team to vaccinate against anthrax. They inoculated either into the abdominal wall or inner hind leg of the sheep. (Reproduced with permission of Pasteur Institute, Paris.)

loud banter and bawdy jokes. Pasteur had a habit of maintaining a calm demeanor when he was nervous, in contrast to a garrulous, assertive manner when he was confident. Betraying his level of anxiety, he entered the barn with deliberate insouciance, to inspect the animals. The sheep were then brought outside and placed on wooden tabletops, one at a time. Roux, Chamberland and Thullier all began the inoculations, swabbing the injection site, then plunging the needle with the Pravaz syringe, named after its French surgeon inventor, under the skin of the abdomen or upper leg, and injecting the inoculum. After completing all injections by mid-afternoon, they marked the right ears of the sheep and the horns of the cows with blue paint, to distinguish them from the un-inoculated animals. Finally, Pasteur led an entourage of interested observers into the farmhouse where he held court, conducting a tutorial on the principles of animal experimentation and the fledgling discipline of immunology.[4] As the day came to an end, he invited all of the attendees back for the second set of injections, scheduled for 17 May.

Despite the diminished likelihood of something newsworthy occurring, the size of the crowd was the same for the second round of inoculations. On this second occasion, to help further boost immunity, the group used a stronger, less-attenuated strain of anthrax. Then, they traveled back to Paris to wait the requisite two weeks while the animals' immune systems did their work.

The big day, 31 May, arrived, in which all animals, except for the 10 controls, were to receive the active, virulent strain of anthrax. Bowing to pressure from some veterinarians in attendance, Pasteur ordered doses of triple the normal strength to be administered to each animal. Pasteur loved any heightened form of public drama, whether a debate or demonstration. Prior to leaving, he calmly announced to the crowd that he would return at 2 o'clock on 2 June, to check which animals would be alive and which ones would be dead, again exhibiting his signature nonchalance. After completing their work by mid-afternoon, the team headed back to Paris, where Pasteur remained for that long two-day wait.

The next day, Roux and Chamberland returned to the farm to check on the animals' welfare. Among the unvaccinated, some perversely good news awaited the scientists. The majority of the sheep held their heads low, appearing listless, refusing to eat, remaining at the periphery of the flock. Some collapsed without any attempt at standing. Within the vaccinated group, however, all was not entirely well. Two sheep were feverish, one refused to eat, while a fourth had inflammation at the injection site.

Upon their return to the laboratory at Rue d'Ulm, Pasteur, pacing back and forth, eagerly inquired about the early results. While the team conversed, a telegram arrived from Rossignol, informing Pasteur that one vaccinated ewe appeared to be near death. With that, Pasteur's pent-up emotions let loose, as though the entire experiment was lost. It was poor Roux who bore the brunt of the Professor's venom. He accused Roux of ruining the experiment through sloppy preparation. His carelessness was jeopardizing the entire future of their work. Pasteur declared that it was Roux who would have to return solo to the farm the next day. Let him alone be humbled before the crowds of Melun. He could put up with the sarcasm of the anti-vaccination forces.[5] Pasteur would not be able to stand the humiliation. Worried that his ambition had finally gotten the best of him, Pasteur experienced a night of very troubled sleep. Then, at 9 the next morning, Pasteur received another telegram from Rossignol. Eighteen of the non-vaccinated sheep had already died and the others were weakening. All of the vaccinated animals were not only standing but appeared to be in good health. Rossignol concluded by declaring it "a tremendous success."[6]

Of course, Roux could not be expected to return to the farm by himself; they would all share in the celebration. When Pasteur, Roux, Chamberland and Thullier arrived in the early afternoon, the entire farm was packed with people, celebrating, shouting to the four men that all of the untreated animals were dead, and the vaccinated ones were alive. Pasteur, still maintaining his calm and imperious persona, as though things had gone exactly as planned, stood in the carriage, exclaiming: "Well then! Men of little faith!"[7]

Next he went through the admiring crowd, accepting congratulations and hearing from many, including Rossignol, who confessed that they had not believed in his methods until now. But Pasteur cautioned them. An autopsy must be performed on at least one of the animals. It was imperative that they confirm anthrax as the cause of death, there at the scene. Later, viewing the tissues from the autopsied animal, Pasteur saw anthrax organisms under the field microscope. The cause of death was evident.

It was a relieved and happy team that left Pouilly-le-Fort, heading back to Paris, amidst the cheers of the crowd. As a result of the demonstration, Rossignol was so strongly converted to the vaccinationists' side that he later changed the name of his farm to Clos Pasteur.[8]

One delayed death did occur in the vaccinated group — the same ewe that Rossignol had warned about in the telegram. She died on the night of 4 June, giving some hope to the few scientists who still refused to believe in Pasteur's methods. A postmortem examination, however, revealed the cause. She had expired from complications of pregnancy — a miscarriage. Since the scientists found no anthrax organisms in her blood, she had apparently been as immune as were her cohorts.[9]

## Further Demonstrations

Given the clear-cut success, the veterinary commission's job was easy. No further experimentation would be necessary. The press feted Pasteur's achievement, both locally and internationally. In the ensuing weeks, he was in demand everywhere. Still, many people scattered throughout France and other countries remained dubious. Responding to that sentiment, Pasteur arranged demonstrations in other parts of France and even Hungary, each experiment being as successful as the first one at Melun. Organizations in countries throughout Europe were interested in learning Pasteur's technique, especially how to produce the vaccine. Pasteur wisely kept control of its production. The chances of some mistake jeopardizing the entire scheme were just too great. Pasteur appointed Chamberland, his trusted aid, to supervise all aspects of commercial vaccine production.[10]

Between 1881 and 1883, with the success of the demonstrations throughout the country, the team began employing actual vaccination programs. Farmers were some of the first converts to this view about germs causing disease. If one could control bacteria, one controlled the disease as well. As a group, farmers saw their vaccinated herds not only resist anthrax but thrive as well. After only two years, Pasteur could buttress his immunological arguments by invoking statistics. Vaccinations had been performed on 85,000 animals, with a mortality rate of 0.65 percent, while it was over 9 percent in an untreated group of similar size. A decade later, 3,400,000 sheep and 438,000 cattle, all vaccinated, had respective mortality rates of 1 and 0.3 percent. At least in agricultural circles, vaccination became the norm.[11] The potential of this new science of immunology had been realized.

## Pasteur's Detractors

Benjamin Bryan, Cobbe's ally, of course saw things differently. In a *Zoophilist* article, "M. Pasteur and the System of Inoculation," he charged that the treatment for anthrax actually made the animals more susceptible to other diseases, resulting in a greater mortality rate than if they had been left alone. He urged that English farmers not subject their flocks and herds to some dangerous and delusive nostrum.[12]

One influential physician in the French Academy of Medicine, Michael Peter, would similarly never be convinced. He remained an effective and vocal critic of Pasteur for years. Ironically, the two were distantly related, since their wives shared a grandfather Loir in common — the great-grandfather of Adrien Loir. Adrien found himself in the uncomfortable position of working in Peter's clinic in the morning and Pasteur's laboratory in the afternoon. Peter's habit of attacking Pasteur and his germ theory at Academy meetings proved emotionally draining to Pasteur. Peter still believed in spontaneous generation. He claimed, "They [bacteria] are worth neither the time spent on them nor the fuss made over them. After so much laborious research, nothing will be changed in medicine, and all there will be are a few more microbes."[13] In an 3 April 1883 letter read aloud to the Academy, Peter described Pasteur's microbicidal methods as homicidal. Peter took advantage of Koch's influence by making reference to the German's criticisms of Pasteur's bacteriological methods. At the same meeting, Pasteur responded to Peter's wearisome criticisms, concluding:

> Meanwhile, you will permit me to point out that in your vain attempt to combat the discovery of the attenuation of viruses and the work of my laboratory, you have found your weapons abroad. My own patriotism, Monseiur, is such that I should be inconsolable if the great discovery of the attenuation of virus vaccines were not a French discovery.[14]

The patriotic Pasteur never accepted any remuneration for his vaccines used in service to France, profiting only from those used outside the country.

An appreciative French government bestowed the Grand Cross of the Legion of Honor upon him, for not only helping to revive French agriculture but for bringing glory to his country. Pasteur was wise enough to recognize that the accomplishment was not his alone. His assistants had arguably saved the day for him with the better attenuated virus. At Pasteur's suggestion, Roux, Chamberland and Thullier each received the Cross of the Legion of Honor.

After his stellar accomplishment at Melun, two different parties encouraged Pasteur to attend the upcoming seventh International Medical Congress in London. Government officials in France were anxious for Pasteur to present his revolutionary work there. He represented a shining example of governmental regime and scientist working together, fostering scientific endeavor. Joseph Lister was equally anxious to bring Pasteur to the Congress. His interest lay in getting Pasteur and Koch together for the benefit of scientific medicine despite their mutual animosities.

# VI

# THE INTERNATIONAL MEDICAL CONGRESS OF 1881

"That this Congress records its conviction that experiments on living animals having proved of the utmost service to medicine in the past, and are indispensable to its future progress. That accordingly, while strongly deprecating the infliction of unnecessary pain, it is of opinion, alike in the interests of man and of animals, that it is not desirable to restrict competent persons in the performance of such experiments."
— Resolution of the Physiological Section of the IMC read by Secretary William MacCormac, 2 August 1881.[1]

CHAPTER 12

# Portents of a Notable Decade

The International Medical Congress, convening at St. James Hall on 2 August 1881, was a resplendent affair, attracting over 3,000 attendees from all over the world. Many were anxious to hear scientists address some of the monumental developments that had been taking place in medicine in the late 1870s. In the plenary session, the Prince of Wales delivered the opening address, followed by William Jenner, president of the Royal College of Physicians. Antivivisectionists often infiltrated such meetings, anxious for new material to use in their attacks on scientists. Sensitive to such dangers, the organizers of the Congress passed a seemingly peculiar resolution which ostracized women from signing on as delegates to the Congress. British scientists, still struggling to incorporate the provisions of the 1876 Cruelty to Animals Act into their working lives, strongly influenced the resolution. Even though 43 female physicians were duly qualified, they remained banned because of a perceived threat: Organizers of the Congress hoped to pass a unanimous resolution as worded in the epigram above, at meeting's end, emphasizing the important role that animals played in scientific experimentation, a statement "deploring any restrictions on their use by competent reasearchers."[1] Given the presumed female proclivity for the antivivisectionists' side in the animal experiment argument, female delegates just might jeopardize the unanimity of that vote.

The speaker following Jenner, Sir James Paget, launched into an attack on the antivivisectionists, pointing out Louis Pasteur in the audience. The Frenchman's work represented a glorious illustration of what could be accomplished by using animals in science, an example that fanatical animal lovers in England were attempting to abolish.

The second major address of the day was delivered by the director of the Pathological Institute in Berlin, Professor Rudolf Virchow, known as the father of cellular pathology. His microscopic work, focusing on diseases at a cellular level, was revolutionary, bringing changes to the entire field of medicine. Wasting little time, Virchow began:

> This congress is taking place in the midst of a wave of agitation. Persons who unscrupulously exploit the average man's love for animals are at work here in London to convince the populace that the British vivisection law of 1876 is inadequate.... It does not satisfy them that all scientific experimentation must be carried out under anesthesia and that animals must be killed at once after the completion of the experiment. Whipped up by vegetarians who would like to forbid all killing of animals, and by homeopaths who hold that they require no knowledge whatsoever of the hidden functions of the human body, these agitators are no longer capable of listening to reason. Although they take it for granted that if they fall ill, medicine will heal their diseases and prolong their lives, they ignore the fact that they owe these blessings to one discovery among others which only vivisection made possible, namely William Harvey's discovery of the circulation of the blood.[2]

Virchow's remarks elicited angry statements from the international anti-vivisection and anti-vaccination groups present. To them, physiology laboratories were still "chambers of torture." Men of science "have the unique desire of inflicting on bound animals, secured on a board, sufferings of which death was the only limit."[3] But it was Pasteur, in particular, that evoked their hatred. He received "numberless letters," mainly from England, filled with insults and threats. Many wanted him to suffer eternal torment for "having multiplied his crimes on the hens, guinea pigs, dogs, and sheep of the laboratory."[4]

Upon completion of the more general addresses, the meeting divided into specific scientific sessions. Lister delivered several talks spanning such topics as pathology, surgery and antisepsis, but he looked forward to his other plan—getting Pasteur and Koch together for the betterment of bacteriology. A social barrier, a persisting effect of the war, still existed between French and German scientists. While they might both attend the plenary sessions, large enough to maintain some space and anonymity, anyone wishing to meet with them personally would be wise to do so on alternate days. Pasteur, on behalf of the French government, spoke on "Vaccination in Relation to Chicken-cholera and Splenic Fever" (anthrax), a presentation Lister called "one of the glories of the Congress."[5] In another gathering, Koch demonstrated his microphotography, illustrating the pathogenic effects bacteria exerted on living tissue. Following that, he gave a practicum at King's College on methods for the isolation and cultivation of microorganisms, in effect a demonstration of his new solid plating technique. Lister, in the audience with Pasteur, was pleased to see, as the demonstration ended, the Frenchman magnanimously shake Koch's hand and state, "C'est un grand progrès, Monsieur."[6]

## Koch's Charges

Pasteur was not yet aware that Koch had been harshly critical of him in the journal *Mitteilungen aus dem Kaiserlichem Gesunheitsamt*, charging that Pasteur had not only contributed nothing towards proving the etiology of anthrax, but had even confused that bacillus with other organisms.[7] Koch further asserted that his own earlier publication had clearly established the anthrax bacillus as the true cause of the disease.[8] Since the article did not come to press until several months after the London Congress had convened, no personal confrontation occurred.

When Pasteur became aware of Koch's criticisms, he organized his favorite form of polemic, a public demonstration. With Pasteur's fine sense of drama, he arranged for the demonstration to take place in Berlin, under Koch's nose. He appointed Louis Thullier to carry out the demonstration, much like the affair at Melun, under the auspices of the Berlin Veterinary School. Rudolf Virchow would judge this event. Although the demonstration had to be executed twice, because of technical difficulties, it proved as successful as any of the previous French efforts. Consequently, the Pasteurian method of vaccination became more widely accepted throughout Germany. Koch, left on the margin, silently observing, never did give Pasteur his due.

Following up on that victory, Pasteur decided to answer Koch's old charges openly at the International Congress of Hygiene in Geneva in August 1882. He had meticulously prepared his talk in anticipation of Koch's presence. Pasteur mounted the rostrum to thunderous applause. As he sized up the crowd, preparing to speak, he noted Koch and his entire team occupying the first row. Undaunted, Pasteur meticulously reviewed his work with anthrax, chicken cholera and bacterial attenuation. "Yet, however blazingly clear the demonstrated truth, it has not always had the privilege of being easily accepted. I have encountered, both in France and abroad, obstinate objectors."[9] He then turned directly to Koch, reiterating Koch's charges against him: Pasteur did not know how to obtain pure cultures, did not know how to distinguish one bacteria from another and was guilty of poor vaccination technique. Pasteur replied:

> The author does not believe that I operated as I said I did, with eighty chickens in certain of my experiments, because that would have cost too much money. But it is true, for in view of establishing the great fact of the attenuation of virulence, my government allowed me not to worry about the expense.[10]

Koch had only a poor grasp of French and Pasteur did not understand any German at all. As Pasteur spoke, an interpreter translating for Koch, made an innocent mistake. Referring to some of Koch's prior work, Pasteur used the phrase, "recueil allemand," meaning "collection of German research." The interpreter innocently misunderstood Pasteur's utterance to be "orgeuil allemand," which translated more as "German arrogance."[11]

Although he was angered by the charge, Koch initially remained mute, wishing to avoid public debate. Finally, he stood to address the audience, stating that he preferred to respond in writing. A debate as important as this one should be conducted in the medical journals. Since neither understood the other's language well, the written word would minimize errors of communication. Three months passed before Koch published *On Anthrax Vaccination: Response to a Speech Given at Geneva by M. Pasteur.* Koch refused to back down at all. Pasteur, he insisted, had brought nothing new to Geneva — the concept of attenuation is a myth — one can only make progress in the study of disease by discovering microorganisms.[12] Furthermore, "although the Congress at Geneva might have celebrated Pasteur as a second Jenner, the members of the Congress should recall that Jenner's triumph did not involve sheep, but human beings."[13] Again, that familiar insinuation: Pasteur was not even a physician.

An irritated Pasteur responded in January 1883 in the *Revue Scientifique*, accusing Koch of owing a debt to French science, apparently referring to his own work. Pasteur would press on. "However violent your attacks, Monsieur, they will not prevent me from succeeding. I am also fully confident that this method of attenuating viruses will have consequences that will help humanity in its struggle against diseases by which it is besieged."[14]

Why had such unnecessary and unbecoming behavior erupted between two great men? Pasteur, at 59, was already the cele-

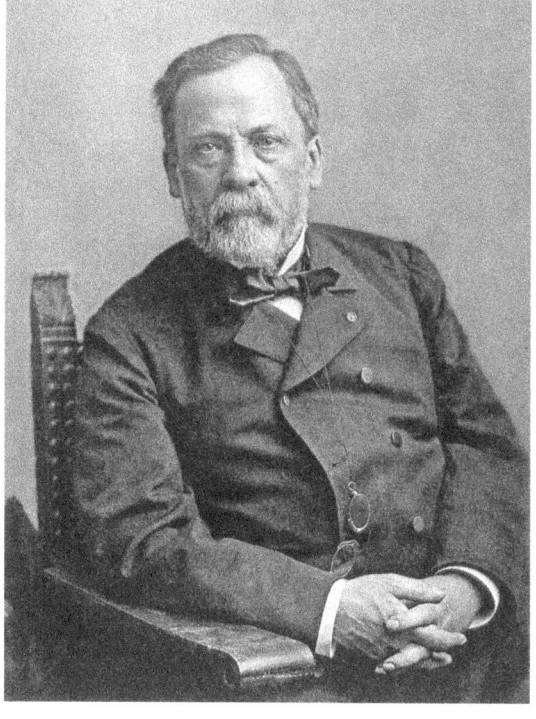

Photogravure of Pasteur in his early sixties by Felix Nadar. In 1884 he was completing his work with anthrax vaccines and just beginning his work with rabies. (Reproduced by permission of the Wellcome Library, London.)

brated scientist, a national hero with little left to prove. Koch, at 38, had just begun his ascendance, based on his publications on anthrax and bacteriological methodology. No doubt, the extreme nationalism of both men primed the pump of mutual resentment. But Koch appeared to be most irritated by Pasteur's chauvinistic penchant for ignoring him and his accomplishments. Even in his everyday discourse Pasteur's attitude was evident, using expressions of French origin, such as "microbes" or "microbiology," while eschewing Koch's terms, "bacteria" and "bacteriology." Even though the latter words had Latin roots, they were tainted with Teutonic usage by the likes of Koch.

But soon, Pasteur would be the aggrieved one, resenting Koch's successes in studying a recurring problem: cholera. Making matters worse, the French government later invited the German to set up his laboratory in France in an effort to rescue the country from the threat of the disease. For centuries, cholera had been limited to the subcontinent of India, where the disease was endemic. Then in the 19th century, it spread worldwide, starting in Asia, spreading to Russia, then northern Europe, England, and most Western countries. In the 1860s, the English anesthesiologist John Snow presciently linked cholera infection to contaminated water, but his warnings were completely ignored.[15] Koch, as a new medical graduate, working at the Hamburg General Hospital, witnessed his first case of cholera. He knew how fearsome the disease could be to the public at large. Many had heard stories handed down through generations of how swiftly a violent epidemic could materialize. The rapid appearance and disappearance of an epidemic was as mystifying as it was terrifying — perceived as a manifestation of God's fury. A person could seemingly be normal one minute and then have a single premonitory diarrheal stool, followed by a fulminating series of pure liquid emissions similar in appearance to "rice water." Dehydration and electrolyte imbalance, conditions of which 19th-century physicians were completely ignorant, became so profound that the patient died of circulatory collapse, in painful spasms of tetany (involuntary muscular contractions) — often within 12 to 24 hours after their first warning stool. Having no clue as to etiology or how the disease developed, the physician dutifully bled the hapless patient and admonished him to drink some useless concoction of herbs and heavy metals as he lay in bed dying.

In 1883, cholera suddenly appeared in Egypt. Frightened government officials there appealed to both France and Germany for help. The French team, organized by Pasteur, included Roux and Thullier, but the chief himself, did not go. Koch gathered a team comprised of himself and two assistants, Georg Gaffky and Bernhard Fischer, plus a chemist, Dr. Treskow. With German precision, they assembled in one week a complete bacteriological laboratory, capable of all contemporary microbiological techniques. With the French laboratory, only animal inoculations and microscopic studies could be performed.[16]

Arriving in Egypt in late August, Koch immediately began examining tissues of autopsied patients and their choleric stools. With the microscope, he consistently saw a small, comma-shaped bacillus in the bowel contents as well as in the intestinal wall. Koch's team tried diligently to grow the bacillus in monkeys, dogs, cats, chickens and mice, failing with each effort. Similarly, all attempts to culture the bacteria in vitro, in the culture plate, were unsuccessful as well. Were those comma-shaped bacteria the cause of cholera, or were they merely concomitants — red herrings? If Koch's team was to have any success at all, it would not be along the traditional line of fulfilling postulates posed by Koch, a series of conditions that must be met before one could conclude that a specific organism was, in fact, the cause of that specific disease. According to Koch's postulates, one must establish that the specific organism is consistently present in the affected tissue. That same microorganism must subsequently be isolated and grown in pure culture. Then, an extract of that pure culture, inoculated into another experimental animal, must produce that same disease in the second generation of animal. If one cannot inoculate animals or grow the bacteria in culture, then he has not proved causality.

Just as the French and German teams were getting well established, the epidemic began subsiding. The French, having experienced even less success than the Germans, continued their studies but also began studying rinderpest, a viral plague of cattle. Koch believed that he could accomplish little more in Egypt. Wishing to continue his research on cholera, he appealed to the German government for permission to travel to India, where a severe outbreak of the disease had struck the city of Calcutta.

While Koch's team awaited authorization, tragedy struck the French camp. Louis Thullier, Pasteur's favorite assistant, who had not worked around cholera for two weeks, reported minor malaise and a loose stool on Monday, 17 September 1883. At 3 A.M. he awoke feeling very ill, experiencing a series of loose stools. After collapsing, he was put to bed by his associates but continued to deteriorate rapidly. By 8 A.M., of the same morning, he was moribund. Doctors were called in immediately, and gave him "frictions" and champagne, but he died approximately 36 hours after the onset of his symptoms, 26 years of age. Koch was not only at his bedside near the end, but later, in an ironic twist, served as one of Thullier's pallbearers. When Pasteur received the news of Thullier's death in Paris, he was devastated. Feelings of sorrow and guilt haunted him for years, since Thullier had been like a son to him. A deflated French team soon disassembled their outpost and returned to Paris.[17] Koch pressed on to India.

In Calcutta, with the epidemic in full swing, opportunities for tackling the disease head on would be greater. In all, the team studied 17 cholera patients plus 22 fresh autopsy specimens. Koch tried to inoculate experimental animals with fresh human specimens. He made efforts to culture pure strains of bacteria from patients' intestines so that he might then inoculate animals with the pure strains derived from those same patients. The team first encountered a young man, 22, who had died from a cholera illness of only 10 hours' duration. At autopsy three hours later, Koch prepared both cultures and stains from the man. He noted that organisms uncovered here looked exactly like those he had seen in Egypt, suggesting that this comma-shaped vibrio was the infective agent. Koch had discovered the reason why they experienced difficulty in their attempts to grow the cholera organism; it had to compete with a plethora of other intestinal bacteria. Acquiring cholera bacilli immediately after death in India, something he could not do in Egypt, seemed more likely. With the recent deaths, one could expect fresh and therefore more virulent pools of bacteria for study. To get that pure culture, these fresher organisms could therefore better rise to the top of all its competitors. With assiduous pure culture techniques, Koch was finally confident that he had successfully grown the cholera organism—the difference did lay in the increased virulence of the cholera organisms residing within the fresh specimens of India.

## Infectious Nature of Cholera

In a journal report of 2 February 1884, Koch was confident enough to conclusively state that the bacteria extracted from the intestines of cholera patients were in fact, the cause of cholera. "In all cases the comma bacillus and only the comma bacillus has been found. These results, taken together with those obtained in Egypt, prove that we have found the pathogen responsible for cholera."[18]

Other parties were not so eager to blindly accept Koch's claim at face value. In a March 1884 editorial, the *British Medical Journal*, following the German effort, stated that Koch's conclusions must be viewed very carefully, and that other scientists must corroborate his findings before making any hard and fast judgments.[19] Pasteur predictably, was dubious as well. Since a series of animals could never be inoculated successfully with cholera organisms, Koch could never technically fulfill his own postulates. Still, his work was ultimately accepted internationally.

Helping to support his claims on causality, Koch's team also carried out supplemental epidemiological studies. In one small Indian village, concrete water tanks served as a source for drinking water, as well as a place to bathe and to wash clothes, including attire from cholera victims. Eventually, Koch and his commission were able to trace 17 deaths, via pure cultures, relating back to one particular tank in which the clothes of a single cholera patient had been washed. Koch cultured the comma bacillus from the tank, establishing the link to the subsequent victims, and corroborating the 30-year-old theories of John Snow. Now, satisfied that they had accomplished what they had set out to do, the team prepared for their homeward journey. It was March 1884, and they had not set eyes on Germany for nine long months.

Setting sail from India, they traveled to Alexandria, Egypt where a severely fatigued Koch was forced to take a break from his travels. He had contracted malaria somewhere along the way. After three weeks, a better rested Koch resumed his itinerary on 22 April 1884. After entering Germany, he traveled to Munich to visit the famed hygienist, Max von Pettenkofer, a germ theory agnostic. He believed that cholera originated in the soil and that bacteria played only a minor role in its pathogenesis. Koch could not persuade Pettenkofer one little bit to change his views. In fact, during a later cholera epidemic in Hamburg in 1892, Pettenkofer, to demonstrate his contempt for the infectious waterborne theory of cholera, procured a fresh culture of cholera organisms from a recent fatal case. He not only drank the culture on an empty stomach, but also ingested a dose vastly larger than one would get in a natural setting. He even consumed some sodium carbonate to neutralize the stomach acid, since Koch had told him that this maneuver would maximize the chances of developing cholera. Aside from a light case of diarrhea, he suffered no ill effects, emphasizing that disease causation is more multifaceted than mere exposure to the bacteria.[20]

The German team finally arrived in Berlin to great fanfare. Koch, now referred to as the "bacillus father," was granted an audience with Chancellor Otto von Bismarck. He also visited with the kaiser, who presented a bronze bust of himself to the scientist. The Reichstag made a grant of 100,000 marks, in gold, to the team. Berlin physicians, proud of their countryman, held a banquet in his honor at the Central Hotel with 700 people attending.[21] Slowly, Koch's life settled back towards normal.

In the summer of 1884, cholera outbreaks occurred in both Marseille and Toulon, France, prompting the French government to request Koch's help. Pasteur and many within the French scientific community were less than pleased with the government's decision to invite a Prussian scientist into their midst. In a conspiratorial tone, Pasteur wrote to Roux and Straus in Toulon:

> He [Koch] has made very strong but premature conclusions, whereas you have been careful and very reserved. What is the story about Koch's bacillus?... I haven't seen this organism. Try to find out the fallacy of his story. How do his microscopic preparations differ from yours? He must have made some sort of great error, if he thinks that in cultures of cholera feces he always sees a bacillus

which is never seen in ordinary diarrhea. As much as possible, work by yourself. Keep your cadavers to yourself. The reports that you have received that tell you how great this Koch is are wrong. His knowledge of cholera is not that good. If your results agreed with his, he alone would get all the credit. Already the German newspapers are crowing.[22]

Pasteur was right about the German press. A Paris newspaper, *La Nouvelle Presse*, cited a claim made by a German paper that the French government invited Koch because Pasteur's Cholera Commission had failed in Egypt whereas the Germans succeeded. *La Nouvelle* reacted:

> It is inconceivable to us that the French government would call into such a mission a Prussian scientist, even one of such scientific authority. France, which has the honor of having in its ranks such eminent savants as M. Pasteur, and which has a faculty of medicine renowned throughout Europe ... does not have any need for the services of a German scientist. M. Pasteur has made a vast number of discoveries of the world of the infinitely small in the past 20 years and is quite able to handle cholera himself.[23]

In Toulon Koch had little difficulty isolating the bacillus from fatal cases. He even gave tutorials to Straus and Roux, two members of the French team. Koch had not brought cholera specimens back to Berlin from his foray in India, fearful that he might start an epidemic in Germany. Apparently having changed his mind, he retrieved fresh cultures from Toulon, to serve as a repository for cholera research in his Berlin laboratory.

In July 1884, a major conference on cholera convened in Berlin. At its conclusion Professor Virchow stood up to announce that, from his vantage point, this vibrio cholera did appear to be the causative agent of the disease — sweet words for Koch from an old nemesis.

Cobbe, of course, offered her own opinion concerning cholera. Since the vibrio could not be cultivated in animals, it proved that animals did not play an indispensable role in experimental science. Elucidation of disease can take place without them. In an 1884 letter to the *Zoophilist*, she claimed that Koch admitted to the uselessness of vivisection in the "real or supposed discovery of the bacillus." There is still no treatment for the ailment — only preventive measures — "small comfort to current sufferers."[24]

Some 15 years after the beginning of their confrontation with experimental scientists, antivivisectionists could still make a consistently valid point, not just about cholera but diseases in general. After these many years of animal exploitation and suffering, physiologists still had no practical treatment to offer the public. It was true that Pasteur had developed a vaccine for anthrax, but that was mainly a disease of animals. Direct medical benefits to humans were minimal. Similarly, Lister had devised a treatment scheme for suppuration based upon germ theory, a doctrine gained through vivisection. But

Cobbe dismissed his theory of antisepsis as well as its clinical application.[25] By the early 1880s, scientists could claim significant gains from vivisection, but only in the field of discovery. They had elucidated the causes of a number of diseases, such as diphtheria, tetanus, anthrax and even tuberculosis, as we shall see, but not one specific curative had yet eventuated as a direct result of vivisection.

But by 1884, the contentious practice of inflicting suffering on a few for the benefit of many could add one definite triumph to its list of accomplishments. Doctor David Ferrier, neurophysiologist, quietly pursued his interests in brain research through the 1870s. At the same London International Medical Congress attended by Lister, Pasteur and Koch, Ferrier played a pivotal role not only in brain research, but also in the agitation between antivivisectionists and experimental medicine.

CHAPTER 13

# Professor Ferrier and His Monkeys

The London Medical Congress proved momentous in other areas besides microbiology. Another decisive scientific meeting of competitors was already creating a certain tension within the physiology section. It featured a face-off between experimental scientists David Ferrier, Professor of Forensic Medicine at King's College, and Doctor Friedrich Goltz of Strasbourg. Each represented different schools of thought regarding brain function. Goltz had spent his early years studying and operating first on the brains of lower vertebrates. He then progressed to dogs, where his experience had become vast. Goltz had traveled all the way from Germany with one of his prized experimental dogs. He had one purpose in mind; to put a stop, once and for all, to this brash new theory of focal brain function. With craters in the animal's skull large enough that one could insert half his fist, Goltz's dog attracted attention wherever he went. This looming battle was not just some confrontation over esoteric knowledge. It involved practical implications for broadening human understanding of brain function and for the feasibility of future surgery on the brain—an organ considered virtually untouchable up to this point. This was to be a big day for Ferrier. The results of his research, over a decade long, made such a confrontation at some point in time inevitable.

Ferrier had been performing brain research in his laboratory on the third floor of the West Riding Lunatic Asylum since the late 1860s. As a younger man, he had been hired by M. Crighton-Brown, a strong proponent of phrenology—a school of thought being slowly exposed as an erroneous science. The founder of the movement, Franz Joseph Gall, claimed that the brain had special functions localized in certain areas, all based on solid anatomical research. But Gall made one huge error. He considered the important focal areas of brain function to be located externally in the skull and scalp rather than on the cortical surface of the brain proper. Even worse, as phrenology gained credence with the public, it gave rise to physiognomy, a belief that one's character could be discerned by the shape of the forehead, jaw and face. Until physiognomy was fully discredited, proponents of racism had "scientific" justification for their views.

After studying all of the cerebral research available up to that time, Ferrier favored the idea that certain bodily functions could be localized to specific sites within the brain, something almost heretical at that time. Starting first with frogs, in the 1860s, Ferrier's studies progressed to operating on the brains of dogs, under light anesthesia. All of his work up to this time gave him no reason to discard the focal theory of brain function.[1]

## Cortical Equipotentiality

The dominant school of thought on the Continent and even in England, however, was totally opposed to Ferrier's views. In the early 1800s, Pierre Flourens, doyen of early 19th-century French physiology, had studied brain physiology in both frogs and pigeons. Removing both cerebral hemispheres of pigeons while leaving their brain stems intact, Flourens allowed the birds to survive chronically. If he progressively sliced away the hemispheres in multiple operations, he noted a uniform gradual decrease of sensory perception and volition. The bird regained the functions within a few days if a sufficient amount of brain tissue had been left intact.[2] Such animals were still able to feed, fly, croak and move about nearly unimpeded. It seemed unnecessary for one to invoke any special idea about cortical focality—a center within the brain devoted exclusively to some unique bodily function. If one removed a specific area of the brain and failed to elicit any demonstrable changes in behavior, there was no need to invoke some theory about centers of function. The brain was exhibiting cortical equipotentiality; all cortical areas exhibit equal functional influences.

If a sphere were composed of numerous small lights, connected by densely arranged wires, much like the New Year's Eve ball in Times Square, one would see uniform lighting throughout the sphere. However, in the case of cortical focality, interwoven into that ball would be well circumscribed areas of brighter lights—the focal centers. Remove one of those areas of brighter lights and they would simply disappear. No other lights would be energized to compensate for their absence. In contrast, with cortical equipotentiality, the sphere would be lit up diffusely and evenly throughout—no special area of concentrated brighter lights. Remove an area of lighting and the other regions would take over, lighting up the darkened area, changing the sphere's appearance very little. In the second case, one could conclude that the brain, acting as a whole, was an equipotential, unitary organ. Flourens and his theory of equipotentiality were sacrosanct. Few scientists had the temerity to rise in opposition to whatever Flourens deemed to be true. Professor Friedrich Goltz was one of Flourens' most distinguished, articulate and influential adherents. Over the last decade, Ferrier and his work had been thrust into the limelight by British scientists, anxious to see this dilemma over brain function possibly resolved.

Ferrier's earlier views had been influenced by Hughlings Jackson and Paul Broca, British and French neurologists, and by two German researchers, Gustav Fritsch and Eduard Hitzig. Broca studied the brain much like Frances Cobbe had advocated — through passive observation of clinical cases. In 1863 he recorded his first case of a patient presenting with right-sided paralysis and aphasia. Aphasia is a higher-associative abnormality. Despite having no demonstrable problems with the sensory and motor parts of speech, the patient with aphasia cannot speak properly, uttering garbled words in naming objects, or even his doctor's name. Broca's patient referred to him repeatedly as "Mr. Such-a-one."[3] When the patient died, Broca noted, at autopsy, a softening of a specific area or mound within the brain called the left third frontal convolution — the lesion apparently responsible for his patient's abnormality of speech. Broca, by 1863, had collected a total of 20 nearly identical patients with right-sided paralysis and aphasia. All but one, at autopsy, exhibited the same changes in the third frontal convolution. Even though the evidence was strong that this locus controlled speech, Broca was not yet ready to make any rash generalizations because of that one exception. Commenting on Broca's evidence, Fritz and Hitzig agreed that Broca's theory suffered from "the faultiness and the difficult interpretations of post mortems as compared with the simplicity and clearness of vivisection."[4] But other clinical observations besides those of Broca's were of value as well.

British neurologist Huglings Jackson, through his years of practice, had observed many patients experiencing seizures — an unpredictable explosion of electrical activity within the brain — which strongly suggested the presence of discrete cerebral motor centers that were responsible not only for limb motion but even for movement down to the individual muscle groups within the limb. A patient's index finger might go into an involuntary spasm, with the process then spreading to all of the fingers, then sequentially to the wrist, to the elbow and then to the shoulder muscles. The seizure might stop at that point or it might progress onward to generalized movements of all four extremities, with or without loss of consciousness. Jackson was convinced that abnormal electrical activity started in that focal area of the brain, the index finger for example, and then spread as illustrated by the progression of the seizure. With time this sequence of events became recognizable enough to be called a "Jacksonian March."

Ferrier's greatest influence, however, came from Fritz and Hitzig, two colorful German physicians. Hitzig later became a renowned psychiatrist with a reputation for "incorrigible conceit and vanity complicated by Prussianism."[5] Earlier, in the Prussian-Danish War, Fritz had taken care of an injured soldier with a traumatically exposed brain. Fritz noted that touching the brain in certain parts produced twitching or tingling on the opposite side of the soldier's body. With curiosity fully piqued, he joined with Hitzig at the Berlin Physiological Institute after the war to study brain function further. Since the Institute had no room for such studies, the two were forced to perform their experiments on a small dressing table in a Berlin home. Their early techniques were crude, but with time and experience their work became elegant for that era.[6] Fritz and Hitzig, by electrically stimulating areas of exposed cerebral cortex in the dog, discovered five areas in the brain which, upon stimulation, consistently resulted in stereotyped movements of the neck, or various muscle groups in the front and hind legs and face. In 1870 they published *On the Electrical Excitability of the Cerebrum*, a classic work that cast the first stone at the equipotential school of thought. The work slowly became so influential that it served as the new experimental paradigm over the next several decades.[7]

Ferrier continued his experiments, progressing from frogs to dogs. He later confirmed the same five cortical centers of Fritz and Hitzig. In 1873 Ferrier announced his success in producing precise movements in muscles by electrically stimulating specific cortical centers in dogs, cats, rabbits, guinea pigs and, later, monkeys. He could also produce seizures electrically. Cortical mapping of sensory areas by electrical stimulation could not work in animals since they are unable to report their sensations back to the observer. Scientists were therefore forced to use ablative procedures, that is, remove specific areas of brain tissue, and then examine the animal for sensory defects after it awakened. Using this method, Ferrier successfully mapped cortical sensory areas as well. He became so accomplished that he could reliably produce various forms of paralysis or numbness at will by removing an appropriate area of the brain. Publication of his work caused an immediate sensation on both sides of the vivisection aisle.[8] To Stephen Coleridge of the VSS, "Even if sanguine anticipation by the torturing [of] a monkey Mr. Bernard Shaw could be preserved to us for 100 years, the issue would still remain whether it is right or wrong to torture a monkey."[9] Professor Rutherford, one of Ferrier's former teachers, was prompted to proclaim, "These investigations constitute the most important work which has been accomplished in physiology for a very considerable time past."[10] The members of the Royal Society were impressed enough to grant Ferrier additional funds, enabling him to extend his studies in primates. Echoing Fritz and Hitzig's work in dogs, Ferrier found 15 specific focal centers in the monkey. Stimulate a precise spot and predictable body movements would result.[11] As August 1881 approached, the lines were clearly drawn between Ferrier's focal theories and Goltz's non-focal position.

When the face-off at the International Congress arrived, Goltz, a rotund man with a round face sporting a walrus mustache, first took to the podium. He appeared about 50 years of age, with a confident affect bordering on arrogance. Speaking in German, Goltz reviewed past research and brought it up to contemporary times. He rejected the method of electrical stimulation as a reliable means for locating the so-called centers. Who knows to what depths those electrical stimuli travel? When a group of muscles is seen twitching, it means little. Reactions of foot muscles can be elicited by stimulating motor nerves, spinal cord, brain or even certain sensory nerves. The only reliable method for proving whether motor or sensory centers exist is through removal of that supposed center. If one were to remove that center and no paralysis ensued, every rational person must regard it as proof positive that the so-called center did not exist. Moreover, Ferrier's ablative procedures were not of sufficient numbers to allow for any conclusions. If the animals were kept alive long enough, any paralysis would surely disappear, proving that the brain does, indeed, function as a whole. Goltz then outlined his method for removing as large an amount of brain tissue as possible while still allowing the animal to survive. His technique consisted of washing the brain substance away with a jet of water under high pressure — much as one might create a line of separation in a snow bank with a jet of water. Although the dogs may be paralyzed, or numb or deaf immediately after surgery, they all recovered those lost functions, proving that Flourens' theory was the correct one.[12] "A dog which was deprived of both frontal lobes of the cerebrum — one that is, which according to Ferrier had lost its psychomotor centers — can move all its limbs, its lower jaw, tongue, tail, eyes and ears. In short, it shows no evidence of muscular or sensory defi-

Friedrich Goltz, German physiologist, championed the unitary (equipotential) theory of brain function. He demonstrated that large portions of the dog's brain could be removed with little demonstrable functional deficit to superficial examination.

ciencies."[13] Goltz's assertions were forceful — cortical equipotentiality was the valid theory.

To demonstrate the veracity of his claims, Goltz informed the audience of his experimental dog that had accompanied him on the crossing from Germany to London. The dog, Goltz claimed, had survived five brain operations over the course of 18 months. Most of his cerebrum was now surgically absent. As Goltz triumphantly stepped down from the dais, he announced that tomorrow he would exhibit that healthy animal, proving not only that Flourens' theory was the correct one but that Ferrier's was wrong.

David Ferrier, appearing slim and professorial with his small wire-framed glasses, gray hair and neatly trimmed beard, moved towards the podium with inscrutable affect, visually engaging no one. Unruffled, he began by stating that he could not dispute Goltz's facts, in that Goltz must be a good observer — but Ferrier did reject his conclusions. He dismissed Goltz's water-jet method of dissecting brain tissue. How delicate could that be? The adjacent tissue had to be significantly injured. Furthermore, Ferrier had learned years earlier that, when it comes to brain function, it is impermissible to draw conclusions about higher animals, much less man, from observations on lower animals. The lower the position occupied by the animal on the evolutionary scale, the less likely will removal of brain tissue affect its behavior. Goltz's experiments only proved how large a role the lower parts of the brain played when one considers the entire behavior of the dog. Ideally, the research of both men aimed to gain a functional understanding of the most highly developed part of the brain in the most highly

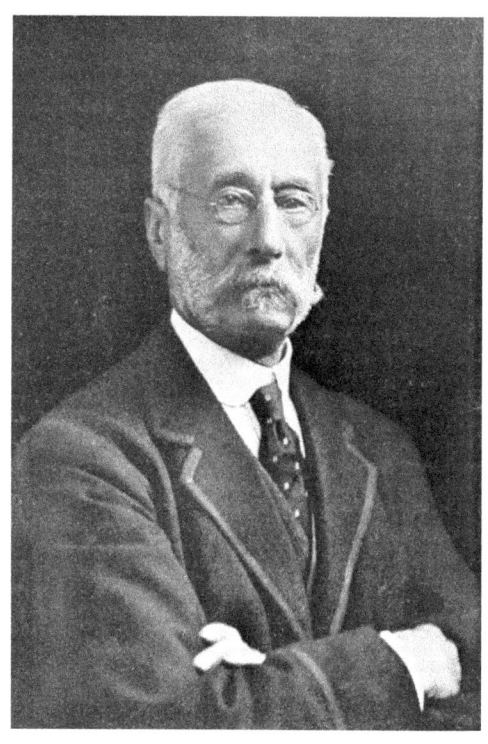

Sir David Ferrier, neurophysiologist, elucidated the theory of focal cerebral function. by removing discrete motor and sensory area of the brain in monkeys. He demonstrated that their neurological deficits corresponded to the area of brain removed. (Reproduced by permission of the Wellcome Library, London.)

evolved brain — that of man. Since man's brain is not available for experimentation, Ferrier had chosen an experimental model as closely related to humans as he could legally get by using the brain of anthropoid apes (monkeys). He then joined Goltz in inviting the audience to Professor Yeo's laboratory at King's College the next day to see two apes, missing certain cerebral centers, meticulously removed several months back. The audience could see for themselves — Ferrier's methods and results contrasted with those of Goltz.[14]

## The Demonstration

Nearly 100 dignitaries convened in Professor Yeo's laboratory at King's College the next day, including Jean-Martin Charcot, world-famous French neurologist; many foreigners; and approximately 70 members of the Medical Congress. Professor Goltz demonstrated his dog first. On the surface of the dog's head, as he had mentioned, were the two large sunken areas where bone and brain had been removed and not replaced, the scalp merely sewn back into place. Amazingly, the dog ran, jumped out of its cage and went through normal movements, with Goltz's prodding, dramatizing his normal state. What argument could Ferrier use to counter this dog, bereft of brain — walking, jumping, seeing?[15] By cracking a whip Goltz demonstrated that the dog could hear. Using pincers on various sites on the dog, he proved that sensation was intact. Goltz then stated that the dog had suffered a loss of intelligence because of the amount of brain removed. The dog would not, of his own free will, chase a cat or even jump out of a cage with low walls. The animal exhibited normal movements, could hear, see, and feel but he had lost much intelligent behavior, proving that Ferrier's theory of localized brain function was wrong. With extensive brain removal Goltz had produced a "canine imbecile" but one with no motor or sensory abnormalities — proof that no focal centers existed.[16]

As Goltz was gathering up his materials to make way for Ferrier, a hush fell over the laboratory. From one side of the room, with the help of a laboratory assistant, in walked a large, sad-faced monkey, standing erect but dragging his right leg behind him, right arm dangling, helplessly. The audience was silent, stunned by the similarities of the monkey to that of a human stroke patient. Finally Charcot gasped, "Why, it's a patient!" Ferrier offered the monkey a banana which it grasped and ate using its functional left hand. When sitting in repose the animal casually lifted the flaccid right arm up with the left. Ferrier then explained how, seven months ago, in a painstaking operation, the motor zone of the brain had been removed. As a long-term survivor, the animal was otherwise completely healthy with no apparent mental deficiencies.

A second monkey, rendered deaf by removal of its hearing centers, was also demonstrated. With the visual impact of the first animal, however, the second must have seemed anticlimactic.

Ferrier announced that his two monkeys and Goltz's dog would be sacrificed under chloroform so that all attendees present could inspect their brains. Surgical results, the preciseness of excision and correlation of motor abnormality to area of brain removed could all be ascertained by anyone wishing to do so. A committee of four eminent physiologists, Professor Schafer, Dr. Klein, Dr. Gowers and Mr. Langley, were appointed to inspect the animals' brains and to later issue a formal report. When the committee issued its report, the conclusions were clear. In Ferrier's cases the excised areas of the monkeys' brains corresponded exactly with the area of the brain that Ferrier had maintained represented the functional centers for movement of arms, legs and hearing. With Goltz's dog, the findings were not so certain. The committee had been unable to exactly define the destroyed portions of the dog's brain, the injuries being more diffuse and random; some areas were destroyed but the dissected areas lacked the discreteness of Ferrier's. A few purported sensory and motor areas had been left undisturbed, allowing his dog to function fairly normally. The victory was clearly Ferrier's and the theory of focal cortical function emerged dominant, reconfirmed both clinically and experimentally innumerable times over the past 130 years.

## Vivisection Is Indispensable

With the meetings of the International Medical Congress concluded, physiologist Michael Foster formally closed the session directing a final Parthian shot at the antivivisectionists present: "this Congress expresses its conviction that experiments on living animals have in the past proved of the greatest service to medicine, and are indispensable for its future progress."[17]

But Cobbe had not been standing idly by, passively observing. Anxious for new or embarrassing information that she might use against the physiologists, Cobbe routinely monitored scientific journals. She hoped to discover mistakes, contradictions or honest disagreements between scientists that she could exploit in her charge that all brain experimentation was useless. The inevitable animal suffering following such experiments could not be justified. In *Pfluger's Archiv*, she noted work from Goltz's laboratory in which 51 dogs had their "brains washed out" and later died of "inflammation of the brain." At autopsy, the scarred brain of one of Goltz's dogs exhibited complete loss of topical architecture due to the disruptive force of the stream of water. Reporting on that finding, the pathologist remarked that the brain "resembled a lately hoed potato field."[18] Intrigued with such vivid imagery, Cobbe repeated the phrase in numerous essays and speeches over the ensuing years, wringing from it every last vestige of drama possible. Following on that, she cited in the *Zoophilist* a Dr. Hermann of Zurich, "one of the greatest foreign investigators," who claimed that making lesions in the brain, the most delicate and complicated organ in the body, was not realistic. Man's operative techniques were so crude that no reliable conclusions could be drawn. Hermann compared these controlled brain injuries of scientists to someone damaging a watch by means of a pistol shot. At best, the injury would be massive and unpredictable. Studying an eloquently organized brain after a similarly devastating injury cannot be justified. Charcot's technique of observing cases of disease with autopsy follow-up still remained the best method of study.[19]

## Pros and Cons of Vivisection

Virchow's antivivisectionist posture at the Congress excited much comment both at the meeting and afterwards, in the press. In 1881, a three-part series of articles entitled "Vivisection, Its Pains and Its Uses," appeared in *Nineteenth Century* magazine — all follow-up arguments favoring vivisection, written by scientists James Paget, Richard Owen and physician Samuel Wilks. Putting vivisection into perspective, Paget stated that the practice was no worse than the caging of birds, placing animals in zoos for public entertainment or allowing bearbaiting or dog fighting. Most animals were strays, already marked for death.[20] Physiologists know that knowledge gained through experimentation far outweighs the usefulness of shooting, hunting or fishing. To subject scientists to legislative restraint, namely the Act of 1876, while the public pursues these other cruel pastimes is unfair.[21] Wilks observed that most vivisection is no more painful or cruel than merely pricking mice or guinea pigs in pursuit of the study of contagion — a process carried out for the benefit of mankind. Those who seek the opinion of all of the leading men of England and Europe will find a uniformity of opinion favoring experimentation on animals. Those opposed are

> certain lords and certain ladies, certain bishops and certain members of Parliament, who, with all the dogmatism of pure ignorance, declare that "vivisection only panders to curiosity, without doing anything for science"; "that it is a detestable practice not attended with scientific results." If history *repeats* itself, we seem to hear the Dominican monks vociferating that the earth does not go round the sun, and to see them putting Galileo in prison to prove their point.[22]

In January 1882, Cobbe answered the three men individually in her essay, "Vivisection: Four Replies." She contemptuously dispatched Paget by accusing him of hiding the truth. He paints a benign picture of experimentation by suppressing the very worst facts of physiology. She criticized Wilks by denying that antivivisectionists ever argued about the inutility of experimental science. It is the moral offense inherent in cutting up living animals that renders the practice intolerable, not whether the results prove to be of any use to mankind or not. She summed up her reply by reiterating the four points against vivisection that she had articulated in the inaugural issue of the *Zoophilist*:

> 1st. Because it is the most cruel of cruelties, and the laboratories where it is practiced are places where torture is not an accident but a business. 2ndly. Because while other cruelties are dying out before the advance of civilization, Vivisection is becoming a new vice. 3rdly. Because it not only involves most pain for brutes, but is most demoralizing to men — because it is most conscious and deliberate. 4thly and lastly. Because the Society is convinced that it is scientifically worthless — a misleading method of physiological research.[23]

## Cobbe's Suit

Never idle, Cobbe had continued faithfully carrying out her practice of reviewing journals and city records, looking for possible infractions by physiologists. In comparing the Medical Congress' records with those of the *British Medical Journal*, she noted a discrepancy. Ferrier had never received a license to experiment. Having scarcely recovered from his victory over Goltz, Ferrier soon found himself facing a summons — he was being sued. Despite warnings from her old confidant, Shaftesbury, Cobbe and the Victoria Street Society (VSS) forged ahead, claiming that Ferrier had willfully and wantonly violated the Cruelty to Animals Act of 1876 by experimenting on animals without a license. It was headline news, of course, as Cobbe had intended.[24]

In November 1881, both parties appeared before Sir James Ingraham at the solemn Bow Street Magistrates Court in Covent Gardens — the same court in which the Artful Dodger from Dickens' *Oliver Twist* had been featured in the 1830s. Professor Ferrier was with his attorney, Mr. Gully, while the opposing attorneys were Mr. Waddy and Bernard Coleridge. The courtroom was stuffed to overflowing with Cobbe and her antivivisectionist allies, plus interested members of the medical community. A large group of medical students had to gather outside the courtroom since they could not be accommodated inside, congesting the sidewalk around the stone building's corner entry.

The prosecutor, Mr. Waddy, led off first charging that Dr. Ferrier had violated the Animal Protection Act of 1876, "an act in favour of the medical profession and in the interest of science." Had Ferrier bothered to obtain a license, he would have been perfectly justified in performing the experiments. It was true that Ferrier did not have a license for experimentation, Mr. Gully of the defense admitted, but it was Professor Yeo, who was licensed, who had actually carried out the experiments. Ferrier had merely observed and advised. A long discussion between Waddy and Gully ensued, centering on what exactly counted as experimentation. Was it the actual operation or the period of observation after the operation? Both sides agreed that the experiment included that time after the monkeys awakened and did not conclude until months later after the animals were sacrificed and their brains examined. Under such circumstances, killing the animals before they emerged from anesthesia would have negated the entire object of the experiment — no information would have been gained. Waddy countered that, were that the case, Ferrier should have either killed the animals before they awakened or he should have had a certificate allowing for chronic survival. Finally, on the witness stand, physiologist Michael Foster offered information that rendered the prior argument moot. He claimed that there were two different groups of monkeys, an older group operated upon by Ferrier and the newer group operated on by Yeo, under the new antiseptic method of Joseph Lister. It was this latter group of Yeo's that had been demonstrated at the recent Medical Congress. Magistrate Ingraham then declared that Ferrier had to have demonstrated some actual "participation in the original Act in order to make this an act of cruelty within the meaning of the Act of Parliament." All evidence pointed to the contrary. Ferrier had only examined the animals on different occasions. Ingraham, who appeared reasonable to both sides, concluded that, for the Act to apply, Professor Ferrier must have participated in the operations in question. Since the operations had been performed by Dr. Yeo, Ferrier had nothing to do with them. "Further, I think the case cannot be carried. The summons will be dismissed."[25]

When the verdict was announced, there were howls of derisive laughter from the medical and scientific men jamming the courtroom, displaying their disgust at the antivivisectionists. Outside, a group of raucous medical students taunted Cobbe and her allies for their obstructionist tactics as they left the scene.

Cobbe, however, was convinced of Ferrier's guilt until the time of her death. In her autobiography she referenced the 1884 *Philosophical Transactions* of the Royal Society stating, "that Professor Ferrier *had* the leading share (his name always appears first) in the experiments."[26]

The physiologists and their sympathizers, chafing over the unjustified attack on Ferrier, covered his legal expenses. In 1882 they formed the Association for the Advancement of Medicine by Research (AAMR) to protect physicians against future antivivisectionist attacks. In a further strategic move, the AAMR negotiated with the Home Secretary to be the vetting agency for all future experimental science license applications, a beneficial move for physiologists.[27]

Although Cobbe denied it, some antivivisectionists had this aggravating habit of asking, "Of what practical use is vivisection? Name one discovery that has led to a medical innovation or benefit." Until the early 1880s, they had a point—one that the physiologists could not effectively counter. Certainly, one should be able to justify vivisection just on the basis of gaining further basic scientific knowledge, impractical or not. Still, some practical consequences would go a long way in making the physiologists' arguments more convincing, their practices more palatable to the public.

Touching on just such a theme, Sir George Humphry, Professor of Physiology at Cambridge University, addressed the AAMR in August 1881. In his speech, "Vivisection: What Good has it Done?" he asserted, much like Bernard and Virchow before him, that virtually every advance in knowledge of bodily function has been gained through vivisection. The way the heart functions, the movement of the blood, the functions of the brain, spinal cord and the nerves that serve the entire body, the glands that secrete have all been elucidated through vivisection. Specific treatments may not have eventuated as yet, but general advances in treatment could be attributed to vivisection.

In answer to the other charge made by the antivivisectionists—animal experimentation hardens the heart and demoralizes the man, Humphry made another point. Such is obviously not the case. Even before the use of anesthetics, we did not consider surgeons, "used to inflicting long, continued severe and horrible pains" on humans, as being hard hearted. It is the motive that reveals the hardened heart, not the act.

Only through vivisection, Humphry argued, can one gain an understanding of bodily function, just as dissection of the human body is the path towards the elucidation of human structure. "What we may call dead structure [anatomy] is pretty much worked out; it is the living processes that need to be investigated, and living processes can only be investigated while life is going on."[28] During the decade of the 1880s, practical advances in studying those living processes began to pay dividends. Information gained as a direct result of Ferrier's monkey experiments helped deliver the first blow.

## Clinical Dividends of Physiology

On November 3, 1884, a 25-year-old Scottish farmer named Henderson was admitted to the Hospital for Epilepsy and Paralysis, under the care of A. Hughes Bennett. Henderson was suffering from disabling headaches and weakness of his left arm and leg. Seizures manifest themselves by a twitching of the left side of his face and tongue that progressed to an involuntary turning of his head and eyes to the left. With time, the seizures increased in frequency, while his headaches became daily and excruciating. When Bennett examined Henderson, he noted a peculiar inflammation of the back of his head and upper neck. On further inquiry, Bennett learned that Henderson's family doctor, out of sheer desperation, had treated him for several weeks with mustard plasters. While under Bennett's care, Henderson's headaches worsened to the point of delirium with the patient screaming wildly, isolated in a room where he would not disturb other patients. Bennett knew that Henderson was suffering from a mass inside his brain—most likely a tumor but brain abscess was also a possibility. It became obvious that this man would die without definitive treatment. It was operation or death.

When Bennett consulted surgeon Rickman Godlee, Lister's nephew and future biographer, he was faced with a dilemma. How could the tumor be located surgically? The headaches were generalized, lending no clue towards localization. There were no external landmarks—only the man's paralysis gave a clue as to location. This was 1884, 11 years before the advent of Roentgen's x-rays and decades before cerebral angiography, the first radiological method for localizing brain masses. To surgically localize the tumor, Godlee would have to rely strictly on clinical manifestations. Since the tumor caused both the seizures and paralysis, it must lie within the motor strip—an area now well known from Ferrier's work on monkeys and Jackson's clinical observations. Having that information gave the surgeon more confidence that motor function could be correlated to a specific site in the human brain. At some time during the pre-operative phase, both Hughlings Jackson and David Ferrier joined the case. They made linear markings on Henderson's scalp, from side to side, with scientific estimates of where the motor strip lay in a front-to-back orientation. Another line, front to back, marked the lateral orientation. They then drew a circle where the lines crossed—where the tumor should lie.[29]

The operation took place in a house converted into a hospital, on a crude wooden table modified for the task at hand. Lacking the proper surgical instruments, Godlee and Bennett borrowed them from King's College. Having trained under Lister, Godlee was already well versed in his antiseptic technique. He procured a carbolic acid nebulizing machine, hoping to kill bacteria in all the critical places. The crew sprayed the air, Henderson's shaved and shiny head, the surgeons' hands and the surgical instruments. Henderson's upper torso and head had previously been soaked in carbolic acid. Towels, similarly drenched, enveloped his shoulders and neck. Although no exact record exists, Bennett, Hughlings Jackson, Ferrier and Victor Horsley, one of the future fathers of neurosurgery, were purportedly all in attendance.[30]

Once Henderson was rendered unconscious with chloroform, Godlee made the scalp incision, followed by several burr holes through the bone. He completed each hole manually with a brace and bit, much like that used to drill through wood. Godlee then connected these holes with hammer and chisel, enabling him to remove a plate of bone. Next he made an opening through the dura mater, a membranous covering, exposing the mounds (gyri) and valleys (sulci) of the brain. Although the bulging brain indicated increased pressure inside the head, no tumor was evident on the surface. Godlee then incised the brain with a knife, enabling him to locate the tumor, discrete and encapsulated, at an unspecified depth. Using dissection techniques considered crude by present standards, he attempted to remove the tumor with a spatula, only to have the tumor fracture in two. Godlee then resorted to dissecting with his finger — an even less delicate maneuver. There was a rapid welling of blood from within the depths of the brain to its surface. Godlee struggled to gain control but measures surgeons use to control bleeding in other parts of the body — vascular clamps and direct pressure, could not be used inside the delicate brain. Several times he tried tamponade — packing the wound to a pressure exceeding the body's blood pressure — and waiting, but that proved futile. Finally, he stopped the bleeding with an electro-cautery device and the essential part of the operation was over. Godlee closed the wound with special carbolic acid-soaked sutures, designed by Lister with the hope of avoiding wound infection. The mass, the size of a pigeon's egg, proved to be a glioma — a tumor composed of primary brain tissue.[31]

Henderson regained consciousness quickly, answering questions within one half-hour of awakening. He had not only come through the operation well, but his left-sided weakness was rapidly improving. Unfortunately, on the fourth post-operative day, while changing the head dressing, Godlee noted a "decidedly putrefactive smell." Over the ensuing days, Henderson's wound opened spontaneously as he deteriorated, with fevers ranging as high as 104°F. Bacterial scalp contaminants related to the mustard plasters were the likely source of his infection. Henderson expired from meningitis 28 days after the historic operation, fully awake until the end.[32]

With Henderson's death, one could hardly claim that the operation had been a resounding success, Still, Godlee and Bennett had crossed a barrier of navigating through the brain — tumors of the brain would not be viewed with quite the same level of futility in the future. Operations had been performed before in which tumors had been removed from both the skull and from the surface of the brain. However, Henderson represented the first case in which a surgeon had deliberately invaded the depths of the brain, guided by physiological knowledge made possible through pioneering operations on monkeys. Godlee and Bennett had demonstrated that the approach and the technique were feasible; man could withstand intentional operative intrusion into his brain without disastrous neurological effects.

But Cobbe was neither impressed with nor did she approve of the accomplishment. She felt that too much has been made of Ferrier's experiments and "how they have enabled himself and others to make out exactly where diseases in the brain were situated." Antivivisectionists continued to cast doubt on the scientists' claims, asserting that many physiologists did not agree completely with Ferrier.[33]

Between December 1884 and January 1885, the *Times* received no fewer than 64 letters relating to the surgery, the most of any non-political topics ever presented by the paper. Antivivisectionists maintained their position asserting that man has no business carrying out such cruel experimentation on animals, let alone invading this part of the human body. However, at the jubilee celebration of the operation in 1934, The *London Times* noted the historic event at the facility which later became Maida Vale Hospital for Nervous Disease, praising pioneers Godlee, Bennett, Ferrier, Jackson and Horsley. By 1934, those dissenting voices of antivivisection had been largely silenced.[34]

Henderson's infection, however, represented a persisting problem. Although Lister's innovative regimen, now seven years in existence, appropriately followed the tenets of Louis Pasteur's nascent germ theory, it was far from a completed scheme. Godlee and colleagues all recognized a serious need for a more thorough understanding of these microscopic beings.

CHAPTER 14

# The Captain of All the Men of Death

Henderson endured his sad episode with operative infection in 1884. A mere two years earlier Robert Koch carried out pioneering work adding further knowledge to the relationship between bacteria and disease. Although Koch's successes could not have transitioned into any practical help for Henderson, his work served to expand the general influence of the germ theory by shedding light on an area of darkness responsible for profound human suffering.

In 1820, John Keats, the young apothecary and a favorite poet of Frances Cobbe, experienced a severe siege of coughing. Tasting blood, he quickly spit into a napkin. As he looked at it, he announced to his friend, "I know the color of that blood. It's 'arterial' blood.... That blood is my death warrant. I must die."[1] Chronic coughs, rampant throughout England, were habitually tolerated with a tinge of optimism, but once blood appeared in the sputum, the die was cast. The only question was, "How long do I have?" In Keats' case, it was only a year. At 14, Keats had watched his mother die of consumption. Then his younger brother, Tom, 19, died of the same illness. Keats had nursed them both through their terminal days. He had already gone through medical training before that eventful cough. He hardly practiced medicine at all before he gave in completely to the compulsion that would define his genius. Hoping to be cured by the clean Neopolitan air, Keats left the love of his life, Fanny Brawne, in England and set sail for Italy, with a newly found urgency to complete his work. Instead, he died there, quietly in his sleep a year later, age 26.[2]

Of all the diseases that have inflicted suffering upon mankind throughout the centuries, tuberculosis stands at the forefront, affecting nations as well as individual lives. In the 18th century, John Bunyon wrote about the devastating consequences of tuberculosis in *The Life and Death of Mister Badman*: "The captain of all these men of death that came against him to take him away, was the Consumption, for it was that that brought him down to the grave."[3]

## 14. The Captain of All the Men of Death

As both Koch and Pasteur had established individually, at least to their own satisfaction, virtually all infectious diseases present with one of several different faces even though one specific bacteria may be the cause common to each presentation. Tuberculosis was one of the most dramatic of such examples, going by such names as phthisis, white plague, consumption, scrofula, white death, and wasting disease. Naming tuberculosis the white plague implied that it was as destructive as the feared black or bubonic plague more common in medieval times. The moniker was apt. Both diseases invaded a community with devastating effects, but the similarities ended there. Bubonic plague entered an area more like a hurricane, producing ugly black buboes, infected, festering lymph nodes, followed by early death by the thousands. Entire communities could be decimated. Those who could afford to do so escaped to the hills to wait out the storm. Like the hurricane that mellows once it makes landfall, epidemics unexpectedly died out as well, due to some nebulous standoff developing between fading bacterial virulence and the level of resistance in the surviving hosts. The black plague then disappeared as mysteriously as it had arrived.

Tuberculosis was different — it was no visitor. It came to stay. As the very picture of insidiousness, tuberculosis could widely infect both the community and individuals with little external manifestation, initially. It silently insinuated itself into a community, causing a mild, chronic illness easily mistaken for bronchitis or the "grippe." In most cases people inhaled the bacillus into their lungs, experiencing no symptoms at all. With time, this smallest of spots in the lung became the early tubercle, causing a minor, chronic cough and low-grade fever. Some people would remain in that condition for years, unaware of their infection, with host and invader reaching some sort of immunological stalemate. In a more common scenario, the tubercle, that bulbous battleground where the confrontation between invader and host took place, would slowly enlarge. As its root word "tuber" implies, this lump looked similar to other tubers, as bulbous as a small potato. With time, the tubercle matured in one of several different directions. It could outgrow its blood supply, degenerating into a white, cheesy (caseous) mass. It might ulcerate as well, rupturing into a bronchus, with consequent lung collapse — or it could erode, à la Keats, into a small blood vessel, resulting in blood-tinged sputum (hemoptysis). Rarely, the tubercle could erode into a large vessel, eventuating in severe hemoptysis and even death. As the tubercles enlarged, in both size and number, replacing almost all functional pulmonary tissue, the individual endured a slow, agonizing death from asphyxia.

The English usually referred to tuberculosis as "consumption," a double entendre, since tubercles slowly replaced or consumed the lungs, while the disease slowly consumed the body. On the Continent, people more commonly used the term "phthisis," derived from the Greek term meaning, "wasting."[4] As tuberculosis passed into its chronic phase, wasting of the body became one of its most striking and consistent manifestations, often leaving a skeleton covered with skin. Haunting pictures of young, previously healthy individuals accented the slow but dramatic changes wrought on the human frame. A little-known ancient physician, Aretaeus of Cappadocia, has given one of the most enduring and pithy descriptions of advanced tuberculosis:

> Voice hoarse, neck slightly bent, tender and stiff; fingers slender but the joints swollen; severe wasting of the fleshy parts leaving the bones prominently outlined; the nails crooked or flat and brittle without their normal rotundity.... The nose is sharp and slender, the cheeks are prominent and abnormally flushed; the eyes are deeply sunk in their hollows but brilliant and glittering.... The slender parts of the jaws rests on the teeth as if smiling but it is the smile of cadavers.... The muscles of the limbs are wasted. Only the nipples mark the breasts in women. One may not only count the ribs but also easily trace them to their terminations for even the articulations of the vertebrae are quite visible as are the connections with the sternum.... The shoulder blades are like the wings of the birds.[5]

In 1844, socialist Friedrich Engels provided another compelling image of consumption in his book decrying the plight of the English working class:

> If one goes into the streets of London, when people are on their way to work, it is astonishing to note how many of them appear to be suffering to a greater or lesser degree from consumption. Even in Manchester one does not see these pale, emaciated, narrow-chested and hollow-eyed ghosts who are to be met with in such large numbers every minute in London.[6]

This was the most common face of tuberculosis, but there were others, depending upon the bodily part infected. Scrofula, meaning pig-like, referred to an infection of the lymph nodes in the neck. The most common manifestation of tuberculosis in youth, the child's swollen neck suggested the porcine image. With further usage, the term "scrofula" took on a more general meaning — a tuberculous soft-tissue infection near lymph nodes. A similar type of tuberculous skin infection, termed "lupus vulgaris" (common wolf), could appear anywhere, but was especially frequent in and around the nose.

Other less common presentations included miliary or "galloping" tuberculosis, in which very small tubercles, the size of millet seeds, became dispersed throughout the entire body, resulting in early death. Chronic tuberculous infections in the gut often broke through the intestinal wall into the abdominal cavity, resulting in peritonitis and death. Hushed and hoarse voices were ubiquitous due to tuberculous infections in the larynx. Infectious involvement of bones and joints were not rare. Pott's disease, an infection of the bony spine, often caused the disfigured, hunchback profile. If the infection eroded into the spinal canal, meningitis and rapid demise followed. Tuberculous infection of the adrenal glands, one cause of Addison's disease, was responsible for Jane Austen's death. Other rare forms of tuberculosis, such as a very painful skin condition and ocular infections, rounded out the many faces of tuberculosis.

The white plague showed no respect for class, status or pecuniary situation. Since it flourished where congestion and filth were common, and in cooler, damper climates, the poor were disproportionately infected. Still, it was the people with celebrated lives who more commonly evoked the pathos caused by the affliction. The poor suffered in the shadows. Most medical authorities, ignoring theories of contagion, thought that tuberculosis was hereditary since it was so strongly familial. Many believed that there was a moral aspect to the disease, as though one who contracted it was somehow lacking in virtue.

But the list of consumptive luminaries was long. John Locke, Baruch Spinoza, Laurence Sterne, Robert Louis Stevenson, all six of the Bronte children, Shelley, Cecil Rhodes, Nicolo Pagannini, Chopin, Louis XIII and XIV all suffered from the disease, to mention but a few.

Tuberculosis evinced a surprising cultural effect through the youthful, consumptive female. She acquired an unforeseen romantic patina. Men found the young blond, blue-eyed consumptive female so fine in appearance and mood and so vulnerable that she was irresistible. As the disease progressed and muscles wasted, bony structures in the face and neck emerged, highlighted. Associated changes in the skin gave a pellucid, blue-gray hue to the face, resulting in a delicate porcelain, doll-like appearance that could evoke a yearning even in the most phlegmatic of males. In England and on the Continent, young healthy women, noting this adulation, began drinking a vinegar and lemon juice mixture in hopes of losing weight and acquiring that porcelain glow.[7] Those close to consumptives noted another irony — their moods remained inappropriately high, as though they did not fully comprehend their own predicament.

This poignant aspect of tuberculosis, coupled with an urgency born of imminent death, provided a different muse than usual for the romantic poets. It was not unrequited love that spurred their imaginations, but rather impending doom, premature involution and death. Poets fed off images of decay and dissolution — crumbling headstones, rotting trees, old, overgrown grottos, abandoned churches. Autumn, with its leaves turning color, the feel of approaching dormancy, became the poets' favorite metaphor. The leaves were falling, dried, discolored and wrinkled.[8] A gloom hung over all. As William Cullen Bryant expressed it:

> The melancholy days have come, the saddest of the year,
> Of wailing winds and naked woods, and meadows brown and sear.[9]

Tuberculosis held such a grip on English culture that the subject permeated both contemporary art and literature. In Puccini's *La Bohème*, taking place in the bohemian Latin Quarter of Paris, Rodolfo falls in love with the flirtatious seamstress, Mimi. The narrative plays off of Rodolfo's guilt for wanting to leave his terminally consumptive lover. In the dramatic closing scene, he runs to Mimi as she lies quietly dying. In novels and plays, consumption served as a poignant and popular mode of exit for the heroine, leaving audiences and readers in tears. In novels such as *Oliver Twist*, Charles Dickens did at least as much to expose the evils of poverty, overcrowding and abusive child-labor practices than did any bureaucratic team surveying social or industrial practices. A well-constructed scene of consumptive children left searing images, not easily forgotten.

While dramatists fed off the pathos of tuberculosis, medical men dithered in feckless activity. The myriad and useless treatment schemes for the malady illustrated the fact that physicians were as ignorant of the disease as their treatments were useless. Some measures made sense: Move to a warmer, drier climate, namely Italy or southern France. However, it was only that small segment of the more wealthy class that could afford a prolonged change of climate. While the move did not provide a cure, it did slow down the process, providing symptomatic improvement, and perhaps a few more months of life. Physicians still offered the more common, general treatments. Anachronistic and dangerous, the practice of bloodletting persisted beyond 1850 before it died out. Another medieval maneuver, cupping, performed over multiple areas of the chest, continued to be employed. Disgusting, pus-like material, those noxious humors, drawn into the cup provided comforting evidence to the physician that the treatment was working. Physicians commonly offered patients drinks of heavy metals, such as antimony or mercury, along with cod liver oil and other potions.

Another dubious treatment consisted of placing a patient into a room to inhale patented gases of unknown content for a prolonged period of time. In another form, much like blowing up a balloon, doctors insufflated air into the rectum, where "it was sure to reach the lungs."[10] Professor Yeo, the brain researcher, incorporated this into his practice. The technique gained orthodoxy by being included in the British pharmacopeia in 1888. Following that same theory, a folk remedy for the poor entailed inhaling the breath of a "healthy beast." Since that treatment could be administered by lay people, it enjoyed some popularity as well.[11] Not surprisingly, charlatans flourished by feeding off the fears of the consumptives, offering them a multitude of different nostrums for their suffering. But the only true relief came from opium, usually in the form of laudanum. As an opiate, laudanum allowed the patient in the latter stages of the disease to sleep, as it helped ease the anxiety that accompanies slow suffocation. It allowed one to die in peace.

Most medical authorities viewed tuberculosis as several different diseases rather than one. This group included Professor Rudolf Virchow, the influential cellular pathologist who had contributed much to the microscopic description of the tubercle. He thought only the solid pulmonary lesion was tuberculosis. To him, the caseating and scrofulous forms were manifestations of cancer or some other disease state. Then there were the Unitarians, like Robert Koch, who rightly considered that all of the disparate manifestations of tuberculosis represented one infectious ailment. Koch had the advantage of knowing, through experimentation, that one bacterial infection, such as staphylococcus, can express itself in the body in different ways.

## Contagious or Cancerous?

A more fundamental question: Was tuberculosis an infectious disease at all — or was it something else, such as a form of cancer? There were hints that favored the infectious etiology. Some groups of people were perfectly healthy until they moved into the congested areas of large cities, such as London, where the majority not only became ill, but became ill at the same time. Other observers of the disease noted that siblings often became sick nearly simultaneously. That seemed unusual for a hereditary disease. The British epidemiologist, William Budd, a non-believer in contagion, finally had to change his views after observing black sailors coming into port, infected. With further investigation, he observed:

> Everywhere along the African sea-board, where the blacks have come into contact and intimate relations with the whites, phthisis causes a large mortality among them. In the interior, where intercourse with Europeans has been limited to casual contact ... there is reason to believe that phthisis does not exist.[12]

He had learned the last fact from none other than the medical missionary Dr. Livingston. After deliberating for over a decade, Budd finally published his views supporting contagion in *Lancet* in 1867.

But proclaiming and proving tuberculosis to be contagious were two very different things. The concept of contagion had been puzzling medical scientists since its origin in the 1500s. Rather than becoming firmly established, contagion's popularity as a concept waxed and waned because it did not have the underpinning of germ theory supporting it. Most physicians did not believe in contagion because they felt it was not supported by the facts. Before germ theory, people viewed the spread of disease as occurring through direct contamination of the healthy by the sick or by dirty air, via some chemical or physical substance, as yet unidentified. Since direct contamination explained only a small part of contagion, that is, over short distances, it seemed inadequate to explain contagion over greater lengths or regional outbreaks of disease. Epidemics often occurred without any relationship to the presence or absence of sick people. Making matters more confusing, a disease might rage in one area of a city, only to leave an adjacent neighborhood completely unscathed. Only when one introduced the concept of living organisms to undergird the theory of contagion did it seem plausible. Diseases could now be explained through long-distance transmission via water, by food supplies, coughing, and by travelers — both human and animal.[13]

Other scientists had attempted to prove an infectious origin for tuberculosis by trying to both culture and transmit the disease from one animal to another. Cohnheim and Solomonsen successfully inoculated the anterior chamber of oxen eyes with tuberculosis, but developed their project no further.[14] In 1865, French army surgeon Jean-Antoine Villemin demonstrated even more convincingly that he could transmit tuberculosis from man to rabbit or guinea pig. He first placed pus taken from a fatal human case and injected it under the skin of two rabbits. At autopsy, several months later, both rabbits displayed widespread lesions in the lungs and lymph nodes. He then showed that he could transmit that disease in an unending string, from generation to generation of animal. Villemin even recognized some "virulent principle" in human sputum that could be transmitted to animals. When he presented his work to the Academy of Medicine, it was met with derision. One critic, Hermann Pidoux, argued that the disease in the poor was due to overcrowding, malnutrition, dirty air and unsanitary conditions. When queried why the wealthy also suffered from the disease, he countered that overeating, flabbiness, laziness and general excess of ambition all played a role in causation.[15] In 1868, Villemin published his experiences, *Etudes sur la tuberculose*. Unfortunately, the reception of his work was tepid, given the skepticism to germ theory at mid-century.[16]

Koch, aware of this experimental work when he made his decision to study tuberculosis, was already strongly inclined to consider tuberculosis an infectious disease. In 1881, he had just returned from his successful demonstration of the pure culture technique at the International Congress in London. Being a peerless microscopist who could utilize all current refinements, such as the achromatic lens, oil immersion and the finest Zeiss microscopes available, Koch seemed a natural to take on the challenge of tuberculosis. He understood microbial culture and the vagaries associated with bacteria, nutrients, humidity, temperature and the like. Koch was one of the few besides Ehrlich who had a sophisticated understanding of organic dyes as they relate to the interaction with the surface of the microorganism — the site that takes on the color.

Koch aimed to prove or disprove that a microscopic organism was the causative agent of tuberculosis. First, he systematically studied material from a phthisis ward in the Berlin Charité Hospital. As Koch came to discover, the tubercle bacillus was small, one-tenth the size of the anthrax bacillus, grew very slowly and was difficult to stain.[17] As he later established, the surface of the tubercle bacillus had a waxy composition, inert to the usual bacterial dyes. Staining it would be like painting a carriage that had a thick coating of wax on its exterior. It is ironic, therefore, that discovering a method of staining the bacillus would be where Koch had his first success. Early in his research, he inoculated many animals with infected material and examined their tissues until he became convinced that he was seeing a consistent living organism in the infected animals but not in his controls. With a fine platinum wire coated with specimen, he streaked the material out on cover glasses. He then systematically applied a variety of stains to the specimens, starting with the standard methylene blue. He consistently saw very tiny rods, about half the size of a five-micron blood cell. But, were these the infectious agents? He could not be sure.

Hoping to take photomicrographs, Koch experimented with different counter-stains and found *vesuvin* (Bismarck Brown) offered a nice contrast to the blue. When photographed in blue light, the brown staining host tissues accentuated the organism as a dark blue. He then discovered that a dye solution, rendered alkaline with ammonia, not only heightened the contrast but made the blue-staining tubercle bacilli brighter and more transparent. Serendipity also played some role. A slide preparation, covered with dyes, had been carelessly left overnight, near a hot stove. When Koch examined the slide the next day, the bacilli were much brighter than usual. After demonstrating by further experimentation that heat intensified the staining of bacilli, heat became an integral part of his staining technique.[18] Koch could now see the organisms relatively easily. He had not only connected the bacillus consistently to the tubercle, but he had also discovered a differential stain capable of distinguishing the tubercle bacillus from all other organisms as well. Ehrlich later refined the technique even further by using an aniline dye and replacing methylene blue with fuchsin.[19]

Having a reliable way to visualize the bacteria was the first big step in identifying the cause of tuberculosis. Armed with his new staining technique, Koch returned to Charité Hospital for new tuberculous specimens. Now, things were different. As a young tubercle developed, he could see a large number of stained bacilli, both in and outside of the cell. As the tubercle aged, the number of bacteria diminished. Koch concluded:

> On the basis of my extensive observations, I consider it as proved that in all tuberculous conditions of man and animals there exists a characteristic bacterium which I have designated as the tubercle bacillus, which has specific properties which allow it to be distinguished from all other microorganisms.[20]

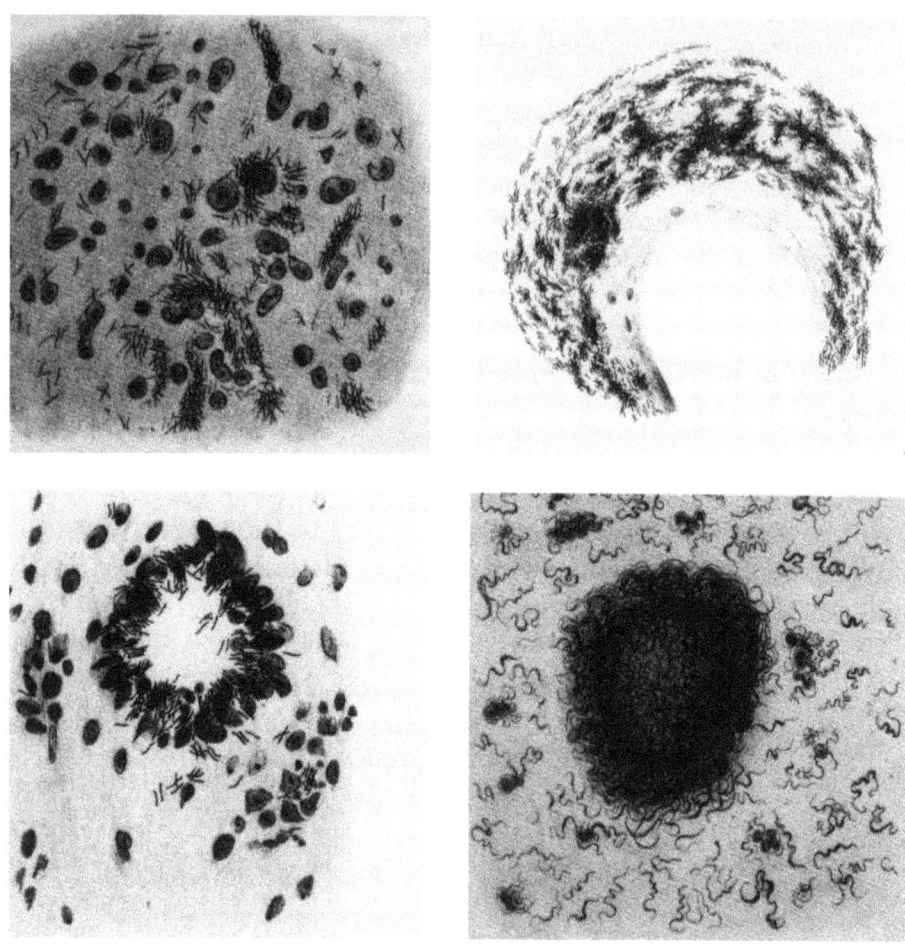

Koch's rendering of tubercle bacilli in different tissues. *Clockwise from upper left:* (1) Tubercle from human lung. (2) Infected tissue immediately adjacent to an arterial wall. (3) Tubercle bacilli in culture. (4) Human lung with giant cell surrounded by tubercle bacilli. (Courtesy of ASM Press and Thos. D. Brock, p. 122.)

## Koch's Postulates

Koch only stated that the bacilli were always found in tubercles, carefully avoiding any claim that they were the cause of the disease. To prove causation he would have to first isolate the organisms in pure culture. Then these bacilli must be injected into other animals and produce the same disease manifestations, both clinically and microscopically, in that animal. In other words, he had to fulfill Koch's postulates to prove causation, something more easily said than done. Culturing the bacillus proved extremely difficult. It would not grow at room temperature at all, while at body temperature his solid nutrient gel liquefied, eliminating the plating method as a useful technique. After many failures, Koch lit upon using coagulated sheep and cow serum, boiled for hours to ensure sterility. By slanting the tubes as the blood serum coagulated, he increased the solid surface area for bacterial growth from a small circle to an expansive ellipse (below). With this technique, he inoculated the serum slants with tuberculous tissue gathered from experimental animals.

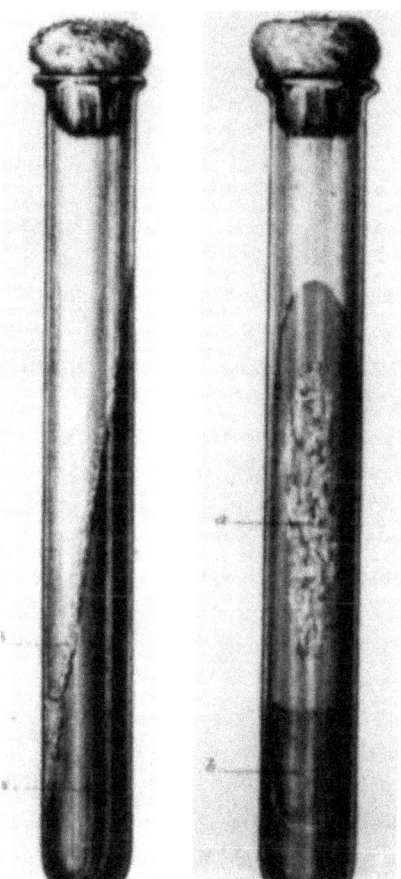

Ordinarily, cultures of most bacteria reveal growth between 24 and 48 hours, but the tubercle bacillus proved different. Under the microscope, Koch could see no growth at one week. Finally, by the end of the second week, after most bacteriologists would have thrown out the cul-

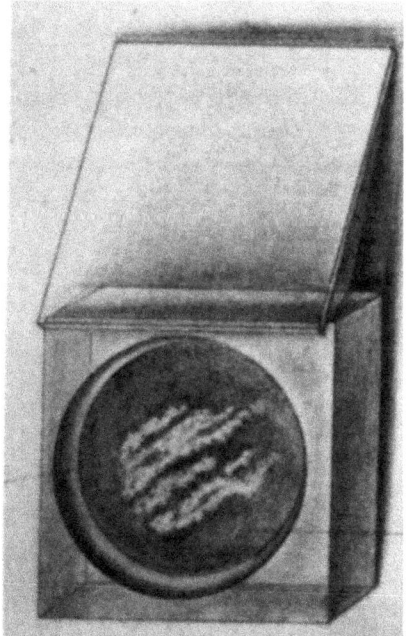

Koch's drawings of cultured tubercle bacilli. *From left:* Side and frontal views of organisms growing on the slanted surface of solidified blood serum. *Right:* A culture of tubercle bacilli growing in a glass box. (Courtesy of ASM Press and Thos. D. Brock, p. 124.)

tures, he noted some sort of growth that he then transferred to a fresh medium. Now, with each succeeding generation of culture, he could not only identify the small bacteria but also purify them.

Next, he had to prove that these pure bacterial cultures caused the disease. The guinea pig proved unusually susceptible to the tubercle bacillus and a wonderful analogue to the tuberculous human, making Koch's task a little easier. When inoculated under aseptic technique, they all developed widespread, fairly typical tubercles, as seen microscopically. All guinea pigs died within four to six weeks. In other words, when Koch inoculated the animals with the pure cultures, they died of the disease with the identical clinical picture as those animals that had been inoculated with human tuberculous material.[21] By fulfilling his own postulates he ultimately proved causation.

Discovering the cause of tuberculosis was Koch's greatest work. Dealing with such small, indolent, chromophobic organisms had forced him to transcend all standard bacteriological techniques. In the process he designed new culture media, new methods of bacterial culture and unique methods for staining bacteria. In all, his experiments included over 100 cases of human tuberculosis and "several hundred animals" of multiple species.[22] Remarkably, Koch spent six years from the time he began his work on anthrax to his solving the riddle of tuberculosis. In contrast, he elucidated the cause of tuberculosis, the greatest bacteriological riddle then known to mankind, in the space of only eight months.

## Koch's Pronouncement

On 24 March 1882, Koch gave a historic presentation to the Berlin Physiological Society, describing his discovery. Ordinarily, this subject would have fallen more under the purview of the Berlin Pathological Society. But Virchow was president of that society. His attitude towards Koch's theories and the Imperial Health Office had remained hostile.[23] With his great influence, Virchow could potentially stifle any ideas to which he did not fully subscribe. Avoiding him altogether was the wiser route. The room in which Koch presented was packed with such personalities as Loeffler; Ehrlich, the bacteriologist; and physicist Helmholz. Due to the smallness of the venue, only 36 scientists attended, a minuscule audience, considering the enormity of Koch's announcement.[24] Not a word of the discovery had been leaked to anyone outside his laboratory. Koch provided as much a demonstration as he did a speech, setting up over 200 microscopic samples, cultures and pathological tissues to supplement his talk. Avoiding dramatic flourishes, Koch delivered his usual methodical, thorough and detailed presentation.

When he concluded his presentation, the audience remained silent with reverential admiration. No clapping, no celebratory backslaps. Slowly, some rose to shake his hand while others milled about or examined the specimens again. They realized that what they witnessed was a historic event. Ehrlich, the dye expert, later observed, "I hold that evening to be the most important experience of my scientific life."[25] So impressed was Sir Robert Phillip, a pioneer in tuberculosis treatment, that he stated, "The enigma of the ages was unfolded ... astonishing for the completeness of the proof, and the perfection of the demonstration."[26] Three weeks later the *Berliner Klinische Wochenschrift* published his lecture, creating a worldwide sensation.

Twelve days later, the British physicist John Tyndall, the same man who had helped Pasteur put the theory of spontaneous generation to rest, received a copy of Koch's work. He was so moved that he summarized it for the general reader, publishing it in the *Times of London*. He could not help but make an argument decrying the antivivisectionists' activities:

> In no other conceivable way [than by animal experimentation] could the true character of the most destructive malady by which humanity is now assailed be determined. And, however noisy the fanaticism of the moment may be, the common sense of Englishmen will not, in the long run, permit us to enact cruelty in the name of tenderness, or to debar us from the light and leading of such investigations as that which is here so imperfectly described.[27]

Within two weeks, the news had spread across the Atlantic where the *New York Times* and *New York Post* published news of Koch's discovery. They, like the *Times*, later wondered how long it would be, through animal experimentation, that a vaccine might be developed to control the disease.

Paul Ehrlich and other dye experts, Franz Ziehl and Friedrich Neelson, added some further refinements to the dyeing process, over the ensuing year. The Ziehl-Neelson stain for tuberculosis, their ultimate refinement, is still used today.[28]

Koch had earlier expressed concerns to Loeffler that it would take as much as a year for the world to accept his findings. Some non-believers did surface, but they proved sporadic and ineffective. Acceptance was so immediate that his laboratory was inundated with scientists over the ensuing months, including one distinguished visitor, Rudolf Virchow. After examining all of Koch's work, he had to admit that the tubercle bacillus could be responsible for all of the manifestations of the disease—an important convert to the Unitarian theory. Maybe there was something, after all, to this theory that a single type of bacteria could cause consumption, scrofula, meningitis and other seemingly different diseases.

Still there were segments of society that would never accept this concept of diseases being caused by specific bacteria. In 1899, 16 years later, Dr. George

Wilson, the noted sanitarian, addressed the British Medical Association in Portsmouth. He excoriated bacteriologists for their research methods, their indiscriminate sacrificing of huge numbers of animals, claiming that scientists pursued vaccination only because of potential commercial interests. And when it came to tuberculosis:

> I say that we can only fight phthisis on the old lines, by improving heritage when that is possible, by improving the homes and conditions of life and labour which are always possible and always call loudly for interference. But this insane hunt after the tubercle bacillus, as if it could be bottled up in a twopenny-halfpenny spittoon and got rid of, is the insanest crusade ever instituted on illogical lines.[29]

Frances Cobbe was similarly unconvinced. In a *Zoophilist* article, "Koch and Tuberculosis," she lamented the enthusiastic crowing of the *Times* over Koch's discovery, as though humanity's problems were over. "Science has thus vindicated forever the right to use the lower creatures for the benefit of man; and those who opposed and shackled her glorious march were ignorant and fanatics, the enemies of true humanity." But anyone familiar with the agonies suffered by the animals knew that they had to wait and see if a cure follows. Months elapsed and people were still dying. Even the vivisectionists had to admit that little practical benefit followed this greatest "triumph" of science.[30]

However, to the world at large, the impact of Koch's discovery was monumental. Tuberculosis would remain incurable until Selman Waksman introduced streptomycin in 1943. Still, by demonstrating the infectious, and therefore contagious, nature of the malady, some of the mysticism surrounding tuberculosis had been diminished. The world would not look at the disease quite as fatalistically. Koch's staining techniques also proved valuable in diagnosing tuberculosis in its incipient stages. Early diagnosis helped diminish its spread. Preventive measures, including public education programs, could now be applied with scientific authority. It made more sense to clean up cities, stop overcrowding, improve ventilation, decrease poverty and improve child labor laws.

Such preventive measures alone benefited the public at large. Despite the protestations of the Frances Cobbes of the world, the worst cases of tuberculosis could now be isolated with confidence, diminishing its contagiousness. Once bacteriologists demonstrated the infectious, bacillus-laden nature of tuberculous sputum, governments began providing spittoons in public buildings. People became more conscious about casually expectorating in public as well as the manner in which they handled their own spittle in private.

Life was good for Robert Koch. He carried out a triumphant tour by lecturing widely throughout Europe, enjoying general adulation for his accomplishment. However, he was carrying on his rancorous debates with Louis

Pasteur during this same time. In 1883, the German Exposition of Hygiene and Public Health convened, with one of the main features being a complete bacteriological experimental laboratory patterned on Koch's own laboratory. With German physicians and international visitors learning Koch's methods, his stature became further solidified, while bacteriological know-how diffused further around the world.[31]

It was now 1883 and the cholera outbreak in Egypt, as noted earlier, interrupted all immediate plans that Koch may have had for tuberculosis. Away from Berlin for nearly a year, he had to endure a hiatus from his tuberculosis work which lasted for several years. Upon his return in 1885, the regents at the Friedrich-Wilhelm University of Berlin appointed Koch Professor of Hygiene, given his successes with cholera and tuberculosis. With his heavy lecture schedule and the required administrative duties of his new post, his research work inevitably entered its nadir.

# VII

## Retreat to Wales

"The permanent and indefensible delights of the country seem somehow to be more indispensable to human beings than the high-strung gratifications of the town. The proof of this fact is that, while *we* can live at home all the year round, Town Mice, after eight or nine months' residence at longest, begin to hate their beloved city, and pine for the country." — Frances Power Cobbe[1]

CHAPTER 15

# Quitting London

In early 1884, with Koch in Egypt, Lister was firmly established at King's, carrying on his campaign of antiseptic surgery. Pasteur was in the earliest stages of transferring his attention from anthrax to rabies when Cobbe and Mary Lloyd "quitted London," moving to Wales.[1] For someone with her political instincts and skills, the move seemed an uncharacteristic tactical blunder. She resigned as Honorary Secretary of VSS and, along with Mary, joined its executive committee. Cobbe admitted that not only was life in London becoming more difficult, but her advancing age and diminishing income played a role as well. She commonly referred to her move as "retirement." Even though she was turning over the "entire charge of the office and of editing the *Zoophilist* to Mr. [Benjamin] Bryan," Cobbe still expected to be consulted on major VSS policy issues."[2] Bryan continued to edit the *Zoophilist* at least into the mid-1890s, exerting considerable political influence with his writings. Lurking somewhere in the administrative shadows was Stephen Coleridge, long-time VSS member and son of old Cobbe ally, the Lord Chief Justice. Cobbe's move to Wales created an opportunistic void within VSS. How long before someone might take advantage of this vacant position of power? How could Cobbe keep an eye on an organization that she still considered to be hers, to ensure that it continued along a proper political path? The eight-hour ride on the new rail line between London and Wales meant that she was too far away to give ready counsel for any new problems that might suddenly arise. Surely her literary efforts would suffer as well. The logistics of writing and sending manuscripts back and forth to London would be less efficient.

Still, Cobbe considered her move to Wales as keeping her end of a bargain. "For twenty years [Mary] lived in London to please me and now I live in Wales to please her."[3] Throughout their entire relationship, the two had vied with each other about how much time to spend in the country versus the city. Mary could have done without the big city entirely. She loved her ponies and the Welsh mountains. Returning to Hengwrt, her childhood home, just outside of Dolgelly, was her dream. But Cobbe, the extrovert, was a creature of the city. How could she function away from the epicenter of feminism, away from social gatherings, stimulating people, debate and lectures — so out of touch from social and political causes? In addition, Cobbe did not function well in the typically cold and damp weather of Wales. At her age of 62, weather loomed as an even stronger negative. Was there some other stronger, if less evident, reason for leaving London?

Certainly the beauty of Wales was a positive for her. But its quietude made it more appropriate as a retreat than a place to live. Hengwrt lay just outside the village of Dolgelly, tucked into the "Y" formed by the confluence of the wild Mawddach and the smaller Wnion rivers, just before their descent into the estuary and the sea at Abermaw.[4] Hengwrt reminded Cobbe of her youth at Newbridge, only on a smaller scale. From the oak-paneled drawing room she and Mary could enjoy a panoramic feast of the entire valley. Their bedroom included a view of the ivy-covered Llanelltyd church and its cemetery where many of the village forefathers had been laid to rest. Hengwrt afforded them both a feeling of peace, a sense of separation from urban strife, amid the luxuriant greenery lining the brooks that fed into the river.

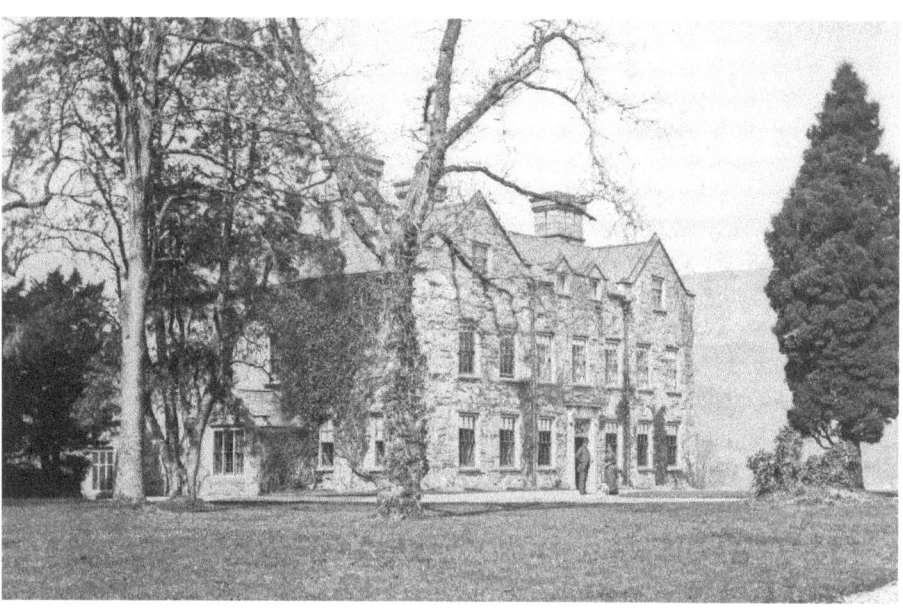

Mary Lloyd's childhood residence in Dolgelly, Wales, taken around 1875. Cobbe and Lloyd spent their remaining years here beginning in 1884. The couple standing at the entrance is unidentified. (By permission of the National Library of Wales.)

## Interpersonal Problems

Another positive, Cobbe would be further away from a legal problem that continued to vex her for another two years — until 1886. Charles Adams, 50, secretary of the VSS and Cobbe's predecessor as editor of the *Zoophilist*, had become romantically involved with VSS employee Mildred Coleridge, 36. In an executive meeting, Cobbe accused Adams of "undue familiarity" with Mildred, having "ruined" the daughter of the Lord Chief Justice in some "darkened room" within the VSS.[5] Cobbe and Shaftsbury inflamed the situation further by plotting to dismiss him. Adams then escalated matters by lodging a suit against Cobbe and the VSS for lack of payment concerning his long string of literary contributions to the VSS. Having the daughter of the Lord Chief Justice involved in a legal scandal with Adams proved great fodder for the press. To ensnare the leading figure of antivivisection, albeit peripherally, added further to the drama. Both the *Times* and provincial newspapers detailed embarrassing charges and counter-charges between the adversaries, causing Cobbe much consternation. As she wrote to her American confidant Sarah Wister, "I am just demented with worry."[6] In Adams' absence from the VSS and prior to Bryan's appearance, Cobbe had been forced to assume editorship of the *Zoophilist*, adding greatly to her already overloaded plate. Even if this legal entanglement seemed interminable, a move to Wales might at least provide some comforting distance for her.

Another rift in the mid-1880s, this one between Cobbe and the Coleridge brothers, was only in its incipient stages — a coup that required 12 years to fully evolve. At the time she left London, Cobbe had not even recognized the danger. While Bryan was leading the VSS, Stephen Coleridge laid in the background. However, through his executive committee position he slowly gained influence. Stephen was Cobbe's junior by 30 years. He and his brother Bernard quietly formulated plans to re-fashion the VSS to more closely fit their vision, now that the lioness was gone. Two factors led the Coleridges and some of the less rigid abolitionists within the VSS to consider a possible change of direction for the organization. In 1877, well before Cobbe's departure, Parliamentarians had made a second attempt to abolish vivisection, but the measure was soundly defeated. Then in 1884, another measure, Reid's Cruelty to Animals Amendment Bill, also failed to get through Parliament.[7] In such an atmosphere, any likelihood of passing legislation that completely banned vivisection in the foreseeable future seemed very remote.

Cobbe first became vaguely aware that something inimical to her interests might be happening within the organization when a friend, M.G.P. Martyn, wrote to her in 1885, warning her to be careful in her dealings with Stephen Coleridge. Although Coleridge sincerely had the Society's best interests at heart, Martyn cryptically indicated that Coleridge was not to be trusted.[8] Cobbe could do little directly except take heed of this warning. With Lord Shaftesbury's death in October 1885, she had lost her most reliable contact within the VSS. As a preemptive move, she did send both Coleridge brothers the second edition of her essay, "The Fallacy of Restriction Applied to Vivisection." Published in 1886, it was intended as a gentle reminder that the two should make no imprudent moves regarding abolition. In her piece, Cobbe argued that the only reasonable course against the vivisectors was total prohibition. Settling for anything less than abolition would be a grievous mistake. She offered four reasons: "Vivisectors are not, and never can be, amenable to humane restrictions." No one could ever design a program of restriction that would cover all of the vagaries of vivisection.[9] Second, gaining the respect and honor of his peers was the vivisector's main incentive. Therefore, through publishing his scientific results, the physiologist realized an even greater level of fame. If the act of vivisection were prohibited, the scientist's incentive would be gone. Third, since the results of vivisection were "worse than *nil*— misleading and injurious to science," closing that path actually would perform a favor to science.[10] Finally, any measure that allowed for vivisection was demoralizing to those who practiced it. Cobbe then concluded that neither a bill of restriction or prohibition had any chance of getting through Parliament in the current political climate. The antivivisectionists' only hope at the present lies in further educating the public to the evils of vivisection. If the restrictionists were ever successful, the vivisecting table will remain a well-used instrument of science. However, if the abolitionists prevail, that horrible instrument

> will be consigned to the museums of chains and "Maidens" and thumbscrews and will be described by the historian of the future as the barbarous invention of Science in his cruel boyhood;— to be bracketed with the Rack of the medieval Judge, and the Stake of the Inquisitor, as things over which men may blush and angels weep.[11]

Thinking that she had put to rest any idea of the VSS turning more towards restriction, Cobbe busied herself with other matters. Her next move managed to alienate a large segment of the Jewish community by innocently trying to recruit them to her cause. In 1891, she published a pamphlet, *An Appeal to the Humane Jews of England*, hoping to improve their views of animals and to recruit their support for the antivivisectionist cause. She boorishly suggested that not only was the Jewish race cruel and corrupt, but compared to Christians, Jews were overrepresented in vivisection, especially German Jews. Incensed, the editor of the *Jewish Chronicle* replied that if excessive numbers of Jews were involved in vivisection, it was because they were restricted from so many other areas of endeavor. Medicine was one discipline in which

Jews could participate. Furthermore, many of these scientists may be genetically Jewish, but they hewed neither culturally nor religiously to Jewish principles. To brand one group by the actions of a few is illogical.[12] Realizing her overstatement, Cobbe later wrote an apology in the *Jewish Chronicle*, but the harm was already done. For many years, a hint of anti–Semitism flavored the antivivisectionist cause.

Not having learned her lesson sufficiently, Cobbe next assailed the Catholics for their tacit pro-vivisectionist views. In an 1895 article in the *Contemporary Review*, she charged that it was anthropocentrism within the Catholic faith that allowed the "vile practice" of vivisection to flourish.[13] One need only look at the Catholic countries where vivisection flourished, such as Italy, France and Spain, to confirm her point. A terse reply in the next issue from the Rev. George Tyrell criticized Cobbe's attempts to vilify the Catholic faith and for her general intolerant attitude. "It is a poor cause that must have recourse to such weapons," he concluded.[14]

## The Nine Circles

Cobbe had no better luck with some of her other publications. She subscribed to the *Journal of Physiology*, constantly monitoring it and allied journals for evidence of scientific cruelty. Trying to be assertive rather than purely reactionary, Cobbe pursued another tactic. She collected a great many examples of perceived cruelty from her journals with the intention of dramatically illustrating to the public just how heartless these men of science were. Patterning the book after Dante's *Inferno* and its circles of suffering, Cobbe titled hers *The Nine Circles of the Hell of the Innocent*. But Cobbe's nine circles included at least 49 imaginative ways in which vivisectors might torture animals through experimentation. The first circle, mangling, itemized anatomical sites, such as the brain, liver, and kidney, where destructive lesions might be created. Artificial diseases comprised the second circle, which included "squirting virus into the brain," inoculations in the eyes, inducing abscesses and the like. The third circle, poisoning, included drugs, curare, snake venom, etc. Fourth circle was suffocation through slow drowning, apnea or "plastering mouth with gypsum." The fifth included burning and freezing while the sixth was starvation. The seventh, flaying and varnishing, included covering the skin with impervious substances or removing the skin from living animals. Cobbe reserved the eighth circle for miscellaneous items, including clamping of natural orifices and the inducement of suicide. Finally, number nine she labeled moral experiments, such as the testing of feelings, amputation of breasts of nursing mothers and so on.[15] All of the items were graphic, designed to induce shock and repugnance. Although each type of "torture" had some semblance of reality, most had been performed in a much earlier era, in other countries by Continental physiologists such as Brachet and Magendie.

Since Cobbe resided in Wales, compiling all of this material in London proved too difficult logistically; she recruited a friend, Georgine M. Rhodes, to organize the data and edit the work. Cobbe rushed the book to print in May so that its release would coincide with the October 1892 Church Congress at Folkestone, where the Anglicans held annual meetings dedicated to public enlightenment. Here, clergymen and invited experts representing the other side of the subject at hand debated various social and religious topics. Up for debate was the query, "Do the Interests of Humanity Require Experiments on Living Animals? If So, Up to What Point Are They Justifiable?" For permanency of record, full tracts of each speech were later published in various literary magazines. Cobbe's VSS published, as formal booklets, those speeches favoring her side. As a non-communicant of the Anglican faith, Cobbe did not attend the Congress, but she was anxious for her book to appear there. The *Zoophilist* featured *Nine Circles* in its May edition, evidently hoping to boost sales. At the June meeting of the VSS in London, the Rev. Canon Wilberforce stood before the audience, reminding all attendees that it was their duty to read and circulate, in every direction, this book, "produced by the prolific pen and the tender loving heart of that great woman, Frances Power Cobbe."[16]

As the Folkestone Congress of 1892 got underway, each antivivisectionist speaker, virtually all clergymen, presented his own case before an overflowing crowd. The Rev. F.S. Arnold stated that vivisectionists consider their work indispensable

Frances Cobbe, age 72. This photograph served as frontispiece for her 1894 autobiography *By Herself*. At this time, her confrontation with Pasteur and his rabies treatment scheme still consumed much of her time. (Reproduced by permission of the Wellcome Library, London.)

to medicine and surgery. But one only need consider the "advances" of Koch and Pasteur to learn otherwise. Koch's bubble burst when his claims of curing consumption with a new concoction failed. One cannot take an argument from animals and apply it to man; the analogy does not hold up.[17] In the case of Pasteur and his new efforts with hydrophobia, the Reverend had similar criticisms.[18] Arnold concluded that "man's interests do not begin and end with his body. Health and knowledge are two most excellent and desirable things, but not even they are worth pursuing at the cost of justice and mercy."[19] Two other speakers supporting the antivivisectionist cause, the Rev. Alfred Barry and physician John H. Clarke, spoke as well. Clarke's generally forgettable comments centered on the fact that any medicine "dominated by the spirit of vivisection" was evil.[20] In answer to vivisectionists' claims, the Reverend Barry thought it absolutely inconceivable "that He should so have arranged the avenues of knowledge that we can attain to truths, which it is His will we should master, only through the unutterable agonies of beings which *trust* in us."[21] He urged the attendees to press for total prohibition of vivisection if they believed that it could not be controlled through regulation.

## Horsley's Response

Towards the meeting's conclusion, Victor Horsley, a neurosurgeon and vivisector, rose from the audience, inquiring if it were not "too much to ask of a church dignitary" to bother to learn the facts regarding scientific experimentation before speaking publicly with such "dogmatic ignorance." Referring to honorable men of science as "morally offensive" and "cruel" was itself an offense. Furthermore, Cobbe's *Nine Circles* was "one of the rankest impostures that had for many years defaced English literature."[22] Horsley then accused her of systematically omitting from her *Nine Circles* any mention of the use of anesthetic agents in 20 of her 26 cited experiments. He asserted that Cobbe had tried such trickery before and was obviously lying once again.[23] Nonplused, the presiding bishops attempted to lighten the mood by making some weak efforts at levity, but the tone of the meeting and subsequent debate had been set.

Cobbe later answered Horsley's charges in the *Times*, admitting that anesthetics had not been mentioned where they should have been. Her only defense was that someone else had compiled all of the material. Horsley replied that those who care for truth and honesty should withdraw "their names and support from the society of which Cobbe was the moving spirit."[24] People within the antivivisectionist movement sprang to her defense. In a letter to the *Spectator*, Georgine Rhodes confessed that she was the person guilty of the omissions. Ironically Cobbe, the fierce and sometime malevolent defender of the voiceless, emerged as the victim. She seemed to find some comfort in her new role as the aggrieved. The *Sunday Times* editor felt that a male scientist such as Horsley should be reminded that in polite society a gentleman should not call a lady a liar.[25] However, Horsley would not back down: "I have documentary (printed) proof that she has chosen for 16 years or more to take an immoral course — namely, accusing medical men of murder, cruelty, falsehood ... while supporting such charges by frauds of the kind I have now exposed."[26] *BMJ* editor Ernest Hart, who had felt the sting of VSS opposition in his 1885 bid for Parliament, spoke out in Horsley's support. Cobbe "has taken refuge when confronted with the facts, and when her falsities are exposed in a plain and convincing manner, behind 'The Privilege of Her Womanhood.'"[27]

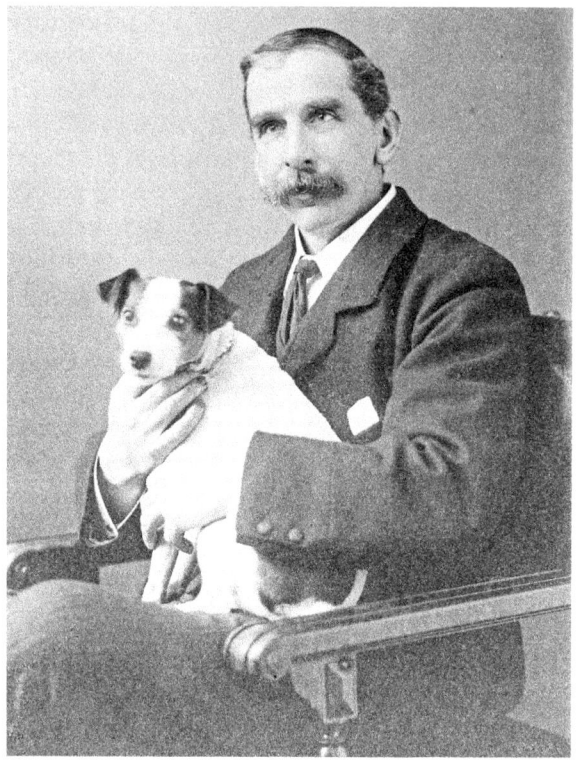

Victor Horsley, vivisector, surgeon and vocal Cobbe critic. His pioneering research performing thyroidectomies in dogs led to a new treatment, reversing the changes of cretinism and myxedema in humans. (Reproduced by permission of the Wellcome Library, London.)

Sensing how deeply her followers sympathized with her, Cobbe finally took full responsibility for the omissions in subsequent antivivisectionist meetings. To make amends, she republished *Nine Circles* in July 1893 with the appropriate corrections, including a profuse apology:

> I throw myself upon your mercy and I hope you will all consider me in the light of an old watch dog who has barked very conscientiously at the tramps for a long time, but once he has given a growl when there was no proper cause for it, and is much ashamed of it — as every good dog would be.[28]

But experimental scientists, still energized by the confrontation, were not yet quite ready to let go. In late 1892, follow-up articles appeared in *Nineteenth Century* magazine, one by Victor Horsley and another by M. Armand Ruffer, paleopathologist and director of the British Institute of Preventive Medicine. Ruffer noted that the Church Congress had been significant, in that few attendees were truly able to make judgments concerning the utility of vivisection, especially the bishops. They are in "utter ignorance" as to how experiments are carried out. When challenged, they merely deferred to "their *lady-champion*" while denouncing from the pulpit men of whose work they are totally ignorant. Should a bishop assert "that man has no right to sacrifice animals because the latter have no power of expressing their opinions, I would reply that animals, having received benefits from man, must help man in his struggle for life."[29] Ruffer contended that if any immorality exists, it occurs when animal advocates place man and animal on "the same footing." Furthermore, if vivisection is useless, then the act would be immoral. But if experimentation is of value in saving human life, then it is justifiable, so long as it is performed with as little pain as possible.[30] Ruffer claimed that vivisectors, though subjected to horrible slanders, were the ones on the side of Goodness. If medicine was ever to take its place among the important sciences, then it could only be advanced by reasoning based upon observation and experimentation.[31]

Horsley took a slightly different slant, pointing out that animals have benefited from experimentation nearly as much as have humans. Cattle used to die by the hundreds and thousands before Pasteur produced his anthrax vaccine. Even rabies victims, previously destined to die when infected, were now saved 14 out of 15 times. Animals, especially dogs, benefit as well since the scourge of rabies was less prevalent than before.[32]

Horsley lamented that a certain amount of "gratuitous injustice" was committed against physiologists by a "superior" set, who felt that they were the only people with humane feelings. They claimed a monopoly on humanity.[33] In addition to being ill-informed they were naive by not only fighting against applied science, but also by refusing to embrace abstract science. It was short-sighted and ignorant to ask, "What is the good of it? How can it be immediately made to serve my ends?"[34] Virtually all biological truths come from a careful collection of scattered facts, not by a sudden, grand revelation. Some obscure fact discovered through abstract research today may seem trivial. However, tomorrow, that same fact might constitute a vital cornerstone of some scheme of applied science. These Folkestone meetings served a great purpose: First, they gave the public a chance to better understand the questions of morality in relation to scientific experimentation. In addition, they "afforded a fresh and very prominent occasion for the renewed demonstration of the unscrupulous methods of antivivisectionism."[35]

If such confrontations at Folkestone left Cobbe dissatisfied and frustrated, her feelings only mounted further. As microbiologists made deeper incursions into their fields, they slowly gained even more credibility. Her next grievance came at the hands of Louis Pasteur. Fresh from his successes producing vaccines for chicken cholera and anthrax, Pasteur planned to confront a disease that uniformly elicited horror in the minds of mankind worldwide — rabies.

# VIII

# Salvation by Filth

"Baptism was never urged by those who believed that it could save Souls from perdition, with such relentlessness as Vaccinationists insisted upon by men whose 'cardinal doctrine ... is Salvation by Filth,' and who insist that it can save Bodies from small-pox." — Frances Power Cobbe[1]

CHAPTER 16

# La Rage

In 1889, Frances Cobbe published *The Modern Rack*, a compilation of antivivisection essays that she had written over the years. In one article, "Mad Dog!," she painted a disturbing picture of the suffering endured by rabid dogs as they passed through the terminal throes of the disease. Her source was veterinarian Edward Mayhew and his book, *The Dog and Its Management*. Dreadful as hydrophobia may be for the human being, rabies is worse for the dog. Its agony is intensified since the disease is not only slower in onset, but it lasts longer with more severe symptoms. In the early phases, the dog expresses an anxious sort of melancholy. He retreats to some area of refuge to avoid personal contact, even from those he loves and ordinarily protects. Being miserable, he usually seeks solitude in a darkened hole, as ambient light causes intense agony. Next comes excessive licking and biting, often including the dog's own paws. He develops a perversion of appetite, consuming rags, hay, excrement, stones and fragments of wood. Often, crossed eyes develop along with a reeling gait, as though maintaining balance has become a problem. Excessive production of thick, tenacious saliva ensues, associated with extreme thirst. But the animal avoids water because it has difficulty swallowing. As its tongue hangs out, a bloody slaver (saliva) drools onto the ground.

In an effort to diminish its anxiety and to avoid social contact, the dog keeps moving, often traveling 30 to 40 miles per day, giving rise to the common image of the rabid dog, head down, tail between his legs, tongue hanging out, trotting along the dusty road. It does not attack, biting only if its progress is thwarted. The animal often emits a hideous cry, beginning as a bark but changing to a howl that suddenly stops midstream.

The dog appears to hallucinate, crouching down, apparently seeing some distant threat coming nearer. Next it lunges forward, biting the air, aiming to tear the threat apart. It then stands looking bewildered, glancing about before retreating back into its hole. This ritual might be repeated 50 times in one hour.

In the final stages of rabies, the dog displays a blind rage, an indiscriminate fury, not out of malice, but as an expression of its torment. Any animate or inanimate object placed in the dog's way will suffer the effects of that rage. Finally, "the eyes ulcerate, the humours escape, and the rabid dog becomes absolutely sightless."[1] Death is a welcome visitor.

## Pasteur as Torquemada

By invoking the imagery of the rack in her publication, Cobbe hoped to equate vivisection to the Spanish Inquisition. Just as in an earlier era, Magendie and Bernard represented Torquemada, the Grand Inquisitor, Louis Pasteur had become its most current embodiment. Cobbe claimed that, prior to Pasteur, rabies had been a rare disease, occurring at a rate of one per year in England. Now, the scientist was increasing those numbers by arbitrarily deciding which animals were to be placed on the rack of vivisection by inoculating them with rabies, making them suffer the agonies of that horrible disease.

She was incensed as she contemplated Pasteur and his team working in his laboratory, violating her code of intuitive ethics:

> Such is the malady which that "Benefactor of Humanity," that "God-sent Healer," as his admirers have styled M. Louis Pasteur, has deliberately produced by injecting the virus from one to another of "innumerable" dogs! A disease which twenty years ago was so rare that only one case at a time was believed to exist in England, now torments scores of unhappy creatures with all its agonies — nay, with somewhat advanced agonies, since instead of being left to perish in their retreats, or quickly put out of misery by a merciful gun-shot, they are now kept in iron cages in the glare of light, and disturbed and prodded with heated bars as fancy may dictate to M. Pasteur's visitors.[2]

It was true that cases of rabies were quite rare. Still, a fear of contracting the disease cast a pall over the citizenry of almost all countries. In most communities stories abounded, fueled by the dramatic picture of rabies — of people suffering bites and dying agonizing deaths. A fulminating case of rabies, whether canine or human, was a terrible thing to behold as it played itself out — something never forgotten by the observer. People knew that once symptoms developed, death was a certainty. Knowing of the infected animal's fear of liquids, some villagers placed buckets of water at street corners as an early warning system. If that solitary animal walking down the street avoided drinking from it, it was suspect.[3]

As the writer and immunologist Patrice Debré suggests, for Pasteur to make rabies the focus of his next project was a strange choice. A childhood experience in Arbois might have played a role. When Pasteur was about eight, a rabid wolf wandered through the village of Arbois, biting eight people. The young Louis had vivid memories of a man suffering from multiple bites being led into a blacksmith's shop, naked from the waist up, covered with bloody slaver. There the proprietor used a red-hot cautery iron on each wound. Screams emanating from the shop left an indelible impression on the young boy. Several other victims of that same wolf died from their wounds, inciting a fear within the community that lasted for generations.

Pasteur was taking on a disease caused by an organism that he would never see. Neither he nor anyone could prove the existence of the virus until 1963, when the electron microscope finally brought its viral structure to light. He felt confident that rabies was an infectious disease since it obeyed the simple rules of contagion. There was that dramatic exposure — the bite — then a latent period of incubation, followed by the full blown malady and certain death. But one could argue that Pasteur's approach was more empirical than theoretical. He aimed to take an organism that he would never see, attenuate it in a process that he did not fully understand, and then subject animals to varying levels of virulence of that organism, in hopes of eliciting an immunological response that he did not fully comprehend. In fact, Pasteur related to Lister, in an August 1880 letter, that he would like to tell him all about the science of attenuating infectious viruses, but

> indeed I cannot do so, not from the vain desire to hide a secret, and hold back an observation which gives me an advantage over others, but from scientific caution and because I am not satisfied with the state of my knowledge. It is too incomplete and too much confused by things I do not yet understand.[4]

Still, the astute Pasteur knew what results to look for, how to evaluate and use them positively, even though he may not have understood the processes behind them. No one did.

## Experimental Models

The ideal disease for a scientist to study is one that is predictable, in which sequelae follow a predictably well-worn path. In the case of an infection, the incubation period of the disease — the time from exposure to the microorganism until symptoms are manifest — should be uniform and predictable. After exposure, the likelihood of developing the disease should be constant. The face of the disease should vary little from case to case, manifesting uniformity of signs and symptoms, in duration, severity and outcome — whether fatal or recoverable. Then, when the scientist deliberately introduces some experimental variable onto that picture, such as exposure to an attenuated organism or a different treatment method, its effects should be more readily identifiable.

Rabies possessed almost none of these characteristics. It was a poor model for study. Only one factor lay in its favor. Since rabies was almost always due to an animal bite, the point of exposure was definite. From that point onward, however, most factors were unpredictable. Often the offending animal bit and ran, nowhere to be found. Confirmation of the disease could therefore be difficult. Even after a rabid dog bit its victim, development of rabies was not a given. The possibility of developing the disease varied per the number and depth of the bites. Quantifying an average risk was virtually impossible. Even Pasteur estimated the overall risk of death at only 16 percent, if a rabid animal bit an individual.[5] The greatest danger for developing rabies came from wolf and cat bites, followed by the bite of a dog. Once an animal bit a victim, the incubation period varied from one to two months. That bitten individual remained in a heightened state of anxiety, not knowing whether he was destined to live or die an excruciating death.[6] Before treatment was available, the desperate victim often fell prey to charlatans offering a multitude of useless treatments.

With bites to the face, the likelihood of developing rabies was 50 to 80 percent — on the hand or arm, 15 to 40 percent. For someone bitten on the leg, chances of developing the disease varied from 3 to 10 percent.[7] Facial bites were also associated with shorter incubation times. As a rule, the further the distance from bite to brainstem, the longer the incubation period, and the decreasing likelihood of developing the disease. Finally, rabies was rare. Only 200–300 people in France died of rabies each year.[8] In England, a country protected by ocean waters, only 43, on average, died annually in the decade 1875 to 1885.[9]

Why didn't Pasteur choose to attack syphilis or tuberculosis instead of rabies? While not as dramatic or fearsome as rabies, they were far more vexing, given their ubiquity, intractability and their impact on society. If he were seeking fame on the level of a Newton or Copernicus, as he sometimes admitted, finding a cure for either of these scourges would have worked mightily in his favor. With Pasteur's affinity for public display and his great sense of drama, as Émile Roux suggested, Pasteur probably saw rabies as that great opportunity. Solving the insoluble would firmly establish immunity as a science:

> If Pasteur chose it as an object of study, it was above all because the rabies virus had always been regarded as the most subtle and mysterious of all, and also because to everyone's mind rabies is the most frightening and dreaded malady.... He thought that to solve the problem of rabies would be a blessing for humanity and a brilliant triumph for his doctrines.[10]

In 1884, Pasteur spoke at the International Medical Congress in Copenhagen. There he offered a slightly different perspective than Roux for making rabies his choice for study. By that time he had been successful in producing vaccines for both chicken cholera and anthrax and was well on his way with rabies. He had a strong desire to extend immune therapy to humans, but he faced one immense obstacle: "experimentation, while allowable on animals, is criminal on man."[11] One must therefore possess a profound knowledge of animal diseases, especially those suffered in common with man such as rabies. If one solved all of the problems related to conferring immunity to animals, he could then apply the identical technique to humans.

## From Centripetal to Centrifugal

In January 1881, physician Henri Duboue, a student of rabies, hearing of Pasteur's interest in the disease, informed him that the crux of the malady appeared to be centered mainly within the nervous system. He wrote to Pasteur that "the morbid agent progresses slowly, in a centripetal direction, from the location of the bite to the *medulla oblongata*, and very rapidly, in a centrifugal direction, from the latter organ to the nerves that originate from it."[12]

Duboue's information has withstood the test of time. As a neurotropic virus, rabies has an affinity for nervous tissue. Its main manifestations are due to encephalitis, a viral inflammation of the nervous system. With the bite, virus is deposited in muscle and fat, where it sits until it invades a neighboring peripheral nerve, beginning the first of the two phases Duboue mentioned. Once the virus begins its centripetal ascent up the peripheral nerve, it invades the neurons of the spinal cord, where it stops to multiply. From there it travels rapidly up the spinal cord to the brainstem (bulb) and the brain proper, where it wreaks its devastating effects. Fevers to 104°F are common. The disease then begins phase two — the centrifugal movement of the virus peripherally into sensory nerves, skin, salivary and lachrymal glands.

In France, rabies is called "*La Rage*" for the fury it typically produces in dogs. In humans, fear is the predominant symptom. The frightening aspects of rabies occur as a result of a bulbar palsy — an infection of the brainstem. Although the picture in humans varies from case to case, the nerves controlling swallowing, speaking, tongue movements, salivation, and facial and eye mechanisms are all affected. Cycles of involuntary crises occur, lasting several minutes, accompanied by great anxiety. Irregular breathing, spasms of the diaphragm and arrhythmias of the heart are common. Like canines, some humans developed a biting behavior, making nursing care hazardous. The rabid crises are most frequently hydrophobic, where the sight or even the suggestion of water can set off severe spasms of the neck muscles, and vocal cords. An increase in salivation, with choking and drooling occur, with a worsening of anxiety, and a feeling of imminent death.

Inflammation of the sensory nerves in the neck frequently occurs, producing a different kind of crisis—aerophobia. In this condition, the nerves and skin are so hyper-sensitive that a gentle breeze or even the breath of an examiner standing too close can set off spells identical to those of hydrophobia. As the brainstem becomes more severely inflamed, the patient mercifully lapses into coma, leaving his family to suffer at the bedside. Death usually ensues between one and two weeks after symptom onset.[13]

## Early Efforts

Pasteur began his work on rabies in December 1880. His early efforts were made somewhat easier by the work of a predecessor in the field. In 1879, Pierre-Victor Galtier, a professor at the Lyon Veterinary School, reported on his successful transmission of rabies from dogs to rabbits. He discovered that if one used serial passages, the incubation time could be diminished from over one month to several weeks. Through his work Galtier established the rabbit as the animal of choice for those studying rabies.[14] Pasteur directed his early efforts towards growing and identifying the organism in artificial media. With rabies being a sub-microscopic virus, of course, he always met with failure. Early in the project he learned that the rabies organism would not grow in the usual in vitro culture media. The living animal itself would have to serve as the repository, necessitating an ongoing presence of rabid laboratory animals at all times.[15] Pasteur worked with various animals such as dogs, rabbits, guinea pigs and monkeys, carrying out serial cultures within a species and from one species to another. In his preliminary efforts he also discovered that he could increase or decrease rabies' virulence depending on the species. Serial passages from rabbit to rabbit increased the virulence when transmitted to dogs, just as serial passages in monkeys decreased its virulence.[16] The always-secretive Pasteur kept silent about efforts expended during these first three years.

The task of conquering rabies placed new demands upon him—different from those he confronted earlier. Anthrax, for instance, infected masses of animals in a wholesale manner. It infected subtly, without warning—with a short period of incubation. Rabies was just the opposite—the dramatic exposure of a bite, then a prolonged and variable incubation time. Rabies was a retail disease, affecting one or a few at a time, while anthrax was wholesale, killing hundreds simultaneously. Anthrax required establishment of pre-exposure immunity, that is, treatment of large numbers of animals before exposure to the disease in that particular community. Rabies treatment, to be effective, was just the opposite — treat one or a few beings only after exposure — to gain post-exposure immunity. Pasteur would need to establish immunity during that critical incubation window of one to two months. This new requirement demanded a refined control of the attenuation process and confidence in the level of virulence of the virus.

Although a paralytic form of animal rabies could be transmitted with an intravenous injection, it would take Émile Roux to come up with a solution for producing a consistently reliable experimental model. Pasteur was repulsed at any thought of open operations on animals. On a day when he was out of the lab, Roux anesthetized a dog, placed a bur hole in his skull and inoculated its brain with rabies virus that had been first cultured in a rabbit. The next day, when Pasteur heard of the operation, he stated. "Poor beast. Its brain is certainly badly wounded. It must be paralyzed."[17] When Roux fetched the animal from the basement, Pasteur was surprised to see the dog running about the lab, sniffing, tail wagging as though nothing had happened. Two weeks later, the animal began displaying signs of rabies. Multiple repetitions of this technique established the practicality of Roux's inspiration. The team now had its experimental model, with consistent incubation times of two weeks, relatively uniform presentations of disease and time to death. Pasteur was most interested in the uniform incubation time since that would serve as his common criterion upon how virulence and attenuation could be judged: The greater the virulence, the shorter was the incubation time. The converse was true as well. In May 1881, Pasteur reported these preliminary results to both of the Academies of Science and Medicine.

These inoculated dogs would serve not only as a repository of live virus for further inoculations but the virus extracted from them would also be used for experimentation with virulence and attenuation — the next major step. Employing animal bodies as their culture medium in place of Petri dishes was a first, something that would greatly increase the number of animals infected and sacrificed.[18] Pasteur sought to employ a highly virulent virus, reasoning that it would elicit the highest immune response in its new host — ultimately humans. As he gained more experience with this method, he noted an interesting phenomenon. When he inoculated each succeeding generation of animal with the virus of the preceding generation, that viral strain became increasingly virulent, occasioning a decrease in incubation time. The usual two-week incubation period produced with a first-generation rabbit could be reduced to eight days by using strains from the 21st-generation rabbit — a near-doubling of virulence. Pasteur confirmed this by inoculating dogs with the more virulent virus, not only producing disease earlier, but also creating a more severe form of the disease.[19]

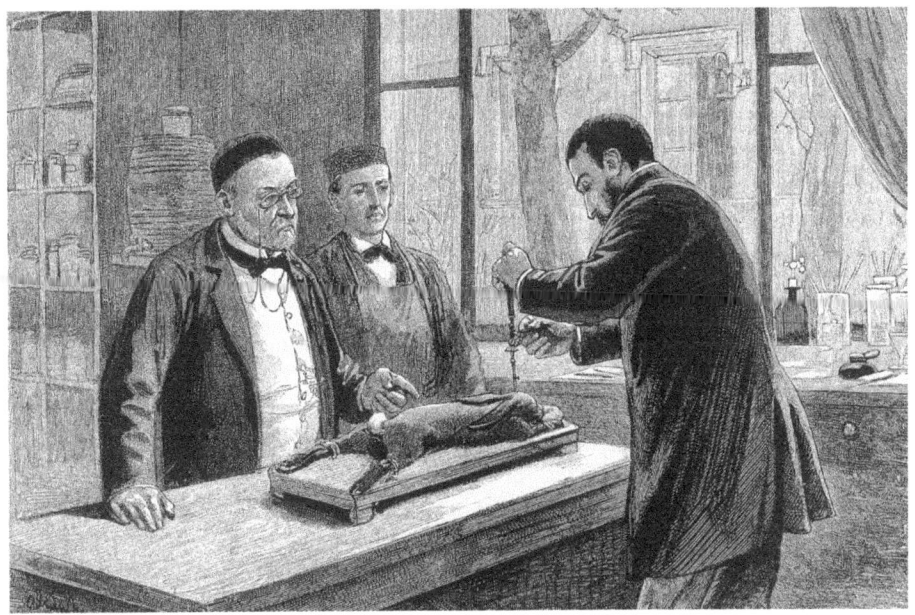

Injection of rabies virus into a rabbit's brain in 1885. Pasteur stands to the left, while an assistant, presumably Roux, performs the trephination. The person in the middle is likely Adrien Loir, Pasteur's nephew and immediate assistant. (Reproduced by permission of the Wellcome Library, London.)

His next goal: To attenuate the virulence of the inoculum at will. Pasteur maintained a supply of infected animals at all times. They were, in effect, his living culture plates. Pasteur used many different species, varying from the rabbit, dog, pigs, monkeys and guinea pigs. He noted one consistent finding. When he transmitted the virus from dog to monkey, the virus consistently became less virulent, manifest by a prolonged incubation time and a less severe form of rabies. In fact, if he administered that virus to dogs previously inoculated with weakened virus, they did not contract the disease — his first refractory subjects. Although this was an accomplishment, Pasteur did not think that this strain of virus would be sufficiently strong for the treatment of humans. In other words, he wanted a more virulent strain so that he might achieve a higher level of immunity.

Pasteur realized that, in essence, he was running a race between conferring immunity and breakout of disease. He must establish immunity more rapidly than the virus could travel from the wound to the brainstem; otherwise it would be too late. He had a window of opportunity, corresponding to the incubation time, of only one to two months. Ideally, the virus used in the vaccine must be what he termed a "weak strong one."[20] The virus had be the most virulent one possible to elicit a rapid immune response, and then, through attenuation, be weakened just to the point of innocuousness for administration to the patient.

## Double-Necked Flask

Pasteur next appropriated a technique from Roux — without his permission and with no later attribution to him — that proved critical to the next stage of development. It was Adrian Loir, Pasteur's nephew, who related how Pasteur purloined Roux's technique. Since Pasteur was partially paralyzed on his left side, Loir performed many of his manual tasks such as his bacterial culturing. Pasteur stood immediately behind Loir — monitoring his moves. On one occasion the two moved into the incubation room for Loir to carry out some task. Pasteur noted several flasks on another shelf, each with two necks (outlets) that allowed for a cross draft of air inside the flask. Suspended inside by a string was a segment of spinal cord. Immediately transfixed, Pasteur picked up one, held it to the light, studying it in detail. He then inquired of Loir as to who might have placed these flasks there. Loir replied that it could only have been Roux. Pasteur left the room, not uttering another word.

Later that afternoon Loir was in the incubation room when Roux happened upon the scene. Seeing the flasks in a different position, he asked Loir who had placed them there. When Loir informed him that it was Pasteur, Roux wanted to know if Pasteur had definitely seen the flasks drying on the shelf. Loir replied that Pasteur had indeed seen them. Without saying a word, Roux turned and walked out, slamming the door behind him, his signature expression of anger, signaling the onset of a great schism between the two. From that point on, Roux and Pasteur worked in parallel lives, virtually never communicating over rabies again. Roux usually worked at night, avoiding any chance of contact with Pasteur.[21]

Pasteur arranged the construction of double-necked flasks, larger than Roux's, in which he suspended spinal cords. Before plugging both ends with sterile cotton, he placed a dessicant, caustic potash in the flask, creating a sterile, dry environment. The spinal cords were, in effect, mummified with time in the warm, dry air. Aging and drying the virus diminished its virulence. Pasteur realized that he now had some control over the process. He not only had his "weak strong one" but, like turning a rheostat, he could control its degree of virulence at will.[22]

Now he could set up his scheme for creating the vaccine. First, he suspended in the flask a spinal cord a day, each taken from a rabbit that died from rabies on day seven after inoculation. Day seven was important — it

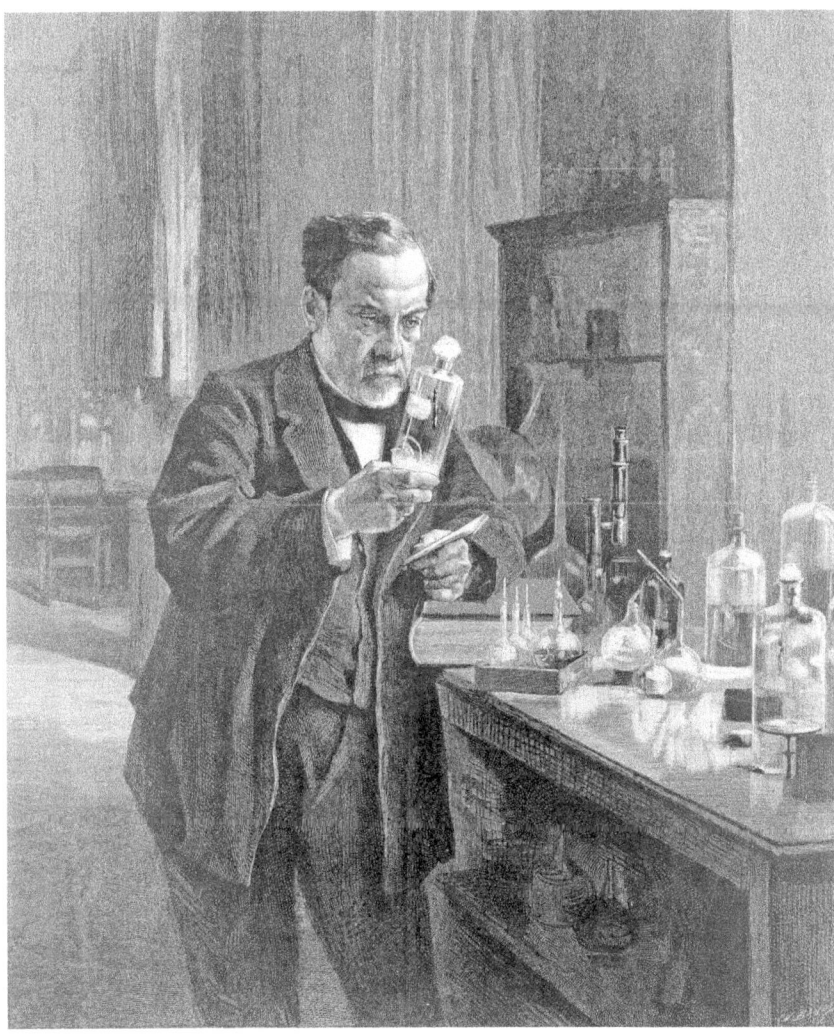

An 1885 engraving by A.G.A. Edelfeldt of Pasteur holding the double-necked flask. The flask, designed by Roux but purloined by Pasteur, provided a warm and dry atmosphere for the attenuation of rabies virus within the rabbit spinal cord. Note the dark strip of spinal cord tissue hanging from the flask's central hook. (Reproduced by permission of the Wellcome Library, London.)

ensured a starting point of uniform virulence for each inoculum. To produce a dog immune to rabies, he began inoculating an animal each day with a suspension of spinal cord in sterile diluent, starting with the oldest (14 days), least virulent, and progressing to the newest and most virulent specimen (1–2 days). In that manner he reached an equilibrium in his production line in which one injection occurred while another specimen of drying spinal cord matured. By day 14, the dog was immune to the highly virulent, one-day-old inoculum. At completion of the series, to prove the dog's immunity, Pasteur inoculated an extract from the rabbit both under the skin and into the brain of an immunized, refractory dog as well as a fresh and healthy dog. As expected, the refractory dog remained healthy, while the non-immune one became rabid.

One can only imagine the number of animals needed to be housed, inoculated, observed and sacrificed in pursuit of this rabies vaccine. Just having a sufficient number of infected animals to serve as a reservoir for coordinating the processes of sacrificing and drying of spinal cords would account for hundreds. Another phenomenon added further to the number of lab animals residing at rue d'Ulm. As word of Pasteur's interest in rabies spread, every veterinarian in Paris knew where to deliver their rabid charges. Soon Pasteur's laboratory was overflowing with all sorts of animals, including 60 dogs — both rabid and refractory. Finally, he moved his entire rabies enterprise to an old chateau with sizeable grounds, Villeneuve-l'Etang, just outside of Paris. Here space was sufficient for his menagerie. Pasteur later moved his household to the grounds there as well.[23]

Even after the team had become experienced and efficient, dealing with enraged, rabid dogs while collecting specimens for culture was an ordeal. Pasteur's son-in-law, René Vallery-Radot, recalled a visit to a veterinarian's premises to inoculate six rabbits using two rabid dogs. To test one bulldog's tendency to bite, a worker poked a metal bar into his cage. Enraged and foaming at the mouth, the dog bit onto a metal bar dripping bloody slaver from his mouth. Strangely when a rabbit's ear was offered through the bars, the dog sat back, indifferent to the rabbit. But Pasteur was determined to infect the rabbits. Therefore:

> Two helpers took a cord with a slip-knot and threw it at the dog as one throws a lasso. The dog was caught and pulled to the edge of the cage. They seized it and tied its jaws together. The dog, choking with rage, its eyes blood-shot, and its body racked with furious spasms, was stretched out on a table, while M. Pasteur, bending a finger's length away over this foaming head, aspirated a few drops of slaver through a thin tube.[24]

Inoculations into the dogs' brains were equally tedious. First the workers killed a rabid dog and then removed the back of his skull, exposing the medulla. Then, with all surfaces sterilized, they aspirated a small portion of the medulla and suspended it in a Pravaz syringe. They next anesthetized the experimental animals to be inoculated. One held the animal down to prevent sudden movements, while the other placed a burr hole in its skull. Now, before closing the wound, one of them, usually Roux, plunged the tip of the syringe into brain tissue for the inoculation. The men wore no gloves but washed their hands after each manipulation. They were not only dealing with infected nervous tissue but also with enraged dogs, always attempting to bite something. One slip of a scalpel or bite of a dog and the man was facing all of the anxieties of impending rabies. Early in their experience, they kept a loaded revolver nearby. If a terrible accident were to happen to one of them, "the more courageous of the ... others would put a bullet in his head."[25] Luckily, no major calamities occurred.

Articles relating to vaccine production at Rue d'Ulm appeared in many magazines, including the *Fortnightly Review, La Paix, L'Illustration, Figaro, The Daily Graphic* and *The Manchester Guardian*. The curiosity of journalists, as well as antivivisectionists, was piqued concerning Pasteur's laboratory and how his animals were treated. If one were to put such a question to Pasteur or his assistants, they received a standard reply. The animals only suffered the pain of a pinprick.

But such assertions about the benignity of injections were not lost on Cobbe. In a *Zoophilist* article, "No More Than a Prick of a Needle," she pointed out the disingenuousness of such remarks. Some equated the needle stick to the pain of a woman having her ears pierced. It was true that injecting something such as the tubercle bacillus was not especially painful, but "what suffering followed."[26] In order to have an abundant supply of vaccine, animals were being injected continuously, sometimes by the hundreds. Observing

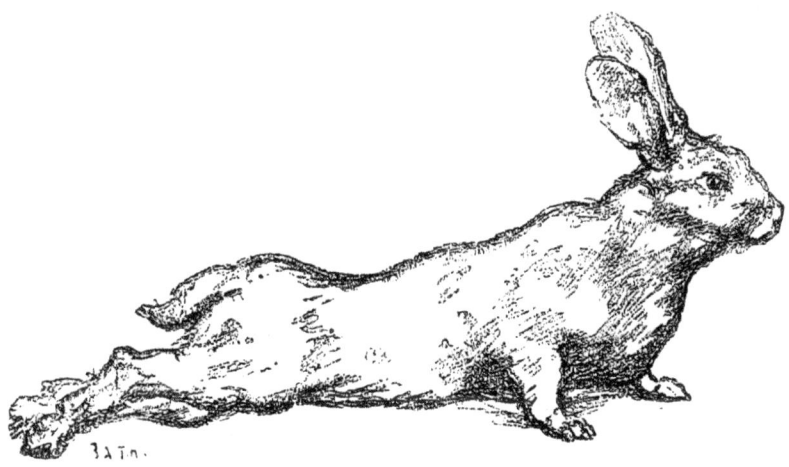

Paralyzed rabbit. Rabbits, rendered paraplegic as infection spread to their spinal cords, propelled themselves forward by using their front legs (from Frances Power Cobbe, *An Institute of Preventive Medicine at Work in France* [London: Victoria Street Society, 1891]).

their fate after the onset of laboratory rabies gave a much truer picture of the misery they endured. One journalist, Charles Mayet, touring the facilities, was aghast at what he saw. Rabid rabbits did not bite like dogs but their suffering was just as intense. Mayet saw them by the score, completely paralyzed in their hind quarters, dragging their bodies forward with great difficulty. Terminally, their eyes became glazed, their breathing labored, until death mercifully ensued. Guinea pigs developed the furious form of the disease, biting at anything placed in their way, enraged and in agony as their end approached.

But the plight of the dogs was most poignant. Pasteur showed Mayet one caged dog with advanced rabies, standing spread-legged, looking imbalanced and bewildered, with tail drooping and mouth foaming. He announced to Mayet that this dog "will die tomorrow." As Pasteur kicked the cage, the enraged animal charged, mouth bleeding, biting the bars of the cage. He then retreated to the rear of the cage, eating some straw while letting out a "piercing and plaintive" cry.

But Pasteur defended his actions in the laboratory to one journalist:

> You ask me, besides my opinion on vivisection. Such a subject ought not be discussed. I condemn barbarity in vivisection as strongly as the most tender-hearted woman. But who is the scientific man, worthy of the name, who can be accused of practicing such barbarity? As to compassionating the death of a few rabbits when the end is to save a life of a man, and as to being sentimental over the sacrifice of a few sheep and oxen to save sheep and oxen by hundreds of thousands — they are only fools who would reason in this manner.[27]

On the practical side, as charged by some reporters, Pasteur "and his clique" found it more expedient to keep these production animals, "as much as possible out of the public gaze."[28]

Around 1887, Cobbe included all of this imagery of cruelty and suffering in her essay, "An Institute of Preventive Medicine at Work in France," her early warning to the people of England. They needed to know that such an institute was being planned in France. If the people of England hoped to avoid such a facility in their country, they should "raise such a storm of righteous indignation, in and out of Parliament, as shall sweep the atmosphere of England clear of such schemes for all future generations."[29]

## Next Therapeutic Step?

By March 1885, Pasteur had completed his immunization plan. He was now confident enough to consider what his next logical step might be. For months he harbored great anxiety about treating that first human subject. Handling animals was one thing, but treating humans represented a major

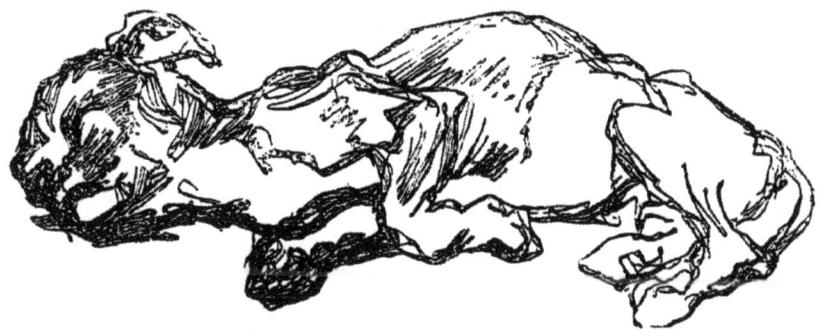

"At Rest at Last." Artist's rendering of the dog's death, a final and welcome state, after the inexorable deterioration from rabies inoculation (from Frances Power Cobbe, *An Institute of Preventive Medicine at Work in France* [London: Victoria Street Society, 1891]).

and terrifying leap. As a chemist, he would have to recruit a licensed physician willing to carry out the immunizations under Pasteur's treatment scheme. Despite his trepidations, he was very close to taking that giant step. He claimed to have produced 50 dogs refractory to rabies "without having encountered a single failure."[30] However, he never backed up his claim with any proof. Still, we know from his memoirs what his thoughts were. He believed that "proofs must be multiplied *ad infinitum* on diverse animal species before human therapeutics should dare to try this mode of prophylaxis on man himself."[31]

However, on 6 July 1885, fate led him in another direction. Pasteur did not have the luxury of a protective circle of personnel surrounding him. Patients could approach him directly with their heartrending stories. Denying treatment under those circumstances was much more difficult than merely refusing to care for a patient through some intermediary. It was in such a setting that nine-year-old Joseph Meister and his mother from Alsace appeared at Pasteur's door, hoping to receive this new treatment. Joseph had recently been bitten by a dog, severely on the middle finger of the right hand, as well as on his thighs and legs — a total of 14 bites. At the dog's autopsy, examiners discovered hay and large chips of wood in his stomach — presumptive evidence of rabies. Apparently Pasteur had no access to the dog's brainstem or even his slaver, so that rabbits might be inoculated for confirmatory tests.

Contemplating his options, Pasteur decided "not without vivid and profound anxiety," that Meister represented a good case for treatment.[32] The boy's bites were deep and fresh. Violating his own plans about further experimentation, Pasteur appealed to Roux, a physician, to carry out the injections.

The conservative Roux adamantly refused to have any part of it. At the French Academy of Medicine meeting the same day, Pasteur posed his dilemma to physiologist Alfred Vulpian and pediatrician Joseph Grancher, both very familiar with his work. After examining Joseph, both physicians felt that the number and severity of the bites made the likelihood of the boy developing a fatal case of rabies sufficient enough to warrant this untested method of treatment.

Therefore, at 8 P.M. on the same day, 60 hours after young Joseph sustained his bites, Dr. Grancher administered his first injection into Joseph's right upper abdomen. The inoculum, harvested from a dead rabbit on 21 June, consisted of half a syringe full of suspended spinal marrow, dried for 15 days in the double-neck flask. Over the next 10 days, Joseph received 13 injections of the spinal marrow, each of decreasing age and increasing virulence. His last injection on 16 July was a highly virulent specimen only one day old.[33] Pasteur trembled at the mere thought of giving this nearly fully active, potentially lethal virus to a human being. In a letter to her children, Marie Pasteur wrote, "This will be another bad night for your father. He cannot come to terms with the idea of applying a measure of last resort to this child. And yet he now has to go through with it. The little fellow continues to feel very well."[34] Joseph tolerated the injections uneventfully, returning home in late July. Pasteur's success was all the sweeter, having successfully applied his pioneering method to a patient from Alsace, Koch's own backyard. Then, Pasteur added to the Meister triumph by successfully treating a second patient, 15-year-old Jean-Baptiste Jupille, in the early fall. In no more than a few months Pasteur had successfully bridged that terrifying chasm separating the treatment of laboratory animals and humans — a gratifying beginning.

CHAPTER 17

# "Whither is Pasteurism to lead us?"

On 26 October 1885 Pasteur presented his work to the Academy of Science, announcing that his new method of prophylaxis was so practical and rapid that it "has already proved successful in the dog so constantly in so many cases that I feel confident of its general applicability to all animals and to man himself."[1] He then proceeded to describe the treatment of both Meister and Jupille. By the end of his presentation, academy members recognized his announcement for what it was — an occasion as momentous as Koch's elucidation of the tubercle bacillus. One member, Henri Bouley, rose to state that this date, 26 October 1885, would be "forever memorable in the history of medicine and forever glorious for French science."[2] Word spread like an explosion worldwide. Pasteur became inundated with requests for treatment from all over the world. He successfully treated four children from Newark, New Jersey, sent to Paris under the sponsorship of the *New York Herald Tribune*. Their story made headlines in many U.S. papers for two weeks, giving further exposure for the Pasteurian method. Then 19 Russians arrived in Paris, having been bitten by a rabid wolf. Two were said to have half of their faces bitten off. Three died, but 16 returned safely to Russia.

Responding to the global need, Pasteur and his team set up treatment centers in London, St. Petersburg, Vienna, Jena and Warsaw. By August 1886, over 1200 patients from France and Algeria alone had been treated, with only three failures.[3]

## Pasteur's Detractors

People the world over were euphoric at the prospect of being rid of rabies — that is, except for antivivisectionists and anti-vaccinationists, those either repulsed by the method of vaccine production or ideologically set against the treatment method. The anti-vaccinationists began targeting Pasteur, in the early 1880s, especially after Claude Bernard's death in 1878. Bernard had earlier countered the antivivisectionists' criticisms of vivisection by stating, "When it comes to that [scientific discovery], one can only cite all the accomplishments of experimental physiology; there is not a single fact that was not the direct and necessary result of a vivisection."[4] In 1881, Darwin had come to Pasteur's aid against the antivivisectionists by stating, "Physiology can make no progress if we do away with animal experiments, and I am deeply convinced that to hold back advances in physiology is to commit a crime against humanity."[5] In 1883, when the government planned to double Pasteur's annual salary to 25,000 francs, pressure against him heightened even further. His biographer, Debré, relates that "an antivivisectionist league" launched a smear campaign against him, labeling vivisection and vaccination equally detestable. In a letter to a French minister, the league president lamented, "Science does not recognize in the great discoveries of M. Pasteur anything but a tissue of dogmatic conceptions and unsuccessful attempts more apt to ruin than to enrich the country that would adopt them."[6] In 1884, just one year before the treatment of young Meister, Prof. Virchow contemptuously answered such protesters in his speech at the International Congress of Medicine in Copenhagen:

> Those who attack vivisection have not the faintest idea of what science is, and even less of the importance and the usefulness of vivisection for the progress of medicine.... No one who is more interested in animals than in science and the knowledge of truth is qualified to exert an official control over scientific matters.[7]

But those words resonated more in the minds of individuals favoring animal experimentation than those against it. To that certain segment of the population, Pasteur's laboratory remained the torture chamber of science. In demonstrations antivivisectionists demanded free access to his laboratory so that they might monitor his activities there. Personal attacks against him took the form of insults, protests and even threats against his life.[8] Some wanted to do to him what he had done to those animals.

Cobbe continued with her attack. In the 1 December 1885 issue of *Zoophilist*, just five months after young Meister's treatment, she argued that his rabies treatment plan defied logic. She posed a great question: If the treatment scheme requires treating rabies before it developed, then how could one know whether the patient would have developed the disease or not? Not only antivivisectionists, but anti-vaccinationists and anti-contagionists had deeper reservations about whether the disease should even be treated. After all, rabies was the consequence of a person being cruel to dogs. Suffering the disease was divine retribution for that sin.[9] Even Cobbe's own trusted medical experts with more orthodox training were of divided opinion on the disease and its treatment. Lawson Tait confessed to holding no opinion of the treatment. But Hoggan was different. Cobbe wrote to a friend that "Dr. Hoggan, less cautious by far!—thinks I am sorry to say that Pasteur is on the right track."[10]

Cobbe had been concerned for several years about the wisdom of protecting against a disease by infecting a patient with an artificial form of that same disease. In an 1882 essay, "The Janus of Science," she attacked Pasteur, inquiring, "Whither is Pasteurism to lead us?" If the public came to accept vaccination, would it be necessary to be vaccinated for every known disease?

> Is it really to be that the order of things has been so perversely constituted as that the health of men and beasts is to be sought, *not* as we fondly believed by pure and sober living and cleanliness, but by pollution of the very fountains of life with the confluent streams of a dozen filthy diseases?... Are we then, our oxen, our sheep, our pigs, our fowls (that is to say, our own bodies and the food which nourishes them), all to be vaccinated, porcinated, equinated, caninized, felinised, and bovinated, once, twice, twenty times in our lives, or in a year? Are we to be converted into so many living nests for the comfortable incubation of disease germs? Is our meat to be saturated with "virus," our milk drawn from inoculated cows, our eggs laid by diseased hens—in short, are we to breakfast, dine and sup upon disease by way of securing the perfection of health?[11]

Cobbe was expressing an anxiety that ran deeper than a mere resistance to the treatment of a single disease. She was questioning the entire concept of infectious diseases and vaccination. The origins of her argument dated back to 1857, when Louis Pasteur proclaimed before the French Academy of Science that specific microorganisms cause specific diseases.[12] Whether she ever fully subscribed, or not, to the notion that minute organisms, invisible to the naked eye, could have such a major impact on one's health is unclear. However, in the 1860s, Cobbe had believed generally in science. In fact, she had praised Edward Jenner for his work with smallpox vaccination in the late 18th century when he convinced parents to rely on vaccination and not just prayer alone to protect their children from the disease.[13]

## Sanitation and Salvation

It was sometime after 1860 that Cobbe became convinced, along with sanitarians and anti-vaccinationists, that disease could be prevented by simple sanitation and salvation—an inner and an outer cleansing—an environmental hygiene and a spiritual sanitation.[14] If one led a virtuous life with clean garments, bodies and minds, contagious diseases would become isolated, unable to self-propagate. Therefore, one need not invoke bacteria to explain disease causation. Nor would any need exist for animal experimentation.[15]

It was the confluence of several forces in the early 1870s that proved pivotal in molding Cobbe's views. First, the discipline of physiology, of which she was so contemptuous, was gaining strength in England as young experimental scientists, trained on the Continent, began returning to their native Britain. This caused her great angst. Second, the animal protection legislation of 1876, so bitterly disappointing to Cobbe, further hardened her views against science. Finally, in 1871, after 20 years of lax vaccination laws, Parliament strengthened England's vaccination statutes, not only forcing immunization on the public, but requiring physicians to report non-compliant patients. Governmental intrusion to this level evoked a strong reaction, not only in Cobbe but also in a large segment of the population. As a result, the anti-vaccination movement became a viable force when several fragmented groups coalesced into one, in 1879. By the 1880s, Cobbe, with her anti-science views solidified, had developed a natural affinity with anti-vaccinationists.

Cobbe now openly supported parents who resisted the government's policy of forced immunization on all English children.[16] To her, providing protection against disease by injecting filth into a person took away the individual's responsibility to live a clean and virtuous life. And then there was the matter of using animals to develop the necessary vaccines. As Cobbe wrote in a Liverpool newspaper, "it would be better for mankind to suffer from epidemics, small and great, for ages to come rather than learn to approve of such sinful cruelty to the brutes, such fatal petrifying of human hearts and consciences.[17] Illustrating her further drift from the mainstream:

> Our bodies are destined to perish sooner or later, and the relief or help which science at its best can ever afford them is a very small matter. There is a greater interest even than the sanitary interest of which we make so much these days — it is the interest of the hearts and souls of men. It is of more importance that tender and just and compassionate feelings should grow and abound than that a cure should be found for corporeal disease.[18]

Cobbe remained as strongly anti-vaccinationist as she was anti-science until her dying day.

On another point, however, Cobbe enjoyed a good deal of unexpected help and it came from the orthodox side of medicine. Even though Pasteur probably acted with the most humane of motives when faced with young Joseph Meister, he paid dearly, in terms of mental stress, for the abrupt manner in which he began treating humans with the vaccine. As Roux had suggested, Pasteur should have performed more animal trials and then extended the treatment to humans only if they were successful. Through the impending confrontation with his adversaries, Pasteur could only count on colleagues Vulpian and Grancher as his defenders. As caregivers, they were nearly as culpable as he, should some patient bring suit.

Whispering campaigns and outright confrontations began in earnest. Hospital staffs, medical students and faculty divided themselves into Pasteurian and anti–Pasteurian camps. As usual, Pasteur's most vociferous critic was that shirt-tailed relative, Michael Peter, who claimed that Pasteur inflated the number of rabies cases and kept inaccurate statistics to further his own cause. In tabulating his results, Pasteur did have a dilemma. If his treated patient survived, his adversaries could always charge that the patient never had the disease in the first place. If the patient died — either the vaccine was ineffective or, worse yet, the patient had contracted the disease from the treatment method itself. Peter, in particular, leveled the charge that Pasteur's treatment gave "laboratory rabies" to some patients, a troubling charge that was difficult to fully neutralize. It was true that a minority of bite victims, when inoculated, did go through a phase of leg weakness much like the laboratory rabbits had — something unusual with the typical human form of hydrophobia. Peter and other critics of Pasteur gained some credibility with this charge. As the treatment numbers soared, naturally failures mounted as well. From 1885 through the early 1890s, anti–Pasteurian articles, especially relating to rabies treatment, dominated each issue of the *Zoophilist*. One recurring feature was a monthly record of Pasteur's treatment failures, a section the editors named "Pasteur's Double Hecatombs." The column, updated monthly, listed items such as patient's name, age, gender, animal involved, dates of bite, treatment and death, cause of death and so on — a running tally of Pasteur's negatives.

## The Rouyer Affair

Pasteur's assistants had to contend with one particularly vexing problem on their own involving Jules Rouyer, a young boy bitten by a dog on 8 October 1886. He was presented to Pasteur 12 days later. After undergoing the full treatment without incident, Rouyer returned home, presumably cured. As he resumed his usual activities, he sustained an injury to his spine resulting in disabling low back pain. On 26 November, the boy suddenly died shortly after being hospitalized. His unbelieving and grief-stricken father, certain that Pasteur's method was the cause of his son's death, lodged a formal complaint with local authorities. At the time, an exhausted Pasteur had retreated to an Italian villa, attempting to recover from the toxic Parisian atmosphere swirling around him and his treatment regimen. Forensic examiner Dr. Brouardel was assigned to perform the Rouyer boy's autopsy. Loir, Grancher, and some Rouyer supporters, including physician and political radical Georges Clemenceau — a natural enemy to the conservative Pasteur — attended the examination. Clemenceau, like Peter, was just waiting for Pasteur to commit some serious blunder. Neither had forgiven him for his triumph over the theory of spontaneous generation. Since the very future of Pasteur's vaccine program rested on what might be found in the brain of Rouyer, Loir had insisted on procuring the boy's brainstem (medulla) for testing. Brouardel's exam revealed enlarged kidneys and opaque urine, due to its high albumin content, possibly related to his back pain. As Brouardel began removing the skull, the room was otherwise silent — everybody waiting to see what the brain might reveal. Despite the high tension, Brouardel merely removed the entire brain and handed it to Loir, making no statement as to its condition. Loir immediately left the premises to deliver his unusual package to the laboratory at Rue d'Ulm. When Roux received the specimen from Loir, he insisted on doing his work alone. He would tolerate no witnesses in the room — not even Loir. After making a dilute paste from some of the medullary tissue, Roux inoculated his concoction into two trepanned rabbits, and the wait began.

Two weeks later, a distressed Loir awakened the sleeping Roux to some bad news. Both rabbits were paralyzed in their hind legs. Incredulous, Roux ran to the lab, only to confirm Loir's assertions. Obviously the Rouyer boy had died from rabies. Roux, the one who wanted no part of Pasteur's treatment scheme in the first place, remained quiet as he pondered the situation. Several days later Brouardel, who trusted Roux, given his well known resistance to Pasteur's regimen, had a conversation with him. Brouardel, whose testimony was vital to the case, was concerned about what sort of consequences his declaration of death might have on Pasteur's entire program. If Pasteur were incriminated, his enemies, including Peter and Clemenceau, would crush him and bring the entire program down with him.

On 4 January 1887, both Brouardel and Roux appeared before the members of the Academy of Medicine, acting much like a tribunal. All present wanted to ensure that a just verdict on the cause of death was rendered. Roux reviewed the events of the past several weeks, including his inoculation of two rabbits with Rouyer's medulla. More than 40 days later, Roux declared before the Academy, the two rabbits remain healthy. Brouardel's verdict? The boy had died from kidney failure, thereby absolving Pasteur of any wrongdoing. The public prosecutor exonerated Pasteur fully.

Peter rose to object. He did not believe any of the testimony he had heard; the boy's clinical picture pointed to a death from rabies. But how could anyone argue? If Rouyer's brain matter had not transmitted the disease, how could rabies be the cause of death?[19] Pasteur, informed of the controversy at sometime while recovering at the villa, remained nonchalant, supremely confident in his method.[20] Whether he knew of Roux's deception or not is unclear.

Antivivisectionists Peter and Clemenceau and other enemies of the savant had to rely on Pasteur's rare treatment failures for their polemical firepower. They could not argue with him on equal terms, scientifically. As a result, Pasteur's team became very vigilant. They thoroughly investigated all failures of treatment and every criticism, no matter how trivial, in an effort to preempt any serious allegation from developing into something more. Pasteur, exhausted by the unending contention, suffered two strokes in late 1887, leaving him with permanently labored speech. Vulpian and Grancher carried on with the argumentation in the halls and in the academies. With time, they successfully painted Peter in the image of a jealous competitor, never able to put the spontaneous generation argument behind him. Similarly, antivivisectionists were seen as the antiquated ones, belonging to an earlier era. Finally, with the help of a friendly medical press, Pasteur and his treatment regimen, portrayed as the protector of the human condition, held sway — his last great struggle a resounding success.[21] Pasteur, like Lister, had the gratifying experience of seeing his efforts come to fruition during his own lifetime.

Increasing age, incessant toil and years of unyielding strife at the hands of diverse adversaries had taken their toll on Pasteur. He carried out no further independent research after 1889. Despite his broken health, however, his legacy was assuming a robust shape. Pasteur Institutes were springing up throughout the world, beginning in Sydney in 1888, then Saigon, Indo-china, in 1891. It would even spawn new activities in some unexpected areas such as England.

## Pasteur's Jubilee

As Pasteur reached his seventieth year, a jubilee celebration convened in the new Sorbonne amphitheater, attended by young students from all over France, government officials, ambassadors and dignitaries from throughout the world. Rixens had memorialized the event in his portrait. In his weakened state, Pasteur is being accompanied to his place of honor on the arm of M. Carnot, president of the republic. After speeches by Carnot and M. Bertrand, Secretary of the Academy, Joseph Lister, representing the Royal Society of London, rose to thunderous applause. Addressing his old friend, Lister acknowledged the great debt that both he and the world owed the savant. "Thanks to you, surgery has undergone a complete revolution which has deprived it of its terrors and enlarged almost without limitations its power for good."[22] Overcome with emotion, Pasteur relied on his son, Jean-Baptiste, to deliver the closing address:

Young men, young men, put your trust in these sound and availing methods of which we still know only the first secrets.... Live in the serene peace of your laboratories and your libraries. Say to begin with, "What have I done for my own improvement?" Then, as you go further, "What have I done for my country?"... Whatever favours life may give, or refuse to a man's work — he ought, as he draws near to the end of it all, have the right to say, "I have done what I could."[23]

On 1 November 1894, Pasteur suffered a severe attack of uremia, rendering him bed-bound for months. He rallied enough by New Year's Day to enjoy seeing the newly discovered bacilli of diphtheria and bubonic plague in a display set up especially for him — his last look through a microscope.[24] In May 1895, the Berlin Academy of Science extended an honorific to him, the Badge of the Order of Merit, for all of his pioneering work. Ever true to France, the resolute Pasteur would not accept any award from Germany, so long as Alsace and Lorraine remained in German hands. As Pasteur grew progressively weaker, he left the Institute in June for the more comfortable environs of Villenueve-l'-Etang. There he became aphasic with near-total paralysis, as he suffered several more strokes. On 27 September 1895, when offered some milk, he weakly uttered his last words, "I cannot." Louis Pasteur died in the afternoon of the 28th, one hand clasping that of his wife's, the other holding a crucifix.[25]

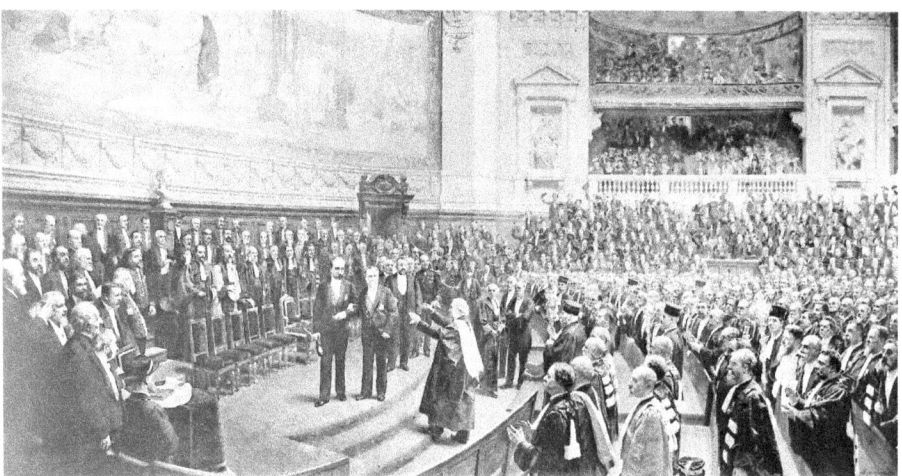

Painting by Jean-André Rixens of Pasteur's Jubilee, 1892. Joseph Lister acclaims Pasteur on the elder's seventieth birthday at the Sorbonne. A grateful Lister is seen giving full attribution to the savant for inspiring Lister's revolutionary scheme of surgical antisepsis. (Reproduced by permission of the Wellcome Library, London.)

An episode, decades later, attested to the reverence still held for him in France. In 1940, as the invading army entered Paris, several German soldiers arrived at the Institute, anxious to visit Pasteur's tomb. They were confronted there by an elderly, white-haired concierge and guardian who refused them entry. It was Joseph Meister, Pasteur's first rabies patient and long time employee at the Institute. He would tolerate no Prussian descendants on such hallowed ground. As Meister began to fully comprehend the sorry state of military affairs in France, he spiraled into a severe depression, finally retreating to his small flat where he took his own life.[26]

In the early 1890s, as the sun was setting on Pasteur's life, the younger Koch remained actively engaged. In his new position as Professor of Hygiene at Berlin University, he stood forth as a prominent public figure, but what he aimed for was anonymity.

CHAPTER 18

# Tuberculin: "Experiment Not Discovery"

In 1889, Robert Koch remained highly visible carrying out his various roles at Berlin University, lecturing, attending meetings and administrating. However, when he retreated to his laboratory, he became the recluse, toiling alone, confiding in no one. From the large numbers of dead guinea pigs the custodians carted off daily, his close associates sensed that something big was about to happen. They did not have to wait too long. On 4 August 1890, addressing the tenth International Congress of Medicine in Berlin, Koch, without making a frank declaration, suggested that he had produced a compound that could cure tuberculosis. As he related:

> All I can say at present is that if guinea pigs are treated they cannot be inoculated with tuberculosis, and guinea pigs that are already in the late stages of the disease are completely cured, although the body suffers no ill effects from the treatment. From these experiments I will draw no other conclusion at present than it is possible to render pathogenic bacteria within the body harmless without ill effects on the body itself.[1]

What Koch had observed must have excited him greatly. All guinea pigs that he had rendered tuberculous, but had intentionally not treated, suffered from swollen glands, fever and weight loss, eventuating in death at eight weeks. At autopsy, each exhibited enlarged spleens and multiple foci of dead tissue within their livers. But when he injected his new therapeutic concoction, a substance he later called tuberculin, into other tuberculous guinea pigs, he noted dramatic improvement. Their fevers and swollen tissues disappeared. They began eating and gaining weight. Their lives were also prolonged. At autopsy these animals displayed none of the findings that he had observed in the untreated group. The tuberculous areas were caseous — clearly degenerating.[2] No wonder the excitement — suddenly there seemed to be some hope on the horizon. Could this be the first step in the treatment of one of man's greatest scourges?

## Koch's Phenomenon

Since tuberculin had never been tried in humans, Koch was naturally concerned about its safety. He therefore first injected himself and his 17-year-old mistress with large doses of the material.[3] In a later scientific paper Koch recounted only his own reaction to the tuberculin. Several hours after his injection, he noted a general feeling of malaise, joint pain and severe rigors (stiffness and shaking), followed by vomiting and a fever of 39.6°C. (103.3°F.) Nearly 24 hours ensued before he fully recovered. Although ignorant of the chemical transformations behind it, he had just stumbled upon the antigen-antibody reaction, later called delayed hypersensitivity, or Koch's Phenomenon.

In September, Koch treated a small number of patients at Charité Hospital with tuberculin — a trial series. While drawing no sweeping conclusions, he soon expanded the trial. Further treatment made him even more encouraged. Just as with the guinea pigs, patients gained weight, their fever curves improved. The most dramatic cases were those with lupus, those ugly, topical skin lesions. Physicians could see the sloughing of the abnormal areas and replacement with fresh scar tissue. Even patients with early pulmonary tuberculosis improved significantly with a decrease in sputum production.[4] Some patients even appeared to be cured. In fact, Paul Ehrlich found himself suffering from the disease in 1888. After spending 1889 in Egypt, he returned to Berlin. After a series of nine injections, he was reportedly cured.[5]

Lister frequently had to deal with tuberculous abscesses in his surgical practice, but he was touched by it personally as well. His young niece suffered from a rapidly progressive, galloping form of the disease. Lister, who was initially very enthusiastic about the therapeutic potential of tuberculin, took her to Berlin for treatment under Koch's supervision. With great expectations, Lister cared for her daily. Unfortunately, he could see her failing in spite of the treatment. She died in Berlin, too weak to endure the return trip to London.[6]

## Early Acceptance

Given Koch's momentous discovery of the tubercle bacillus and his past triumphs with cholera and anthrax, he enjoyed a high level of credibility. The world accepted his claims about tuberculin uncritically, virtually overnight.[7] The *Lancet* gushed about "glad tidings of great joy."[8] The *Review of Reviews* devoted its entire December edition to tuberculin. Its editor sent writer and physician Arthur Conan Doyle to Berlin for a firsthand look. Conan Doyle reported back, with guarded optimism:

> Koch has never claimed that his fluid kills the tubercle bacillus. On the contrary, it has no effect on it, but it destroys the low form of tissue in the meshes of which the bacillus lurks. Should this tissue then be sloughed off in the case of lupus or be expelled as sputum in the case of phthisis then it might be possible to hope for a complete cure.[9]

Although Koch refused to reveal the details of his concoction at this early point in time, what he had prepared was a sterile protein extract from tubercle bacilli.

Inquisitive reporters and physicians anxious to learn about Koch's "lymph," streamed into the city of Berlin and Koch's institute. But most of all, it was the suffering patients from around the world that inundated the city, coughing and full of optimism. Those tuberculous enclaves of Italy and southern France emptied as patients sought transportation to Berlin. Consumptives, anxious to receive the treatment, filled hospitals, hotels and boarding houses.

## Initial Trials

Koch worked diligently to satisfy their treatment demands. Beginning in November 1890, his institute and the health ministry dispensed tuberculin to physicians for widespread treatment of patients. They were poorly equipped intellectually to evaluate the efficacy of any treatment method. For a discipline barely emerging from theories of humoral disease causation, any ideas concerning treatment protocols would have been in their most nascent stages. Beyond the measures that Pasteur had used at Melun, no systematic method for studying the efficacy of tuberculin or any other product existed in the 1890s. It is true that James Lind, in 1747, solved the puzzle of scurvy in English sailors by using a crude form of trial. He administered lemons or limes to one group of sailors, while contrasting the outcome of that group to a second, untreated cohort. In the late 1700s, Edward Jenner carried out a similar study for small pox. However, formal trials, in which clinicians make an effort to control the variables of both disease and patient, are a product of the early 20th century. Such strategies as randomization and stratification of patients or blinding and double blinding of participants were not introduced until well after 1890.

It is therefore not surprising that physicians acted too indiscriminately in addressing the soaring rush of consumptives, treating virtually all patients suffering from any manifestation of the disease. Some were questionably tuberculous while others were moribund. After two months of such activity, physicians outside of Koch's circle began experiencing difficulty duplicating the other group's results. By late 1890, most were openly questioning the therapeutic efficacy of tuberculin. Although a minority of patients noted moderate improvement, most appeared unaffected by the injections. The general elation of November evolved into perplexity by late December.

In January 1891, Koch's old adversary, Virchow, delivered the first definitive blow to this new hope for mankind. He presented pathological specimens from patients treated with tuberculin that revealed fresh tuberculous tissue surrounding the older necrotized (dead) areas.[10] Even if old diseased tissues had died or degenerated, the new tuberculous areas demonstrated that the disease was very much alive. This was no cure.

Spurred by the dubious therapeutic results of tuberculin, the Berlin Medical Society staged debates and more formal trials, trying to resolve this dilemma. That study extended into early 1891, but its results were still far from conclusive. Finally, researchers from all Prussian universities that had participated in the treatments compiled their crude statistics: A total of 17,500 injections had been administered to 2,172 patients. Less than 10 percent appeared to have been even moderately improved by the injections.[11] No one could claim that Koch's fluid was even remotely as successful as anticipated.

How could Koch have committed such a blunder? For him to even imply in a speech that he had developed a cure for tuberculosis without the supporting facts was completely out of character. This was the man who was meticulous to a fault, who agonized over questions of finality before announcing any type of conclusion. In the fall of 1890, American bacteriologist Harry Russell, while visiting Koch's laboratory at the time of the grand announcement, discovered that the German government was to blame. Russell's diary revealed, "Koch announced his so-called cure for tuberculosis by means of tuberculin in Oct. [sic] 1890. Was *forced* to do

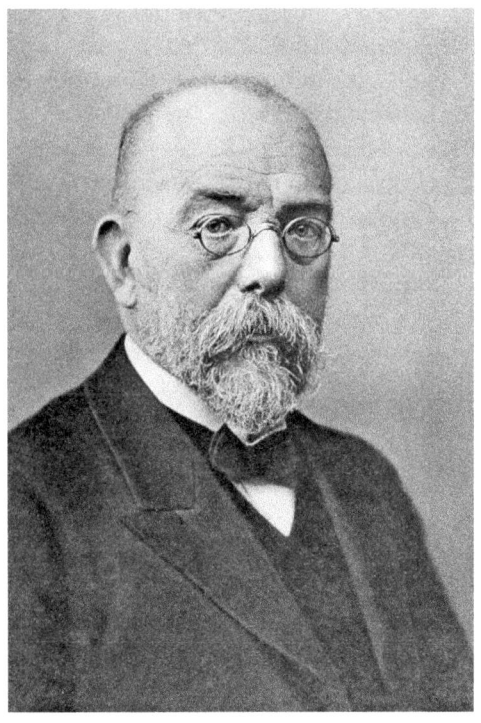

Robert Koch, age 69, near the end of his research career. (Reproduced by permission of the Wellcome Library, London.)

so by pressure from the Emperor (Wilhelm II)."[12] Still, other writers such as Christoph Gradman, Koch's Norwegian biographer, makes no mention of such governmental pressure upon Koch.

However, one beneficial effect did emerge from this debacle. Tuberculin did appear to have some future as a diagnostic tool. A positive reaction to the injection proved to be a very sensitive indicator of an individual's prior exposure to tuberculosis. The PPD (purified protein derivative) injection remains in use today. Still, with the failure of tuberculin as a definitive remedy for tuberculosis, Koch and the German Health Ministry had suffered an international embarrassment of major proportions. With his reputation badly bruised, Koch withdrew, traveling to Egypt for a mental defervescence lasting three months.

## Antivivisectionists' Response

Legitimate microbiological breakthroughs accumulating through the 1880s forced Cobbe into a reactionary position. Her polemical efforts had been reduced to exploiting, in the press, any failed medical expectations or genuine differences of opinion existing between scientists. Antivivisectionists were energized by Koch's embarrassing episode. Benjamin Bryan, secretary of the VSS, published "Kochism: Experiment Not Discovery" in VSS's own *Zoophilist*, deploring the whole tuberculin debacle. He charged English doctors who had traveled to Berlin to study tuberculin with promoting not only the "boom" of the remedy but of attempting to promote their own personal interests. He mentioned the decidedly negative experiences of several Continental researchers who had used the preparation, including that of Viennese Professor Theodore Billroth. In three of his patients, the reaction to tuberculin had been so extreme that Billroth discontinued any further treatments. Bryan felt that it was "little less than criminal" to continue using the remedy. Since so many of the patients treated were poor and from charity hospitals, he claimed it his duty to protest in the name of humanity.[13]

In a June 1891 issue, the *Zoophilist* lamented Koch's vivisection of 4,000 guinea pigs in pursuit of his treatment. Now this second Pasteur, this other great "Benefactor of Humanity," has managed to get a patent medicine, soon to be declared by physicians as "inefficacious and probably dangerous," accepted by the state as a panacea. "But think of the misery, the suffering, the blighted hopes, the ruinous expense that this heartless sham has inflicted upon hundreds and thousands of consumptive patients and their friends all over the world."[14]

Hoping to capitalize on this scientific icon's stumble, Cobbe set out to prove a larger point: the ultimate aim of doctors was to experiment on humans. She charged in a pamphlet, *Cancer Experiments on Human Beings*, that surgeons were grafting cancer onto the breasts of poor patients, rendered senseless with chloroform.[15] *The Zoophilist* then featured a large number of similar cases discovered in European hospitals. Rather than working to cure the patients, the materialist physicians were satisfying their curiosity by following the cancer's development throughout the body.[16] Charges that sounded baseless may have contained some element of truth. Walkowitz, in a study of Victorian prostitution, similarly asserted that physicians were conducting such experiments on the hospitalized indigent. Doctors were inoculating such unwitting patients of both genders with syphilitic and gonorrheal pus to better elucidate the course of the ensuing illness.[17]

Just as Cobbe and other antivivisectionists had been preaching, "cruelty begets further cruelty." No longer satisfied with dissecting live animals, doctors were pursuing further scientific experimentation in the corridors of charity hospitals, or so Cobbe claimed. As one *Zoophilist* article complained, "the poor working man or woman who seeks the shelter of one of our public hospitals, will henceforth be — if the doctors can have their way — actually a prisoner."[18] This scientific medicine was going too far.

Cobbe foresaw a disturbing evolution taking place in Britain, a dystopic society headed in the wrong direction, a natural outcome of experimental medicine's ascendency. Scientific influence was growing like a cancer within the body politic. In *The Age of Science*, she described her nightmare, a projection of Britain in 1977 in which science reigned supreme over all human affairs. In her vision, science had become so dominant that it caused the Church of England to fall. All cathedrals and churches had been converted to accommodate scientific pursuits.[19] Physicians comprised the entire governmental Upper House, while apothecaries occupied the Lower House. These physicians had been appointed Ministers of the Body, through governmental decree. Only through these caregivers could one's health be salvaged. With the scientific spirit so strong, each citizen's primary aim had become the prolongation of life at all costs. Society accorded special places of honor to scientists who discovered causes of such scourges as cholera, plague, leprosy and consumption. Doctors still experimented on patients in the hospital. All patients willing to be subjected to painful experimentation were fattened up on good food — just compensation for their impending pain and inconvenience. Children were still used for vivisection.[20]

Most lamentable were the ethical changes wrought upon society by the materialistic scientists. There was a time, she claimed, before this Age of Science, when an Invisible Being watched over men, encouraging them to do good deeds for a variety of reasons. First, they had a faith in the Lord and

Master called God. Men, as well, adhered to a sacred internal guide called Conscience. Finally, people still trusted in a peculiar sentiment called Honor.[21] Now, in the Age of Science, God was unknown or unknowable, Conscience was merely a quaint prejudice from a bygone era. Even Honor had fallen out of vogue. Science had extracted the very soul from a society now ruled only by the edicts of Criminal Jurisprudence. Some said that one should "labour for the good of Humanity in future generations," as though that would substitute for the "old Historic Religions."[22] But astronomers had informed us that our planetary solar heat was rapidly exhausting. Therefore, man could not inhabit this earth for too much longer. Cobbe must have had secular humanists in mind when she continued:

> Therefore, when the day comes — as come it must — when the fruits of the earth perish one by one, when the dead and silent woods petrify, and all of the races of animals become extinct — when the icy seas flow no longer, and the pallid Sun shines dimly over the frozen world, locked like the moon in eternal frost and lifelessness — what, in that day predicted so surely by Science, will avail all the works, and hopes, and martyrdom of man?... No mind in the universe will know or remember that there ever existed such a being as Man. This is what Science teaches us unerringly to expect — and in view of it, who shall talk to us of — "labouring for the sake of Humanity?" The enthusiasm which could work disinterestedly for a Progress destined inevitably to end in an eternal Glacial Period must be recognized as a dream, wherein no man in a Scientific Age can long indulge.[23]

Her essay ends abruptly as though she had suddenly awakened from her worst nightmare.

# IX

# Triumph and Descent

"There were many years of my life which I regarded it [science] with profound, though always distant admiration. Grown old, I have come to think that many spirits in the hierarchy are loftier and purer; that the noblest study of mankind is Man, rather than rock or insect; and that, even at its best, Knowledge is immeasurably less precious than Goodness and Love." — Frances Power Cobbe[1]

CHAPTER 19

# Nearly Universal

While Cobbe contemplated the dreadful changes wrought by science, Lister continued advancing along his professional path, rising through the academic ranks of the surgical world. He left Glasgow University in 1869, after being appointed Professor of Surgery at Edinburgh University, beginning what was arguably the most contented period in his career. The general atmosphere in Edinburgh was so collegial that he felt at home there. His tenure at Edinburgh spanned nine years.[1] During this time his antiseptic scheme continued to gain acceptance in an ever-widening sphere. Still, it was in the provinces more than the larger medical centers where physicians looked favorably upon his methods. Lister enjoyed his lecture schedule at Edinburgh where he regularly attracted over 200 appreciative medical students, eager to hear him expound on this novel way of treating patients antiseptically. He also enjoyed the use of an expansive ward for his patients in the infirmary. He treated a large number of individuals with abscesses, later recognized as being mainly tuberculous in origin after Koch's contributions. Since these individuals, as a group, were some of his sickest, they required longer hospital stays. Therefore, the number of beds available to him was an important factor.

In 1877, the regents of King's College, a much smaller university in London, offered Lister a professorship in systematic surgery. Given his level of comfort at Edinburgh, the proposal forced him into a period of intense soul-searching. He even endured pleas and formal petitions from his loyal students to remain in Edinburgh. Happy as he was there, he had to admit that, in his heart, he remained a true Londoner. More importantly, London still represented a problem to him. As one of the last bastions of the unclean, the unconverted, the big city was a natural place for him to continue his campaign.[2] London physicians would prove the most difficult to change. Joseph and Lady Lister made their move to King's College in September 1877. Boarding the train to London, Lister personally carried his precious flasks of sterile urine with him. He could entrust the care of these teaching aids to no one else. He spent the next 15 years at King's until forced into retirement at age 65. His prescribed work schedule at King's proved much less demanding than in Edinburgh, but he maintained the rigors of his research unabated, centered mainly on antisepsis, germicidal agents and the perfection of catgut suture.

Compared with the atmosphere in Edinburgh, Lister noted a significant and uncomfortable difference. Everything about King's was smaller, from the campus, to the number of students, to the number of beds under his care. Rather than overt opposition, Lister detected among the medical students and nursing staff an attitude of indifference, a feeling of passive resistance towards him. Although his relationships with physicians were generally cordial, he could sense, as well, that some were against him and his method. In a city so large, with a multiplicity of universities and disparate medical factions, advancing a revolutionary form of treatment would require something irrefutable such as demonstrably superior results. Despite the dubious beginning, he was resolute. Converting Londoners to his antiseptic method would take some time.

## Lister's Inaugural Lecture

Lister gave his first introductory address for winter term, a class designed for students, but attended as well by some leading scientists and distinguished physicians and surgeons. To those unaware that germ theory represented the foundation of his antiseptic system, his subject, "On the Nature of Fermentation," must have seemed a strange choice. In a demonstration before the class Lister employed his old teaching technique of using an analogy to elucidate the cause of infections in living beings. His desk was stacked with beakers, flasks and other lab paraphernalia. He had previously rendered some milk samples either sterile by heating or sour by inoculating with *B. lactis*. The sterile milk in the first flask was a liquid analogous to human blood. The glass of the flask represented a protective barrier analogous to human skin. If he filtered the air as it entered the flask, the fluid remained sterile, demonstrating that air, filtered free of impurities, was incapable of producing infections. However, if the glass neck were broken and free air entered, infection (souring) of the milk (blood) ensued.[3] Therefore, the infectious elements were something that resided in ambient air. Just as a bone fragment alters the integrity of skin by puncturing through it, an analogous loss of integrity to the flask, such as breaking its neck, resulted in growth of bacteria in the milk.

In another demonstration he diluted small volumes of fermented milk 500,000 times. At this dilution, each drop of sour milk theoretically represented one microorganism of *Bacterium lactis*. When he placed that single drop into sterile milk, it resulted in fermentation.[4] Lister hoped to illustrate the power and specificity of a few microscopic organisms in producing fermented milk and how other microorganisms might play an analogous role in human infections. According to John Stewart, one of four dressers to accompany Lister to London from Edinburgh, this speech represented Lister's first salvo in a campaign for converts.

Seeing the apathy in members of the audience, Lister's four Edinburgh trained assistants could sense his disappointment. Despite the clarity and simplicity of his analogy, many in his audience still had difficulty accepting it. Older physicians did not believe in, or were agnostic towards, the existence of germs. Others, still clinging to the theory of spontaneous generation, scratched their heads wondering what the souring of milk had to do with surgery. To them any argument using flasks was so far removed from clinical conditions that it was meaningless. However, one writer from the *Medical Examiner* was impressed enough to call Lister the "apostle of the surgery of thought," as opposed to the older, medieval artisan's approach of "the surgery of action."[5] Over the ensuing weeks, Lister's house surgeons wandered around the wards of King's, perplexed by the refusal of otherwise enlightened men to open their eyes. "In these wards the air was heavy with the odour of suppuration, the shining eye and flushed cheek spoke eloquently of surgical fever." They longed for the enthusiastic participation of the Edinburgh school with its hundreds of eager students. Instead, "our hearts were chilled by the listless air of the twelve or twenty students who lounged in the lecture at King's."[6]

Some fellow surgeons could be overtly critical, as well. In October 1877, Lister performed an open operation, wiring a fractured kneecap, as he had done many times before. One indignant surgeon, ignorant of Lister's system, remarked how the risk of infection made such an operation unjustified. "Now when this poor fellow dies, it is proper that someone should proceed against that man for malpraxis."[7] Of course, no infection ever developed.

## Exemplary Results

Despite such inauspicious beginnings, Lister's situation at King's slowly improved. Physicians from around the world still visited, observing his methods. As his practice grew, he performed more operations, some uncontroversial, some "unjustified." As both students and colleagues at King's began noticing Lister's superior results, they discussed it among themselves. Good outcomes begat good reviews. Nor did the cleaner wards and absence of putrefactive aromas go unnoticed. Slowly, more by example than by polemic, he gained converts locally, within the hospital. The older surgeons, more artisans than scientists, again proved the most resistant to this new scheme. Through attrition, their numbers decreased while a newer cadre of younger converts emerged. Lister and his dressers noted a slow but gratifying improvement in the learning environment.

From the beginning Continental surgeons had been more receptive to Lister's regimen than were the English. Much had to do with how they were educated. In an earlier era, 1867, out of 64 surgeons affiliated with London hospitals, only seven held medical degrees; the remainder had been apprentice-trained.[8] European surgeons, particularly the Germans, all held university degrees. With a solid grounding in science they were better prepared to evaluate more esoteric scientific theories. Still it was on the Continent where some of the worst environments for hospitalism existed. Most of the great institutions, such as the Hotel Dieu in Paris, Charité in Berlin, and Allgemeines Krankenhaus in Vienna, were near-pestilential.[9]

Before Lister began his antisepsis campaign European surgeons had been just as perplexed by the problem of sepsis as were the English. As they visited Lister's wards and learned of his method of wound care, most left inspired

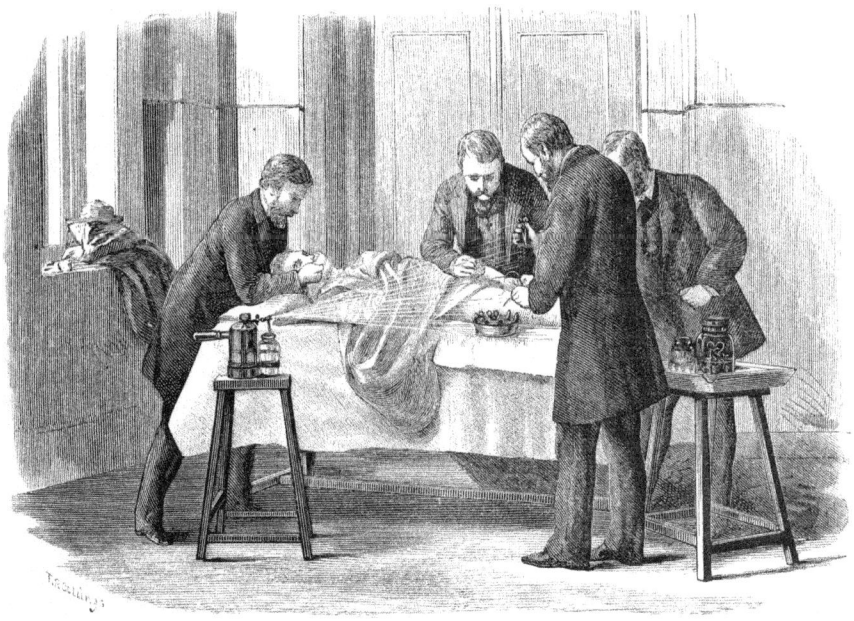

Lister's spray of carbolic acid in use during an operation in 1882. The illustration is self-explanatory. Surgeons who were chronically and repetitively exposed to the spray suffered from skin and airway ailments as well as numbness in their fingers. Lister abandoned the spray in 1887, much to the relief of his assistants. (Reproduced by permission of the Wellcome Library, London.)

enough to consider bringing the program to their own hospital. They were also sufficiently influential in their own country to help spread the word of antisepsis more rapidly. During Lister's Glasgow days, Carl Thiersch, from Leipzig, became one of Lister's earliest and most fervent converts after his visit. Richard von Volkmann, who had gone through the military campaigns of 1870 in Sedan and Paris, returned to Halle to find German veterans ensnared in the filth of sepsis at their local hospital. Just as in England, any operation meant almost certain death. After thoroughly learning Lister's method, he began an antiseptic program with results that he termed "magical," another instant and ardent convert.[10] Such stories could be repeated in multiple countries with many different surgeons such as Prof. Saxtorph from Copenhagen, Carl Reyher from Russia and Just Lucas-Championnière from Paris, to name but a few. In 1876, the Parisian surgeon delivered the first comprehensive accounting of antisepsis in a 150-page book. The Paris of 1875 saw few physicians practicing antiseptic surgery. However, by 1880, it enjoyed wide acceptance. In his book Lucas-Championnière happily concluded: "A few years ago Paris hospitals were reckoned amongst the very worst, even by some of their own surgeons. Now surgery may be as well carried out in them as anywhere else. You may even see a patient recover after Caesarean section."[11]

Americans were even slower to adopt the antiseptic method than were London physicians. Since American medical education was patterned on the English method, surgeons were apprentice-trained with little grounding in science. Lister had made one trip to address the International Medical Congress in Philadelphia in 1876, which helped broaden exposure to his scheme. Still, it was only after 1877 that surgeons began using his scheme. Surgeons complained that it not only entailed a belief in germ theory, but the regimen was just too complicated to deal with.[12]

Foreign surgeons continued to visit Lister after his move to King's in 1877. But not all were practicing surgeons. In November 1877, a highly interested Dr. Burdon Sanderson visited Lister's wards, followed a week later by physicist John Tyndall and John Simon, surgeon. Even the *Lancet*, which had been resistant to Lister, seemed to be softening. Their editors published an article in July 1878 illustrating a series of cases treated successfully with the antiseptic method by J.C. Will, Aberdeen surgeon. Will remarked, "There is something more in it than careful drainage and absolute cleanliness."[13]

So varied were attitudes about antisepsis in the 1870s that Lister could get two entirely different receptions, only a few weeks apart, depending on the circumstances. William Savory, surgeon at London's St. Bartholomew's Hospital, attacked him at a BMA meeting in Cork in August 1879. As an advocate for "clean water, adequately used," Savory claimed an admirable mortality from sepsis of only 1½ percent at Bart's. Challenging Lister, Savory wanted statistics demonstrating that the antiseptic method was superior to his own. But Lister had an innate distrust for statistics, given the vagaries of diseases — from their manners of presentation, to their responses to treatment. Savory would never get them.[14] Only a few weeks after Cork, Lister traveled to Amsterdam to speak at the September 1879 meeting of the International Medical Congress. Here he was received with boundless enthusiasm. As recorded by the *British Medical Journal*:

> When he stepped forward ... the whole assembly rose to its feet; and with deafening and repeated rounds of cheers, waving of hats and handkerchiefs, hailed the distinguished Professor from King's College with acclimations renewed ... until Professor Donders, the President ... taking Professor Lister by the hand, as he stood overwhelmed by this magnificent ovation, obtained a moment's silence, and addressing him said: "Professor Lister, it is not only our admiration we offer you; it is our gratitude, and that of the nations to which we belong."[15]

As his fame grew, the decade of the eighties involved greater demands for lectures, appearances at more scientific meetings and memberships in professional societies. Although his topics for speeches might vary from discussing patellar operations, to vascular procedures, to his latest on catgut, it was his updates on antiseptic wound care that evoked the most interest. By 1890 the acceptance of Lister's antiseptic method was nearly universal.[16]

## An Institute in England?

Another pursuit that began to occupy a great deal of Lister's time, a testimony to the government's growing reliance on scientific medicine, involved the question: Should some type of institute for preventive medicine be established in England? Since rabies remained a problem in England, an institute along the lines of what Pasteur had been working on for France seemed a reasonable proposal to scientists and government officials. In 1887, English authorities appointed a committee to investigate the feasibility of such a venture. Committee members included Victor Horsley, Sir James Paget, Lauder Brunton, Burdon Sanderson and others. While Horsley remained in London, repeating many of Pasteur's rabies experiments, the other members traveled to Paris. There they reviewed all of Pasteur's work, scrutinized his notebooks and even visited the homes of 90 patients treated by the Pasteurian method.[17] In their July 1888 official report, committee members fully validated Pasteur's claims, citing "perfect accuracy" of his records. They believed with certainty that Pasteur's inoculations of patients bitten by rabid animals had prevented the development of hydrophobia. Moreover, had the victims not been inoculated, they would have died of the disease.[18]

Offended by such findings and their implications, VSS secretary Benjamin Bryan published "Reasons Why the English Committee's Report on Pasteurism Does Not Settle the Question," even before the committee had publicized their final conclusions. Bryan asserted that, since not one antivivisectionist sat on the committee, the entire investigation represented a "pitiful effort by a packed committee" to maintain a discredited method.[19] He then invoked the usual arguments against Pasteur, alleging shoddy record keeping and the deliberate under-reporting of deaths. For further support he also identified the many scientists, such as Billroth, from other countries who vehemently disagreed with Pasteur's method. Bryan then argued, strangely, if the committee believes so thoroughly in Pasteur and his method, why are they not recommending a Pasteur Institute in England?[20] Of course, the English committee had been considering that very item, whether it be a duplication of the French institution or some uniquely British version. Cobbe, at least, had been well aware of such plans.

One other recommendation by the English committee concerned the muzzling of dogs. With England's very controllable borders, a muzzling program should ensure a slow dying out of rabies through attrition. England could avoid the entire expense of an anti-rabies program. But Cobbe and her allies were dead set against such a move since muzzles do not allow a dog to get rid of bodily heat through panting. In another defeat for Cobbe, the proposal passed.

In a larger sense the English committee was ineffectual. It dithered for 10 years before an actual proposal for a British Institute of Preventive Medicine materialized. As a first step, the board merely moved to incorporate. Alarmed by such plans, antivivisectionists reacted. Numerous antivivisectionist leaders composed a letter to Michael Hicks-Beach, chairman of the Board of Trade, expressing alarm that an Institute of Bacteriology would exist within the larger Institute. That meant a "vast amount of experimentation with all manner of diseases, some painful, some loathsome, on a large number of animals.... It will place in our midst ... a gigantic vivisection laboratory in which the worst experiments ever made might be repeated." They "humbly prayed" that the honorable board would withhold such licensure.[21]

After a delay of months, Lister, as chairman of the institute, finally interceded with a letter to Hicks-Beach, reminding him that England, for the good of its citizens, merely wanted the same sort of high quality institute as those existing in France and Germany. He requested that the board support medicine in its struggle against "prejudice and ignorance" by authorizing incorporation.[22] In June 1891, Hicks-Beach acceded to Lister's request, allowing incorporation to move forward.

Much like the Pasteur Institute, the board resolved to prevent and cure infectious diseases in man and animals, and to educate students, physicians and veterinarians in the science of disease prevention.[23] As the institute expanded, it assumed the functions of surveillance and prevention of diphtheria, typhoid, tuberculosis and other infectious diseases by testing milk, blood and sputum. Lister, who began serving as chairman of the board in 1891, took an active interest in the institute's ventures. He became fully engaged in both its scientific pursuits and logistical functions, including its anti-serum production. In 1903, the facility officially became the Lister Institute of Preventive Medicine, a fitting honor given his accomplishments and his tireless dedication over so many years. He served as president of the institute until 1910, when physical infirmities of age prevented further involvement.[24]

## Chapter 20

# Lister's Retrospective

During his active career Lister delivered virtually all of his speeches to fellow physicians and scientists, but in his role as elder statesman, one of his final utterances on antisepsis occurred before a general audience. In 1896, as president of the British Association, a lay society devoted to the promotion of scientific advancement, Lister gave an address on "The Interdependence of Science and the Healing Art." In essence, he delivered a retrospective on the great strides in medical science, achieved through scientific investigation, in the short span of one man's career. There is no record that Cobbe was in the audience, but Lister's methodical recapitulation of scientific achievements taking place in the latter half of the 19th century would have offered her another nightmare scenario.

Lister began with the 1895 discovery of Roentgen's x-rays, occurring less than one year before. One could only speculate about the huge diagnostic and therapeutic implications of this new discovery. He then progressed on to Louis Pasteur, the science behind fermentation and his elucidation of germ theory. Then there was Lister's own revolutionary work controlling suppuration and putrefaction in the care of wounds, one of the greatest examples of basic science being exploited by an applied scientist. Another historic microbiological contribution by Pasteur was his attenuation of viruses, eventuating in a new science — immunology. It was 1896, only one year before the centenary of Jenner's work with smallpox. At the very time of Lister's speech a smallpox epidemic raged in Gloucester, a consequence of neglect by city fathers. Despite a general awareness of the risks before the epidemic, only 600,000 out of 900,000 citizens had bothered to undergo vaccination.[1] As the epidemic erupted and the officials recognized their error, Gloucester became, belatedly, the best vaccinated city in England. But, sadly, as Lister pointed out, "They cannot recall the dead to life, or restore beauty to marred features, or sight to blinded eyes. Would that the entire country and our Legislature might take duly to heart this object lesson!"[2]

Lister had in mind certain people of influence, confirmed anti-vaccinationists who resided in Gloucester. One was future Cobbe ally, Walter Hadwen, M.D., who, at the height of the epidemic, still railed against the evils of vaccination. "Sanitation did for Prussia what 35 years of compulsory vaccination was unable to accomplish. At the present time in Prussia smallpox is almost extinct. It is not that people are being vaccinated more; they are vaccinated less."[3] Gloucester city fathers wisely ignored Hadwen's observations when they ordered widespread smallpox inoculations.

In his address, Lister next proceeded to Koch's pioneering accomplishments, followed by Albert Neisser's isolation of the gonorrhea organism in 1879, and Carl Eberth's discovery of the typhoid bacillus, *Salmonella typhi*, in 1880. The disciples of both Pasteur and Koch made significant contributions as well. In 1883, Friedrich Loeffler, from Koch's laboratory, discovered the causal agent of diphtheria, one of the greatest killers of children worldwide.

## Birth of Serotherapy

In 1889, Shibasaburo Kitasato isolated the tetanus organism (*Clostridium tetani*). He and Emil von Behring subsequently discovered that tetanus produced a neurotoxin, which wreaked its effects via the nervous system. Severe tetanic spasms affect all of the bodily musculature, little different from what Magendie observed with the strychnine-containing *upas tiute*. After first isolating tetanus toxin, Kitasato and von Behring discovered that if a toxin, such as that of tetanus, were given to animals in a safe dosage, the animals developed an immunity unique to that disease. That infected or inoculated animal produced a substance the researchers named antitoxin. In addition, that serum, if injected into another animal, provided protection against that respective disease. They could thus achieve two ends by its administration. First, giving any animal the antitoxin rendered it immune to the disease. More importantly, if it were given to an animal suffering from all manifestations of the disease, it reversed the symptoms, effecting a cure.[4]

Then further progress came from Roux and Alexandre Yersin at the Pasteur Institute. Learning of von Behring's and Kitasato's work with tetanus, they duplicated much of the Germans' work in a similar pursuit of a remedy for diphtheria. Roux discovered that a comparatively small number of bacteria exerted, out of all proportion to their numbers, systemic changes in the victim. He correctly sensed that those effects must be due to the bacterial release of a toxin. In essence, the bacteria establish an enclave within the body, releasing a toxin into the general circulation that caused both the suffering and dangerous bodily changes that define the illness. In 1889, Roux and Yersin isolated the toxin produced by the diphtheria bacillus.⁵ In parallel with the work on tetanus, Roux developed diphtheria serum that neutralized the effects of the disease. With an eye towards treating humans, Roux administered the serum in successive doses to minimize any hazard to the animal that would be supplying the serum for treatment. It was Roux who first conceived of using a large animal with a huge blood volume for serum production. Only an animal the size of a horse could provide the volumes required if humans were to be treated on a large scale.⁶

As a consequence of their work, von Behring in Germany and Roux at the Pasteur Institute had independently created the field of serotherapy, a method constituting one leg of this new discipline called immunology. Referring back to an old medieval term, they realized that immunity could be conferred to an animal on a "humoral" basis — from chemical constituents residing within the serum.

In his retrospective on medical accomplishments, Lister neglected to mention Victor Horsley's revolutionary work with the thyroid gland. Horsley continued some of the work begun in Florence by Mauritz Schiff, the same work that had drawn Cobbe's ire in 1863. After removing the thyroid glands from dogs, Schiff saw the animals become lethargic and gain weight, followed by death in 6–8 weeks.

In 1884, as Director of the Brown Institute, Horsley studied the relationship between cretinism and the thyroid gland, believing that the thyroid was an important secretory organ.⁷ In a series of famous Brown lectures over a six-year period, Horsley outlined his revolutionary work. Congenital cretins presented a dramatic image, with dwarfism, mental retardation, a dull and vacuous expression, with swollen tongue protruding through an open mouth. Cretinism was the youthful form of hypothyroidism, while myxedema represented the adult form. In both states a mucin-like material resided in between cells, causing swelling of soft tissues. When Horsley removed the thyroid glands from monkeys, he observed them huddling in their corners, disinterested in their surroundings. They then progressed on to coma and death around two months after thyroidectomy. In their autopsies he found mucin, a viscous protein, in the muscles and blood. He along with others, were able to causally connect myxedema, cretinism and cachexia (emaciated state) to thyroid deficiency.

Some, such as Horsley and Swiss surgeon Emil Kocher, attempted to treat this deficiency with transplants of thyroid glands, but most glands were rejected or resorbed over time. Finally, George Murray, a pupil of Horsley's, established a landmark in endocrinology. He injected "thyroid juice," an extract of sheep thyroid suspended in glycerin, under the skin of myxedematous adults and cretins with gratifying reversal of signs and symptoms.⁸ Another disease was in its early stage of resolution.

Of course Cobbe and her allies were critical of all such research. A *Zoophilist* article, "Vivisection and the New Treatment of Myxedema," decried the use of animals at all, arguing as though vivisection and clinical research were mutually exclusive. With all the human clinical material available, why should vivisection be necessary at all? She then suggested that this "thyroid juice" was part of a "craze these days for treating all [maladies] with animal extracts."[9]

## England's First Diphtheria Cure

In 1894, the British Institute for Preventive Medicine became intimately involved in the production of diphtheria antitoxin in England. Charles Sherrington, future iconic neurophysiologist, and Armand Ruffer, director of research at the institute, were in charge of producing the antitoxin on a large scale for human use. They had been injecting Tommy, their first production

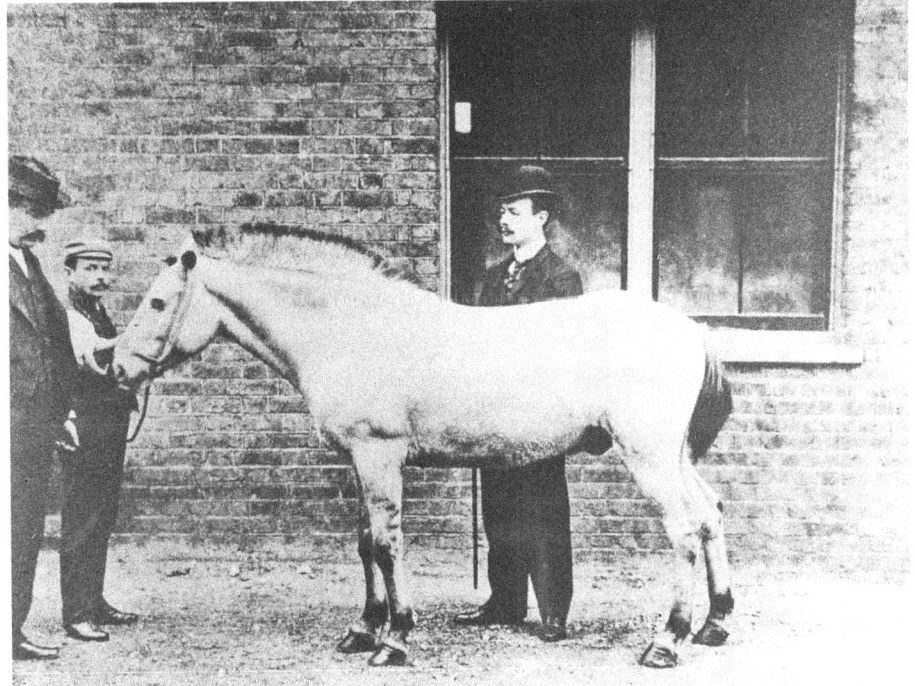

Production pony, "Tommy," was the first English horse used for producing diphtheria vaccine. Charles Sherrington, in the bowler, stands behind the horse while Armand Ruffer, director of the British Institute, stands at its head. An unidentified aide is petting the horse's nose. (Reproduced by permission of the Wellcome Library, London.)

horse, only a short period of time, still struggling with concerns over technique and proper dosing. One Saturday in August, around 7 P.M., Sherrington received a wire concerning his seven-year-old nephew, who lived in Lewes, 30 miles outside London. Sherrington's brother-in-law stated, "George has diphtheria. Can you come?" Since time would not allow for shipment of antitoxin from France, Sherrington had to make a quick decision. Should he use Tommy's serum despite Ruffer's assertions that "it is not yet ripe for trial"? Given his choices, he did not have to ponder for too long. Sherrington traveled to the institute, where he bled two liters from the horse by lantern light, then let the blood cells settle with time and gravity. Returning at midnight, he decanted the serum onto ice for his trip to Lewes.

Carrying all of the requisite pipettes, syringes and serum, Sherrington boarded the train to Lewes early Sunday morning. It was a solemn Dr. Fawssett, the family physician, who met Sherrington at the Lewes depot. With downcast eyes Fawssett muttered, "You can do what you like with the boy. He will not be alive at tea-time." Sherrington entered the home to find a frightened and silent household, clearly aware of the situation. The boy was weak and displayed labored breathing. Both doctors began injecting serum, emptying their small syringes, "time and again." Remaining at the boy's bedside, Sherrington began noting signs of improvement by early afternoon. From that point on, progress continued unabated.

On Tuesday an elated Sherrington returned to London, informing Ruffer of his experience. Ruffer insisted that they immediately inform Lister, who, as head of the institute, was heavily invested in the antitoxin project. When they located him at his home in Park Crescent, he was entertaining Continental surgeons in his drawing room. Upon Lister's insistence, Sherrington related the entire episode to them all. Sherrington later recalled that, although the boy had a severe paralysis for some time, he matured into a six-foot man and received a commission during the first World War.[10] Such pioneering work helped to bring one of the country's most heart-wrenching and fatal childhood illnesses to an end. No longer would parents and physicians have to sit by passively, agonizing as their child suffocated before their eyes. In a stellar year for experimental medicine, 1894, Alexandre Yersin identified the organism causing bubonic plague, arguably the most feared disease in human history. Waldemar Haffkine followed that triumph in 1897 by developing a vaccine against the plague.

In Paris, under the guidance of Roux, the Hopital des Enfants became the French epicenter for the treatment of diphtheria. Roux's results proved so effective that in September 1894, he presented his early treatment experiences to the International Congress of Hygiene and Demography in Budapest. Its benefits were so obvious that worldwide use ensued rapidly as word spread.[11]

In the United States, the mere announcement of the antitoxin's efficacy, in 1894, caused the beginning of the antivivisection dormancy there. According to government physician, J.J. Kinyoun, if the antitoxin had been available in the preceding five years, "at the lowest estimate 150,000 lives" would have been spared. This beneficent treatment scheme was attributable completely to the systematic programs of vivisection in Germany and France.[12]

## Cobbe's Position

Predictably, Cobbe remained unconvinced. To the claim that Roux's serum treatment was saving lives, she charged in an 1894 article that no such evidence existed. But the best she could manage was to introduce uncertainty into the argument. She claimed that diphtheria had an inordinately high death rate in children under the age of two. Therefore, without stratifying for age within the treatment series, how could anyone draw any sort of conclusions about its efficacy?[13] In 1901, she demonstrated continuing resistance by stating that faith was weakening for this treatment that used serum from a "poisoned horse" as a remedy for a delicate child struggling with diphtheria. The horse does not get the disease with a membrane over its throat. Why would any man who cares for the truth continue to use such a nostrum? The remedy is a "wretched delusion" maintained like other quack remedies for commercial purposes.[14] Even Stephen Coleridge, her old ally, in a 1902 letter to *The Morning Post*, joined in. He took issue with the claim that the antitoxin greatly diminished the severity of the disease and the need for tracheotomy. Since he did not believe in its efficacy, he claimed that he would not permit the use of the serum in his own case or for that of his own child.[15]

In 1897, the queen honored Lis-

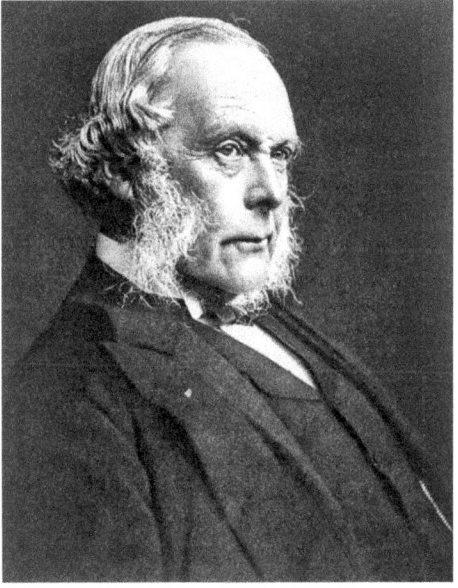

The Right Honourable Baron Lister by R.A. Bickersteth. This photograph, at the time of his election to the peerage in 1897, served as the frontispiece to Rickman Godlee's 1918 biography of Lister. (Reproduced by permission of the Wellcome Library, London.)

ter with the peerage in recognition of his service to mankind. Such institutional validation of his 30 years of work was a blow to Cobbe, who bitterly denounced the queen's actions. Other governmental moves such as granting financial support to research hospitals for cancer and allied human afflictions was a declaration of the state's approval of scientific medicine. In 1899, shortly after Cobbe organized the BUAV, the British Colonial Office founded the London School of Tropical Medicine, a specialized institution concentrating on diseases such as malaria and yellow fever. Nineteen years earlier, the physician Charles Laveran had discovered plasmodia, the protozoan residing within red blood cells of malarial patients. By century's end, Dr. Ronald Ross supplemented Laveran's contribution by elucidating the full life cycle of the plasmodium organism. Ross discovered plasmodia residing in the salivary glands of the *anophyles* mosquito, the carrier of human malaria. Cinchona bark, of course, had been used empirically in the treatment of malaria for decades. While not a curative, it did lessen the suffering. Both Laveran and Ross received the Nobel Prize for their contributions, the mechanism of one more disease elucidated.

## Cellular Immunity

It was a Russian, Elie Metchnikoff, lured into Pasteur's Institute around 1890, who ushered in the second leg of immunology. Robert Koch had previously given Metchnikoff and his theories an icy reception, reminiscent of Virchow's treatment of a younger Koch decades earlier. When Metchnikoff came to Paris, Pasteur recognized his potential. As a researcher in Odessa, Metchnikoff had become intrigued with the manner in which amoebas devoured their food particles by engulfing them. Wondering if certain of our white blood cells might function in a similar manner, he began observing starfish larvae, an ideal model for study. Since their bodies are completely transparent, they provided a perfect window for investigating physiological phenomena. Metchnikoff gathered thorns from his own rose garden and systematically inserted them into the larvae. He was elated when, under his microscope, he observed host cells immediately surrounding these foreign invaders, setting up a wall of resistance.[16] This seminal observation evolved into Metchnikoff's discovery of the phagocytic process — the act in which white blood cells destroyed foreign material, such as bacteria, by engulfing them. Metchnikoff demonstrated that immunity was not just a chemical (humoral) process but a cellular one as well. Lister, in particular, was enthralled by Metchnikoff's work. He experienced a sense of fulfillment since "Metchnikoff's researches, while they have illumined the whole pathology of infective diseases, have beautifully completed the theory of antiseptic treatment in surgery."[17]

This revolutionary shift in attitude about that other world of microscopic organisms did not just include scientific disciplines. Even within most households one could detect a civic realization: We live within a world of germs. Just as Cobbe had predicted, a general awareness of bacteria had wrought changes in human behavior. However, the changes resulted in improvement, not decline. People became more aware of cleanliness and hygiene. Women wore shorter dresses, hoping to avoid dragging organisms from the street into the home, while men shaved their beards and long hair in the name of better hygiene. Homeowners changed their heavy drapes, carpets, upholstered furniture, anything that might serve as safe harbors for organisms, to lighter, more streamlined fashions.[18] The rising tide of public opinion combined with expanding state policies that incorporated scientific theory into their institutions was stronger than any countermovement could withstand. It was the birth of medical modernity.

Chapter 21

# Descent

Cobbe, of course, failed or refused to recognize these general advancements or the specific ones recounted by Lister, continuing on with her confrontations — now centered upon her current concern, people's health: Individuals became ill because they did not follow the natural laws of cleanliness and sobriety. Instead, they placed their trust in scientific theories concerning microbes and contagion, allowing their bodies to be polluted with the filth of vaccines just to avoid some disease. She was convinced that the average person preferred to bear the pain and malaise of disease rather than obtain relief via some remedy gained through animal experimentation. It would be better to suffer epidemics than resort to cures found through the cruelty of vivisection.[1] In an 1895 pamphlet, *Controversy in a Nutshell*, Cobbe observed,

> Our bodies are destined to perish sooner or later, and the relief or help which science at its best can ever afford them is a very small matter. There is a greater interest even than the sanitary interest of which we make so much these days — it is the interest of the hearts and souls of men. It is of more importance that tender and just and compassionate feelings should grow and abound than that a cure should be found for corporeal disease.[2]

In a similar vein, Cobbe's old ally R.H. Hutton pointed out so "magnanimously" that he would prefer to observe his wife suffering from a painful disease than have her obtain relief from any treatment that had been gained through animal experimentation.[3]

## Increasing Marginalization

Rather than gaining converts to her views, both friends and strangers began viewing Cobbe as more alienating and increasingly rigid. She and her lot cared much more about animals than they did humans. Some writers suggested that not just Cobbe but the entire antivivisection movement was filled with unmarried and unfulfilled women who, through their ignorance of science, took out their dissatisfactions in life on the men of experimental medicine. In one *Zoophilist* letter, a writer complained "Why does our silly contemporary the *Times* publish letters of the stupid old maid, Cobbe?... It is enough to make one's gorge rise to hear these fools of dog fanciers speak as if hydrophobia were a trifle, and the life of a human being of less value even than the life of a nasty, rabid brute of a dog."[4]

Others whose profession included caring for the ill, contending with their suffering on a daily basis, approached this increasing fanaticism from a different angle. One nurse suggested that these antivivisectionists should spend some time caring for the infirm

> and see the recovered and lessened suffering (the result of knowledge gained by experiments), and then compare the treatment and comparative ignorance of the alleviation eighty years ago, they may perhaps then feel inclined to direct their energies to a more profitable theme than the discussion of a subject on which they think they know a great deal, but in fact know nothing, showing that "a little knowledge is a dangerous thing."[5]

One activity, however, did bring Cobbe some much needed respite from her fading relevance, some buoyancy to her life. Her friend Blanche Atkinson suggested that she write her autobiography. The necessary research and writing, which occupied much of 1893 and into 1894, provided her with a pleasant review of her life. Whether she was being coy or truly humble, Cobbe expressed the thought that people in Britain might think her too arrogant in writing her autobiography. She therefore arranged for an 1894 publication not in Britain, but rather in Boston, through Houghton Mifflin. American sales proved so brisk that her book was soon being printed in Britain as well. Hearing from old friends and new admirers from around the world who read her book provided a great source of pleasure to her, lifting her for a time out of the doldrums.

The winter of 1895 proved to be unseasonably cold, coinciding with the beginning of Mary's deterioration. Temperatures dropped so low that vegetation froze and livestock died in the field. Both Cobbe and Lloyd developed bronchitis, pulling through only "with a new medication called 'Codein' which magically stops paroxysms of coughing."[6] Even after her bronchitis resolved, Lloyd never regained her full strength. In one of her frequent letters to an American friend, Sarah Wister, Cobbe expressed her deep concern over Lloyd's health. Only a few months later, October 1896, Mary died from heart disease, at age 77. In a follow-up letter to Wister, Cobbe revealed how Mary died "bravely resting on my arm & telling me we should not long be separated."

She was buried in the Llanelltyd churchyard, visible from Hengwrt. "It is a most lovely spot with a great view of Cader — & this place & woods — & the whole estuary down to the sea."[7] Cobbe chose a double plot with a headstone for two — one side left blank, awaiting the uncertain arrival of its second occupant.

With Mary's death, Cobbe's loneliness and depression remained a near constant. As she confided to an old friend Millicent Fawcett, it was "almost a mortal blow, & I have yet to learn how I am to live without the one who has shared all my thoughts & feelings so long."[8] It was not until early 1897 that Cobbe was able to be out among friends in Barmouth, Wales, beginning to resume her writing.

With her move to Wales it seems that Cobbe spent at least as much time extinguishing peripheral brush fires as she did carrying out constructive moves for her cause. Earlier in 1892, members within the VSS attempted once again to push an abolition bill through Parliament, only to meet with failure. To reasonable people, the point seemed obvious: Agitating for abolition at this time was as unrealistic as it had been a decade before. Some forces within the VSS felt that perhaps a new face on an older organization would be helpful. In May 1897, at a VSS meeting instigated by Stephen Coleridge, members changed the title of the VSS to the National Anti-Vivisection Society (NAVS).[9] Other meetings in the summer brought a change to the rules of governance and added members to the executive committee of the NAVS.[10] If Cobbe was suspicious of these changes going on in what she still considered to be her organization, it was not apparent. Then in February 1898, with Cobbe absent, Stephen Coleridge held a special council meeting to vote on a new resolution. He declared that the abolition of vivisection was still the ultimate aim of the NAVS; however, "the Society is thereby not precluded from making efforts in Parliament for lesser measures, having for their object the saving of animals from scientific torture."[11] The measure, effectively ending the practical pursuit of abolition, passed 29 to 21.

When Cobbe received the news of this radical change in policy, she angrily threatened to resign from the society and to renege on her promised financial endowment to the NAVS. Coleridge countered her protest observing that, at present, there was no hope of getting abolition legislation through Parliament. It was time to change tactics "as opposed to the hopeless sterile policy of the last twenty years." He and other members of the society admired Miss Cobbe "for her stainless and beautiful life. But at this point of our path we believe that her judgment is astray."[12] On 14 April 1898, Cobbe issued a pamphlet objecting to the NAVS's decision and to Coleridge's reference to the "sterile policy." Coleridge answered in a letter to the *Zoophilist* dated 24 April, re-asserting his views:

We have been told that to endeavour to mitigate the abominations of vivisection, during such time as its entire abolition is impossible, is a base acknowledgement of the necessity of vivisection.... The National Society can afford to regard Miss Cobbe's efforts in these directions [abolition] with perfect good will for it has never received more hearty and generous support than during the few months since it decided to abandon what I still venture to call its sterile Parliamentary tactics.[13]

Cobbe's attitude towards abolition was obviously in the minority. Sensing a deadlock, she severed all relations, leaving the society accompanied by a small coterie of friends. Conspicuously absent from Cobbe's group was her influential and trusted medical advisor, Lawson Tait, who remained with the NAVS.

Cobbe was as sad as she was angry over the split, already experiencing feelings of uselessness residing in her mountain home, far removed from the action. Here was a new and younger order taking over, ideologically less rigid and determined to wrest change through the minds within England's political structure. From her painful experiences of 1876, Cobbe knew how easily the best laid plans of people could be derailed through the Parliamentary process. She knew better than these upstarts at NAVS; the only hope for abolition rested with changing civic opinion about vivisection. Surely, once the public fully appreciated the seriousness of this scientific cruelty, they would demand change.

## Forming the BUAV

The next spring found Cobbe re-energized, planning another society committed entirely to the abolition of vivisection. Calling it the British Union for the Abolition of Vivisection (BUAV), she convened her remaining friends and supporters in Dolgelly to lay its legal foundation in early May 1898. Those present designed the BUAV to be a consortium, to act independently on local concerns, but to organize as one unit for larger national issues. This time Cobbe was wiser. The charter stated that no one could hold office unless she was totally committed to the abolition of vivisection — there would be no room for half measures, no incrementalism. Cobbe appointed herself president and packed the hierarchy of the BUAV with nieces, nephews and old supporters from the NAVS. Still, it lacked the luminaries that were so abundant in the old VSS. Despite enlisting many different antivivisection societies within its structure, the BUAV could never match the old VSS in its level of influence. Through a 10,000-pound legacy, Cobbe began publishing the *Abolitionist*, which functioned just as the *Zoophilist* had for the VSS. Borrowing the title from the anti-slavery movement, she loved the fact that just one word, *Abolitionist*, conveyed the intent of her organization.

Not one to exit NAVS quietly, Cobbe wrote a pamphlet, *Why We Have Founded the British Union for the Abolition of Vivisection*, to explain her departure from the organization. She decried "half measures." Abolition was the only reasonable course. The responsibility for her departure from NAVS rested solely with those who had changed its policy to one of restriction. Cobbe suggested that perhaps her former society's vote for restriction rather than abolition had not been a fair one. Since the members' names and how they voted had not been made public, how could anyone know if the vote had been fair or not? Predictably, when Stephen Coleridge read her pamphlet, he believed it to be a personal attack upon him. Defending himself in *Step by Step*, he called Cobbe an "irrational old woman, doomed to fail." She was "cocooned in North Wales, too isolated from Parliament and public opinion, unable to gauge the best future for, and hold credible command of the antivivisection crusade. She was illogical too, if she refused to concede to lesser measures as stepping stones for more radical ones."[14]

But given Cobbe's moral outlook, her stance was predictable. For the author of *Intuitive Morals*, reversing her lifelong positions would have been completely out of character. She complained that in the early years of the controversy, Parliament was on the side of the antivivisectionists. Now the Home Secretary is indifferent "to us while the Premier loads the most notorious Vivisectors with baronetcies and knighthoods."[15] Although she may not have expressed her angst to anyone directly at this time, she was too perceptive to overlook the signposts pointing to the defeat of her cause. The antivivisection movement sat on increasingly unstable ground, with the lapping tides of scientific progress continually eroding its base. On the other hand, experimental medicine, floating around for decades in a sea of medieval fecklessness, had fastened on to stable bedrock, gaining credulity.

The British government left little doubt concerning its faith in medical science by bringing medical theories and practices progressively into its institutions. In 1889, Parliament passed an Infectious Diseases Act, astutely avoiding the inflammatory word, "contagious." This measure ordered the head of each household to report to authorities any case of infectious disease such as smallpox, cholera, erysipelas, diphtheria, typhus, typhoid and other lesser known ailments. Even though specific chemical treatments were not available, except for smallpox and rabies prophylaxis, beneficial programs of isolation and quarantine could now be enacted with confidence, based upon solid scientific evidence.

Then in 1891, the International Congress of Hygiene and Demography, meeting in London, formally incorporated germ theory into its platform. Germ theorists were no longer marginalized, looking in from the outside. They had won their rightful place not only in science, but within these British institutions. All future public policy directed towards preventing or curing contagious diseases would be guided by the principles of that theory — a fitting recognition of the validity of bacteriology as a discipline.[16]

Cobbe's remaining years were characterized by a progressive quietude. She still contributed to the *Abolitionist*, but her days as the central figure, addressing crowds of admirers and strategizing with other antivivisectionists, were over. Even though she had lost much of her base of antivivisectionist followers, Cobbe remained a moral authority when it came to religious or feminist issues. However, as the century turned, she still devoted much of her energy pursuing her dream of abolishing vivisection. Her days were occupied by answering a steady volume of letters from all over Britain and America. Despite her ebbing strength, she continued to experience a burst of energy between 2 and 6 A.M., which she reserved for writing and corresponding. Otherwise, she spent time indulging her menagerie of old and unwanted animals, feeding bread or apples to an old pony that she had saved from the knacker's yard, or tending to her devoted Pomeranian, Browny, named after her friend and fellow dog lover, Elizabeth Barrett Browning. Much as she had done in her youth, she gained spiritual renewal in her forest sanctuaries where she observed the flora and fauna beside the tributaries of the Mawddach. As walking became more difficult with age, Cobbe often spent hours at Mary's graveside or in her verdant garden with its beautiful azaleas.

Another in a diminishing array of bright spots occurred on 4 December 1902, with the arrival of her eightieth birthday. She received a congratulatory birthday card that day signed by 346 admirers from both Britain and the United States. Prominent among the signatures were Mark Twain, Florence Nightingale and Julia Ward Howe.[17] Cobbe's heart was temporarily warmed by the good wishes of such eminent people. Another event, watching her BUAV expand, gave her some satisfaction. Still, it grew more difficult for her to maintain much sense of optimism as she witnessed the power of her pen diminish along with her ability to concentrate on topics she previously considered important.

## Cobbe's Successor

As Cobbe grew older, she realized the need for a reliable successor at the BUAV. She had heard of the physician Walter Hadwen, known all over Britain as "Hadwen of Gloucester," for his independent stand against smallpox vaccination in that city's epidemic of 1896. From afar, she had admired his independent spirit and his talents as a firebrand orator and trenchant writer, but she did not really know him. Cobbe therefore sent a private investigator to

Gloucester to learn more about the man.[18] She received nothing but good reviews. Locals described him as clever and honorable. He enjoyed a fine reputation professionally, outside of the orthodox medical community. As an innate contrarian he opposed many standard medical theories even though he had received a traditional medical education. It was almost a given that he had earned some bitter enemies. Dr. Hadwen had also edited a book, *Premature Burial and How to Prevent It*. Since Cobbe had always feared such a fate, the book must have resonated with her. After studying the man, she learned that not only was he already an antivivisectionist, he did not even subscribe to germ theory, describing it as "witchcraft — a fetish."[19] He believed that the practitioner was much wiser to rely on cleanliness and hygiene in dealing with disease. He was so independent that he did not even revere the ordinarily sacrosanct Edward Jenner, father of vaccination. Why would anyone hold Jenner in esteem? He had been Pasteur's inspiration just as Pasteur was the current guiding light of the vivisectionists. One man was no more scientifically pure than the other. To Cobbe's mind, Hadwen held all of the proper views. Confident that she had found her man, she made him honorable secretary of the BUAV. Over the ensuing years he proved as strong and reliable as she predicted, continuing to lead the BUAV long after her death. For 20 years he also edited the *Abolitionist*, anonymously and gratuitously.[20]

With a solid successor in hand, Cobbe could indulge in more personal concerns. In a 1903 letter to Sarah Wister, Cobbe spoke of her loneliness, imploring Wister to visit her. Cobbe presciently declared that it "must naturally be —, if not my last summer, but almost so. I have no reason to regret that it should be so. My 80 years have been very rich and full. Now they are poor & of no value to anybody."[21] She dreaded the cold and loneliness of the approaching Welsh winter. In an unpublished essay written early in 1904, she concluded that "the griefs of youth bring despair, for all life lies before us in which we shall suffer from them. The griefs of age bring desolation; but we know that there is only a little time in which we shall feel them."[22]

On the morning of 4 April, Cobbe arose as usual, wrote letters and enjoyed tea with a visitor. The next morning she was found dead in her bedroom. Long-time admirer, the Vicar John Verschoyle, wrote,

> On the morning of her death she rose very early in the cold gray dawn, opened the shutters to let in the light, and as she walked across the room the gates of the unseen world opened to her with the merciful swiftness that she had hoped and prayed for, and she passed the threshold, perhaps to find her loved ones waiting to receive her in the new life.[23]

On her bedside stand were telegrams to notify extended family members of her death, apparently placed there by Cobbe each night before retiring. A second one addressed to Dr. Hadwen made a specific request.[24] In her updated will she offered Hadwen 20 guineas "to perform on my body the operation of completely and thoroughly severing the arteries of the neck & windpipe (nearly severing the head altogether) so as to render my revival in the grave absolutely impossible."[25] Hadwen complied with her request.

Cobbe welcomed her departure from this world of desolation and pain. Even in death, as in life, she displayed her independence of spirit, eschewing convention. In her will she specified that her coffin not be made of oak or any more durable wood, but of something "merely sufficient" to transport her remains to the grave. She wanted no ornamentation, no inscriptions.

> I desire to be carried to Llanelltyd Cemetery not on a funeral hearse or on men's shoulders; but in one or other of my own carriages driven by my coachman, at his usual pace. And I desire that neither then nor at any time may my friends or servants wear mourning for me.[26]

The cortege was purposefully small, with mourners limited to family and old friends. A large arrangement of red roses adorned her coffin. As a cold wind blew up the valley, the Rev. J. Estlin Carpenter conducted services, reviewing Cobbe's life, her selfless devotion to feminist and humanitarian causes, and her associations with many of England's great. Backed by the strains of "Nearer My God to Thee," Cobbe was laid to rest beside her beloved life partner, Mary, completing that other half of the headstone.[27]

The Reverend Verschoyle recalled that, upon returning to Hengwrt after the services, he sensed that Cobbe's animals were "dimly conscious" that she would tend to them no longer. Her old pony, neighing, looked in all directions for his friend. Her little Pomeranian ran up and down the stairs in a futile search of each room for her mistress.[28]

Thus ended the life of one whose name was synonymous with antivivisection. To Cobbe's adversaries, who reviled her for her obstructionist and anti-scientific attitudes, it was perhaps none too soon. She had become the embodiment of blind opposition. While recognized as a forceful spokesperson for her cause, they considered her duplicitous if not untruthful to the end, one who would subvert any scientific effort in favor of lesser beings. She *did* love animals more than mankind.

But to her devoted friends and followers she would always remain heroic and selfless. Despite her triumphs for the oppressed, the ragged school children, the battered wives, the disenfranchised, she died a tragic figure. She was so dedicated to the cause that, early in her crusade, she vowed never to go to bed until she had done everything possible in the name of animal protection. Ironically, Cobbe had never asked for this job fighting the physiologists. She had hoped to spend her life in her favorite pursuit — the study of religion. After one such religious discussion with the Reverend Verschoyle, she confided to him, "Oh how different it is to think of these sublime subjects and our sad work; whenever I revert to them, or look into these books my heart yearns to dwell again in such a pure atmosphere."[29] It was by default that she heroically led the battle against a method of science she considered so cruel. No one else would do the work. She remained true to the moral scheme she had laid out over 50 years before in *Intuitive Morals*. Virtue is an act of selflessness, given without regard to any future reward. Happiness, itself, is not a goal — one's soul progresses only through virtuous acts. Although she seriously bent some rules of ethics in her pursuit of abolition, she held true to that code throughout her life.

Over time, Cobbe learned to quietly accept with resignation the fact that she would never see her antivivisection efforts bear any fruit. Only in the last days of her fading life did she confide to intimates, such as Verschoyle, her deep disappointment with the failure of her crusade. "I have sacrificed everything to it and it is a failure."[30] In her own life, Cobbe easily compartmentalized her multifaceted humanitarian efforts. However, history would grant her no such luxury, using her least illustrious facet as the major criterion — judging her harshly by the one pursuit in her life where she had given her all and failed — the abolition of vivisection. Verschoyle sensed this tragic element when he observed, "There is something infinitely pathetic to those who knew her well in the dreary discouragement of this last period of her life."[31]

Some would argue that Cobbe, with ample doses of nobility and obtuseness, had pursued the wrong ideal, tilting towards the wrong windmill. Despite her many intellectual and spiritual gifts, she, like most headstrong and tragic figures, had become a victim of her own *hamartia*, her congenital intellectual flaw. Cobbe's rigid morality was as much her undoing as it was her source of strength and security. Early in her efforts to protect animals, hers was the humane position. She fought from that moral high ground a brand of scientific medicine considered by many as crude and inhumane. But she was blinded by an immutable sense of that moral security, combined with a visceral hatred of vivisection. In her world, science should ever burn in the shadow of religion. Untempered by religion, the materialistic science of medicine could never evolve into anything altruistic. To her own peril, she refused to reevaluate the scientists' gains or to reconsider her own moral or scientific views. Under her own unseeing eyes, science had metamorphosed from its early primitive and cruel condition to a state of beneficence. It had evolved into mankind's greatest hope for combating the scourges of disease. Guilty of tragic oversight, Cobbe failed to recognize those warning tremors signaling a tectonic shift — a complete reversal of positions. In the new order, science reigned. Cobbe, the tragic figure, had evolved into the personification of "Fanatic and Obscurant."

# X

# Update

"Science must go on and on, seeking for more. It is the lack of knowledge that makes the world unhappy, not the converse. In the pursuit of knowledge concerning the human race, the lower creatures are lending their help." — James Peter Warbasse[1]

CHAPTER 22

# Science Must Go On and On

During the height of the 1874 agitation to control experimentation, Edwin Lankester, the pro-vivisectionist zoologist, made both an unwise and impolitic statement in a letter to the *Spectator*. His utterance would be exploited repeatedly by the antivivisectionists. "If you allow experiment at all, you must admit the more of it the better, since it is very certain that for many years to come the problems of physiology demanding experimental solution will increase in something like geometrical ratio, instead of decreasing."[1] He could not have had any idea just how prescient his statement would prove to be. In 1880, 311 medical experiments were performed in Britain. By 1910, the figure had increased to 95,731 and by 1938, to 958,761.[2] Today, in both Britain and the U.S., many millions of animals, primarily mice and rats, are used annually for biomedical experimentation (BME), to say nothing of the numbers used in toxicological studies, cosmetic research, and agribusiness.

While the use of experimental animals continued to increase, the antivivisection movement passed into a period of comparative dormancy related to the two world wars. Around mid-century, the antivivisectionist effort resurfaced, but in a different, more broadly based form. The term "animal rights activist" (ARA) gave a more accurate representation of their concerns. Activists began questioning the use of animals not only for BME, but for other enterprises such as toxicity testing for drugs and cosmetics, and industries producing such items as fur and leather. The admittedly poor living conditions of all animals raised for their meat proved to be an easy target as well. While these ancillary forms of animal use may still remain a cultural concern, for the sake of this argument, I will limit consideration to the subject of this work — biomedical research, both basic and applied.

As the 1950s rolled into the '60s and '70s, the social turbulence caused by a divisive war produced a general mood of rebellion. In the more libertine era that followed, people questioned all established norms, traditional religion, cultural mores and the entire Western way of life. While Cobbe's Victorian movement had been propelled mainly by evangelical Christians, the current animal rights movement sprang from a more secular origin. Current advocates tend to reject traditional Western philosophical thought as it relates to human relationships with animals. It was into such an environment, in 1975, that Australian Peter Singer, animal rights philosopher, entered the American scene with his seminal work, *Animal Liberation*. Singer proclaimed that all animals, including humankind, are equal, and it is only "the selfish desire to preserve the privileges of the exploiting group — for refusing to extend the basic principle of equality of consideration to members of other species."[3] By resurrecting some old opinions dating back to Humphry Primatt, Singer provided a new template for contemporary animal advocates grappling with what they perceived as a great problem — the unfair exploitation of animals by humans. Over the ensuing 40 years, their war on scientific experimentation has continued unabated. A variety of animal rights activists and theorists have emerged, all of whom possess views differing from the traditional relationship of man and animal.

## Roger Scruton

It is useful to examine the traditional Western philosophical view of the human/animal relationship to better understand where the ARAs parted from it. Modern philosophical theory concerning animal ethics has existed, minimally unchanged, since the time of Aristotle. The later advent of Christian dogma, placing man at the head of the animal world, naturally melded in well with the older philosophical views, fortifying it further. I have extracted the following scheme from the philosopher Roger Scruton, who articulates well the traditional view in the animal rights debate.

Western philosophy evolved, over centuries, into a structure of moral or natural law that guided mankind in society. With respect to human-animal relationships, that traditional structure remained essentially unchallenged until the 1960s. Humanity accepted this code so broadly that its principles even served as a pattern for our modern legal systems. For a person to be morally relevant, he must be rational, that is, he must possess the ability to reason, and to make judgments between good and bad. He must also be a free agent, capable of assessing different options and making informed decisions of his own free will. A rational being must not only possess the ability of self-recognition (self-consciousness), but also have a moral perspective — the capacity of seeing himself within a greater moral community.

In belonging to this moral community, each rational entity possesses rights which are inviolate and universally respected by others within the community. These rights can be taken away only with that being's permission. Along with rights come the equally important obligations, both to other moral beings within the community and to certain causes, such as justice. In following the principle of moral equality, the considerations which justify or impugn one person will, in identical circumstances, justify or impugn another. For the moral community to function under this natural law, each being must uphold the following principles:

- Rights are to be respected.
- Obligations are to be fulfilled.
- Agreements are to be honored.
- Disputes are to be settled by rational argument, not by force.
- Persons who do not respect the rights of others forfeit rights of their own.[4]

## Richard Ryder

Scruton, the American philosopher Carl Cohen and others have described such a moral framework as it relates to animals, but not all agree with such a scheme. Among the earliest dissenters from this traditional view was Richard Ryder, British psychologist. In 1969, he began his quest to rid the world of what he considered an evil—"speciesism." His book, *Victims of Science*, opens by declaring man to be just one animal species existing among many others. All of the traits defining man as different from animals, such as superior intelligence, are morally irrelevant. "For too long man has arrogantly exaggerated his uniqueness."[5]

Ryder believes that both man and animal have the capacity to suffer equally and therefore each is in the "same moral category." When it comes to a consideration of species, he argues that the entire classification system is one of "descriptive convenience," based upon appearance.[6]

> I use the word "speciesism" to describe the widespread discrimination that is practiced by man against the other species, and to draw a parallel with racism. Speciesism and racism are both forms of prejudice that are based upon appearances—if the other individual looks different then he is rated as being beyond the moral pale.... Speciesism and racism (and indeed sexism) overlook or underestimate the similarities between the discriminator and those discriminated against and both forms of prejudice show a selfish disregard for the interests of others, and for their sufferings.[7]

To further his argument, Ryder invokes the British evolutionary biologist Richard Dawkins and his view of the human fetus. Completely ignoring the developmental potential existing within every human fetus, Dawkins, in *The Selfish Gene*, states:

> A human foetus, with no more human feeling than an omoeba, enjoys a reverence and legal protection far in excess of those granted to an adult chimpanzee. Yet the chimp feels and thinks and — according to recent experimental evidence — may even be capable of learning a form of human language. The foetus belongs to our own species, and is instantly accorded special privileges and rights because of it.[8]

Other representatives of the ARAs including Ingrid Newkirk, founder of PETA, have made similarly irreverent statements, equating all species with the simple statement, "A rat is a pig is a dog is a boy." Michael Fox, former senior scholar of the Humane Society of the United States (HSUS), expresses a similar sentiment with "the life of an ant and the life of my child should be granted equal consideration."[9]

## Peter Singer

Just as Ryder is identified with the concept of speciesism, the idea of equal consideration of species is more associated with Peter Singer. He elevates sub-human species based more upon philosophically utilitarian lines. It is only man's "selfish desire to preserve the privileges of the exploiting group" that prohibits the extension of equality to members of other species.[10] Singer then takes a slightly different slant than Ryder, by declaring all beings equal, relying heavily on parallels from racial and women's rights movements. Just because a difference exists between two beings does not mean that they are not equal and deserving of equality, he argues. Women have the right to vote because they are as capable of making a rational decision as are men. Lower beings, such as dogs, are not as capable of making that decision and therefore cannot have the right to vote. To say that men and women are very similar and that dogs and humans are very different explains their possession or lack of possession of rights. But Singer claims that those differences are insufficient for denying rights to lower animals. Men and women have different rights, such as the right to an abortion, something granted to women but not to men. "Since a man cannot have an abortion, it is meaningless to talk of his right to have one. Since dogs can't vote, it is meaningless to talk of their right to vote."[11] Singer asserts that granting the principle of equality to two different groups does not mean that they must be treated in exactly the same way. He claims that the concept of equality does not mean identical *treatment* of an individual, but rather identical *consideration*. But traditionalists would argue that if a being deserves equal consideration, he should inherently receive equal treatment. Separating the two is tantamount to cleaving one from his shadow.

To my view, Singer grants equal weight where he should not. Two analogous reproductive functions between genders — the ability to get pregnant or not, cannot be given the same polemical weight as two hierarchical functions between two species — the differing mental capacities for understanding or not understanding the vote. Singer has equated two "equal" but differing capacities based upon genders within a species, with two "unequal" abilities between human and nonhuman. He and Ryder accuse the scientific side of displaying prejudice against animals. However, the scientific side could just as easily charge them with bias against humankind. Blurring or dissolving that natural interface existing between human and animal species is their intent. In their zeal to protect animals, they aim to destroy those privileges currently enjoyed by humans. Both claim to desire equal consideration between species, but equal treatment appears to be their aim.

In *Animal Liberation*, Singer expresses one last concern about animals enduring pain during biomedical experimentation. He cites scientific authorities who claim that animals do indeed, experience pain, a fact already evident. Except for their cerebral cortex, Singer claims, the nervous systems of animals are "remarkably similar" to ours.[12] That is analogous to claiming that a Model T Ford is "nearly identical" to a modern Mercedes Benz. Putting that point aside — do animals experience pain to the same degree as do humans? Singer would seem to answer in the affirmative, since, "there can be no moral justification for regarding the pain (or pleasure) that animals feel as less important than the same amount of pain (or pleasure) felt by humans."[13] Singer places infants and retarded humans in the same moral category with nonhumans, which allows him to then inquire: If one is to allow painful experiments on nonhuman animals,

> we have to ask ourselves whether we are also prepared to allow experiments on human infants and retarded adults; and if we make a distinction between animals and these humans, on what basis can we do it, other than a bare-faced — and morally indefensible — preference for members of our own species?[14]

## Tom Regan

Another philosopher reasoning along the same lines is North Carolina State University professor Tom Regan. He argues for the abolition of all forms of animal exploitation, including animal agriculture, the fur industry and any scientific experimentation involving animals.[15] As we shall see later, through some detailed philosophical apologetics, Regan concludes that all sentient animals possess rights on the same level as do humans. No one, including the medical researcher, is "morally authorized to override the *basic rights* of others" no matter how laudable his purpose.[16] A "science that routinely harms animals in pursuit of its goals is morally corrupt."[17] Regan dismisses utilitarianism by declaring that a scientist cannot justify harming a single rat by citing the benefit society might derive from such research.[18]

Regan declares that animals have rights on par with humans because his entire position rests upon that claim. He begins by agreeing with the views of Immanuel Kant, 17th-century German philosopher, but he later parts from Kant's line of reasoning. Just like the modern scheme of Scruton, Kant taught that, for living organisms to warrant rights, they must be morally responsible, that is, they must be both sentient and capable of making decisions freely concerning both moral obligations and rights within a moral community. Since animals are not moral agents, in Kant's scheme they cannot possess rights. Consequently, he believed that the world could be divided into "persons and things," or as Regan states, "somebodies and somethings."[19] By Kant's reasoning, animals belong in the "things" category. Continuing with this line of reasoning, Regan argues that, even under Kant's scheme, demented humans, such as the anencephalic, are not free moral agents and therefore do not possess the same rights as normal humans. Anencephalics theoretically lie in that grey zone between species — less than a person but more than a thing. By exploiting this nebulous status of the impaired human, Regan gains a new polemical handle. He resolves this exclusion of the mentally impaired from moral agency by building a new, all-inclusive philosophical scheme. Regan argues for a new category of being called "subjects-of-a-life." His scheme excludes plants but includes most living beings since such organisms are sentient, "experiential," and are "somebodies." In short, any "being with a biography" belongs in this category.[20]

But with this one devolutionary step, Regan has bypassed considerations of whether a being is a human or an animal. By creating this new, more generic entity, Regan has rendered superfluous any distinctions that might exist between the two categories, human and animals. To individuals, such as ARAs, who believe that mentally incompetent humans have been wrongly excluded from the moral community, this new entity may appear to be a desirable concept, since all humans, both normal and demented, now belong within this new entity. But if one allows the mentally blighted human into this new circle, then intellectual consistency demands that he allow the sentient animal in as well, since they also fit the criteria of the "subjects-of-a-life" category. All experiential beings, such as mammals, even birds, suddenly fit into this new "subjects-of-a-life" category. By inventing a more generic definition, Regan has accomplished his goal of combining humans and sentient animals into the same category where, by "definition," they can all be declared equal. The net effect of Regan's reasoning is the lowering of normal humans into a category in which, to his reasoning, both animals and demented humans belong. It is critical to his argument to have all such entities above included in this new taxonomic entity because, per his scheme, every being within that category has inherent value.[21] Suddenly, all beings within that circle are equal and have rights. By using the mentally blighted human being as a common link between normal humans and the less intelligent animal, Regan has managed to "equate" them all — humans and animals.

It is only through interpreting traditional logic differently that ARAs such as Regan, Ryder and Singer are able to justify their agenda of terminating animal experimentation. In their zeal to grant equality to all beings, each is overly generous to nonhumans and excessively parsimonious to mankind. Their views are every bit as much anti-human as they are pro-animal. By superimposing in mirror-image fashion, the extreme right side of the nonhuman bell-shaped curve onto the extreme left hand side of the human bell-shaped curve, they can then declare those two bell-shaped curves as being essentially super-imposable. They compare the least able of humans to the most able of nonhumans and, not surprisingly, find them nearly equal.

## Declaration of Great Apes

So far, all arguments in favor of limiting the use of animals for research could be considered philosophical in nature. However, another threat to BME comes from at least two legal sources. Their stances are arguably even more threatening than the philosophical ones in that, if the legal principles were ever enacted, it could, in one stroke, become the law of the land by judicial fiat. The first of these is the Great Ape Project, introduced in 1993, by Singer and an Italian philosopher, Paola Cavalieri. Backed by such ARAs as Jane Goodall and Richard Dawkins, they present *A Declaration of Great Apes*, defining a "community of equals," that is, a moral community to which, at present, only human beings belong. Singer and his group "demand" that not only humans but all great apes, such as chimpanzees, gorillas and orangutans, be included in this community of equals. Their declaration asserts that anyone residing within this community has the protections of:

- The Right to Life: No member may be killed except for very rigidly defined reasons.
- The Protection of Individual Liberty: No individual may be imprisoned without due legal process. Only if the individual is a danger to himself or to his community can this rule be circumvented.

- The Prohibition of Torture: Torture is wrong. It is defined as the deliberate infliction of severe pain "either wantonly or for the alleged benefit of others."[22]

Clearly this group of activists considers animals to be every bit as morally relevant as humans. But are they justified in making such a declaration? Even the most sentient of primates has no concept of a legal right, let alone an obligation. Do chimpanzees know how to honor an agreement or settle a dispute through rational discourse? In reality, even the most highly evolved sub-human primates mete out their code of justice by some variation of "might makes right." Obviously, these non-human primates are incapable of existing within the traditional moral community — that is, without someone else representing them.

But lack of representation would not appear to pose a problem for Singer's group. If they are successful, these animals will be provided lawyers to articulate their grievances in court. Presumably a scientist could be charged with murder if an ape died during the course of an experiment, unless the scientist had strictly followed the rigidly defined criteria expounded in the *Declaration of Great Apes*. Their second rule against imprisonment appears to grant the condition of *habeas corpus* to animals, carrying with it the prolonged and expensive sequence of legal maneuvers currently available only to humans. Equally disturbing, in the Prohibition of Torture clause, is the activists' deliberate inclusion of the phrase "for the alleged benefit of others," aimed specifically at experimental scientists. If these edicts ever become law, a lethal chill will blow through scientific communities, bringing much valuable work to a halt. The Great Ape Project might begin with apes, but it will incrementally spread to include many other species if the ARAs ever achieve their first step.

## Gary Francione

The second legal argument against animal use is one espoused by Gary Francione, animal rights theorist. After seeing his views expounded below, the reader might think that Francione's theory could just be summarily dismissed, but it is not that easy. He enjoys a certain level of moral authority within the animal advocacy movement. As a Rutgers Law School professor, he has an ample platform for expounding upon his views. Francione's scheme is even more pernicious than the Great Ape Project because of the completeness of the changes mandated under his plan. He argues that all of the evils associated with animal exploitation originate from one human attitude: We consider animals to be our things or property. For support, he cites the 19th-century British philosopher and legal scholar Jeremy Bentham, who proclaimed that all animals are sentient. Since they are sentient, all are also morally significant.[23] Therefore, it is imperative that we, as humans, treat animals with more respect. Even though Bentham's views already form the basis of our Western legal criminal code for animal treatment, the philosopher did not go far enough for Francione. In the early 1800s, when Bentham was promulgating his legal theories, he should have challenged society's long-held tradition of considering animals as property. In any dispute over rights, if animals are considered to be mere possessions, the odds will always be stacked against them. The owners will always win, Francione argues. Echoing the other ARAs, he also believes that animals will only stand a chance of being treated equally when they are able to enter that moral community currently reserved exclusively for humans.

Francione's prescription for correcting this problem is on par with Regan, and even more draconian than those of Ryder or Singer. He considers all forms of human activity involving the use of animals, when considered in relation to the rights of that animal, to be comparatively trivial and therefore unjustified. Nothing but total abolition of all such activities will solve the problem. Any enterprise in which animals comprise the essential element must be abolished, including the meat industry, rodeos, racing, horseback riding, circuses, any many types of toxicological and cosmetic testing, as well as biomedical experimentation (BME). The changes forced upon society would be so destabilizing that the Western way of life would cease to exist. Cattle and sheep ranches would become a thing of the past. Shearing sheep, an atrocity to the ARAs, would be prohibited. Perhaps few would lament the disappearance of pig farms or chicken and turkey enterprises, considering their aroma, but they too would be gone forever. If Francione's plan were ever fully enacted, all humans would eventually be forced to adopt veganism, forgoing not only meat but also all dairy products such as eggs, milk and cheese. Since eating all flesh is a transgression in Francione's scheme, the existence of fish hatcheries or ocean industries that gather fish and sea food could no longer be justified. Leather and fur industries would become a distant memory. Sport hunters and fishermen would have to look for less "cruel" pursuits, never mind that such hunts often serve a purpose by trimming overgrown herds.

Francione questions whether society might ever be justified in treating animals in a manner different from man. Citing Charles Darwin and cognitive ethologists for support, he argues that animals and man differ only quantitatively, not qualitatively. All sentient species possess the same qualities; we just differ in the quantity of that characteristic accorded to each. To Francione, man's facility with calculus and other mental gymnastics are no better inherently than an animal's superior perception of scents, or its ability to fly. Human traits are only better because we dominant humans deem them to be.[24] Therefore, he asks: If no qualitative differences exist between species, why do we think it is morally acceptable to use nonhumans in experiments while we exclude humans?[25]

Francione's claim that no qualitative inter-species differences exist is certainly an arguable point. Even though his claim might not withstand closer scrutiny, let us assume for a moment that it is true — all differences are merely quantitative, not qualitative. Quantitative discrepancies in skills between species, if sufficiently great, should still count as a valid criterion for determining how one considers or treats them. ARAs, with their anthropomorphic point of view, frequently romanticize the comparatively limited intellectual skills of animals, while ignoring if not denigrating man's more highly developed intellect. These advocates celebrate the great ape's simplest use of sign language for a primitive form of communication, or their use of rudimentary tools, such as twigs, to drag out insects from underneath bark. At the same time, ARAs barely mention man's great triumphs — human accomplishments so great when compared to that of even the most highly evolved sub-human primates (SHP) that it is analogous to equating a cave-bound existence to a life spent soaring in the stratosphere. Only man possesses sufficient brain power to elevate inductive reasoning to the levels of a Newton or a Darwin, moving humanity forward with revolutionary generalizations. When one weighs human accomplishment against the best that animals can achieve, the differences are so profound that it becomes academic as to whether the defining characteristics of species are qualitative or quantitative. Equating man and chimpanzee by minimizing human accomplishment while romanticizing animal sentience is not a tenable argument.

It is extremely difficult to accurately assess quantitative differences between species in, for example, intelligence because of the uncertainties inherent in experimental design. As philosopher Niall Shanks observes in his book, *Animals and Science*, any experiments that assess animal cognition must be tightly controlled to exclude experimental artifacts, such as the Clever Hans effect.[26] Clever Hans was a horse with seemingly amazing computing skills. Using one hoof to tap out the correct answer to all forms of arithmetic, he was correct nearly 90 percent of the time, vexing the skeptics in the crowd. It took a panel of experts to finally discover how the horse determined the number of taps to make to deliver the correct answer. It was not the horse's facility with numbers that led to the right response. He could sense an unconscious tension in his handler's body language, giving the horse a clue as to when to stop his tapping. Citing the work of several experimental psychologists, Shanks asserts that, if one rigidly excludes such experimental artifacts, accords equal weight to unsuccessful as well as successful responses, eschews anecdotal data, field observations and "untutored common sense," the cognitive performance of even the highest of the SHPs falls off dramatically. Uncertainty of explication exists as well. Even under the most ideal of conditions, different scientists, while observing the same experimental data, will occasionally render varying interpretations and arrive at differing conclusions.[27]

## Qualitative Differences?

Further refuting the claims of Francione and other ARAs, there is some evidence that a qualitative difference between species does exist and that it is centered upon facility with language. As explained by Shanks, researchers such as E.M. Macphail claim that a "Cognitive Trinity" exists within the animal kingdom, consisting of feeling-consciousness, self-consciousness and the ability to use language.[28] Only man clearly possesses all three of these qualities. Although the higher SHPs exhibit comparatively sophisticated methods of communication, their best representatives, chimpanzees, cannot use language even remotely comparable to a human for several reasons. They possess neither the appropriate neural circuitry nor sufficiently developed peripheral speech apparatus, such as tongue and larynx, to allow for speech. Without even considering differing forms of consciousness between species, one could argue that facility with language alone meets the standard of a qualitative interspecies difference.

Macphail further contends that a cognitive discontinuity separates humans from both SHPs and pre-verbal children.[29] In all probability, a language-specific organ exists within the human nervous system, analogous to a language chip in a computer, that accounts for this discontinuity.[30]

Consciousness, the other consideration besides language, is of two types. First is feeling-consciousness, the subjective or affective awareness of internal emotions, such as pleasure or pain and suffering. The other, self-consciousness, is objective — the awareness of self in an outer world. It is most commonly discerned by an organism's ability to recognize itself in a mirror. Even among SHPs, only the chimpanzee, bonobo (pygmy chimp) and the orangutan have this ability. While many animals are feeling-conscious, most are not self-conscious.[31]

Consciousness and facility with language are useful criteria for differentiating cognitive abilities between species. They provide some guidance to the person in a laboratory setting pondering the question as to whether it is moral or not to use animals in scientific experimentation. No matter how rigid or loose the experimental controls may be, it is difficult to make accurate generalizations about the existence or non-existence of self-consciousness or feeling-consciousness. In this regard, Shanks speaks of the principle of cognitive charity.[32] No scientist has yet proved that animals do not possess consciousness. Until such factors are certain enough to allow for definite conclusions, he argues that it is prudent to err on the side of benevolence, giving animals the benefit of the doubt.

## Jeremy Bentham

Shanks suggests that we consider animals as possessing moral status consistent with the views of Jeremy Bentham. Choosing Bentham's moderate views as a guide is not an unreasonable choice. His position lies between the more radical contemporary animal rights theorists, such as Singer, and the 18th-century philosopher Immanuel Kant. Kant believed that only humans are capable of belonging to a moral community. When it came to judging whether an act was moral or immoral, he considered the motive behind that act to be the prime determinant between evil and good. But Bentham, arriving on the scene 50 years later, took a different tack. One of his famous statements concerned animals and vivisection. "The question is not, Can they reason? Nor, Can they talk? But, Can they suffer?"[33] He considered it irrelevant whether an animal was capable of behaving morally towards another. The question was rather, "How should humans treat any being of any species capable of experiencing pain and suffering?" Bentham asserted that all living creatures are subject to two morally relevant characteristics — pleasure and pain.[34] In determining whether an act is moral or not, he employed a "Felicific Calculus" in which the pleasures and pains of a particular act were quantified in juxtaposition. One arrived at a net result only after adding up the opposing columns. If good outweighed bad, he concluded that the act was morally good.

Since all sub-human sentient creatures experience pleasure and pain, they were morally relevant in Bentham's eyes. They should therefore reside within the moral community. Bentham's actions, however, suggest something different. He only partially included animals in the moral community since he defended slaughtering them for their meat — the infliction of pain and suffering *with a purpose.* In his own words, animals "had none of those long-protracted anticipations of future misery" to which humans were subject.[35] He clearly viewed animals as existing at a lower level of morality than humans. In effect he allowed animals to partially reside within the moral community — one foot in and one foot out.

Still, Bentham, a utilitarian, clearly did not sanction wanton cruelty, that is, the deliberate infliction of pain and suffering with no purpose except for the entertainment of the perpetrator. Considering the above, it would appear that Bentham's attitude allowed for the act of vivisection as long as it was carried out with a distinct purpose in mind, and in as painless and humane a manner as possible. But Bentham was also a consequentialist — he took the resultant good or bad consequences of an act into consideration. Robert Koch's work with tuberculosis was so momentous that he received the Nobel Prize in 1905. Before his efforts conquered tuberculosis, approximately one in every seven deaths in the developed world was attributable to the disease. Although he undeniably made guinea pigs, cattle and sheep suffer by the hundreds if not by the thousands, it would be difficult for one to defend a charge that Koch's "cruel" acts outweighed the ultimate good of solving man's greatest scourge.

In that same vein, another contemporary philosopher, arguably the most important to the current debate is Bernard E. Rollin, Ph.D. He recently added to his prolific list of works with his intelligent and witty book *Putting the Horse Before Descartes*. Rollin has spent his entire career on the faculty of Colorado State University School of Veterinary Medicine fighting for more humane treatment of all animals used in agriculture, industry and scientific research. Unlike the other philosophers above, Rollin's positions are more difficult to refute. His efforts have resulted in many improvements in animal care, some as prosaic as employing anesthetics during castration or getting rid of confining cages for livestock and poultry. Others are more estimable such as making euthanasia a less onerous experience by ensuring that animals slip into a symptomless coma from true hypoxia rather than suffering the agonies associated with an excess of carbon dioxide.[36]

Rollin has been a prime force in bringing Institutional Animal Care and Use Committees (IACUC) into operation.[37] It was through his determination that legislation amending the Animal Welfare Act passed in 1985. Another law, the National Institutes of Health Reauthorization Bill forced the NIH to enforce the provisions of animal welfare legislation, giving teeth to previously empty rhetoric.[38]

Through invoking the old Greek concept of *telos* (the unique nature of each organism) into his argument, Rollin's line of reasoning makes eminent sense. Not only humans but animals possess natures, "a unique set of functions, needs, and interests specific to each kind of animal — the 'pigness' of a pig, the 'dogness' of a dog." Every being of all species deserves to live up to their full potential — to self-actualize. With humans it is our natures that determine our possession of rights, granting us legal and moral protections. Similarly, animals deserve analogous protections corresponding to their degree of nature. Rollin asserts that "we should also protect the fundamental interests of animals as dictated by their *telos* even as we use them."[39] I am not aware of Rollin protesting the use of animals for science or other uses. In fact, he has worked in concert with abattoir owners, scientists and cattlemen to improve conditions for the animals in their charge. Much like the Bentham of old, Rollin appears to accept the fate of animals in science and the meat industry, objecting only to the manner in which animals are used or misused by humans.

Other ARAs, such as Francione, unrealistically criticize the practice of extrapolating data acquired from animals and applying it to humans, asserting that it "would still be more efficacious to use humans as experimental subjects," thus obviating any need for extrapolation.[40] Similarly, Regan argues that using animals in place of humans offers "very little hope of benefits for humanity because of the by-now well-established difficulty of extrapolating results from animals [sic] tests to the species *Homo sapiens*."[41] It must be only among the ARAs that such misinformation is "well-established." As the preceding chapters attest, medical history is replete with examples of great scientific progress resulting from just such extrapolations.

But contemporary readers not already convinced would probably not be swayed by further examples from the modern era, such as the development of polio vaccine in the mid–20th century, or the modern advances in HIV-AIDS research. Such projects have relied heavily on monkeys in particular. In the area of basic research, there is the work of Dr. Eric Kandel and his elucidation of the chemical changes explaining the acquisition of short- and long-term memory. His discovery of how memory forms, including the role of protein synthesis in long-term memory, is truly epochal. One would be accurate in asserting that his subject, *Aplysia californica*, the giant marine snail, is barely sentient.[42] Still, as experimental successes mount, the natural progression in subjects beyond *Aplysia* would be inevitably up the phylogenetic scale, ultimately to primates.

## Legislation

Legislation regulating animal research has also progressed immensely over the past 50 years. Animal welfare advocates, despite their anti-scientific outlook, have contributed positively to the general debate by helping to force the issue of humane treatment to the forefront, thereby elevating public consciousness. Similarly, they have helped contribute positively in the passage of legislation favorable to experimental animals. Since their animal welfare act of 1876, Britain has continued to lead the world in legislation aimed at minimizing painful exploitation of animals used in experimentation. Parliament followed with more modern and detailed regulations in the 1960s. In the U.S., similar laws establishing the regulatory structure have been passed, most notably in 1966, but the subsequent Health Research Extension Act of 1985 (Animal Welfare Act) has been the most comprehensive. The Office of Laboratory Animal Welfare (OLAW) administers the plan according to the concept of Animal Welfare Assurance. A tract, *Guidelines for the Proper Care and Treatment of Animals*, serves as the organization's Bible.[43] By law, any institution planning to maintain facilities for carrying out experiments must establish an Institutional Animal Care and Use Committee (IACUC) to oversee its functions. This committee, made up of at least one veterinarian, one active scientist, one nonscientist and one person with no other formal affiliation with the institution, ensures that all laboratory personnel are adequately trained in animal care and that a veterinarian administers care through all phases of an experimental process. In addition, IACUC must report to its parent institution biannually and to OLAW once per year. Prior to any experiment the scientist must submit a complete description of her project, including the number and type of species used. Assurance must be given to the committee that she will use the minimum number of animals in the most efficient and painless manner possible. The experimenter must also provide an outline specifying the drugs and dosages planned for pre-operative sedation, anesthetic agents to be used, and the post-operative treatment plan if long-term survival for the animal is planned. IACUC is empowered to shut down the entire experimental program if its members feel that the institution does not measure up to OLAW standards.

As if those regulations were insufficient, another private, non-governmental organization, the Association for the Assessment and Accreditation of Laboratory Animal Care (AAALAC), conducts, as its name implies, thorough inspections of facilities in which animal experimentation is practiced.[44] Institutions seek AAALAC out as a sort of underwriters laboratory for institutions involved in research. Its seal of approval gives outside institutions, unfamiliar with a particular facility, assurance that the program in question is run professionally and humanely.

## The Three Rs

Scientists can minimize animal suffering by continuously improving their own level of expertise and the environment in which they work. A practical guidebook, *The Principles of Humane Experimental Technique*, written in 1959 by W.M.S. Russell and R.L. Burch, expound upon this topic. After making a systematic study of British laboratory practices, these two men suggested that scientists could reduce the "inhumanity" of vivisection by practicing the "three Rs," that is, replacement, reduction and refinement.[45] In any experiment, wherever scientists might *replace* sentient animals with less sensitive experimental material, they should do so. Utilization of tissue culture techniques in place of animals in such disciplines as virology or cancer research is just one such example. Secondly, a scientist can *reduce* the number of animals he uses by carefully following "deductively inspired research" rather than trial-and-error strategies.[46] Claude Bernard was as shining an example of the former as Francois Magendie was of the latter. Experimental *refinement*, the most difficult goal to achieve, can be accomplished on multiple fronts by becoming a better scientist. With time and effort, one improves his technique by becoming a better surgeon, by minimizing infections and by using better instrumentation. A scientist who keeps abreast of pharmacological advances can better treat his subjects before, during and after operations.[47] Over the decades, more potent analgesics and better paralyzing agents have undoubtedly decreased the mental stress and physical pain associated with an operative procedure. Newer pre-operative medications that chemically ablate memory, erasing it for as much as an hour or two before an operation (retrograde amnesia), can even wipe away any recollection of the experiment.

Science must continue to use animals to exploit the biological systems they possess in common with man — systems available only in living animals, whether it be their immune or nervous systems, their respiratory reflexes, their genomes or another of their myriad bodily functions. Scientists should, as ARAs suggest, use animal substitutes such as computerized systems as mockups of the biological systems they are studying, if it is at all possible. But how can one build a complex biologic system when he does not fully comprehend the system that he is learning about in the first place? Could Pasteur have built some artificial immune system for vaccine production when he was empirically using an animal's immune system to fashion his vaccines? Pasteur could crudely manipulate the systems for effect, but, despite his genius, by modern standards he had a marginal understanding of how the immune system actually functioned. Similarly, in contemporary times, when scientists delete and interject genetic particles into chromosomes in the study of disease, they are merely introducing variables into a process. They must still rely upon incompletely understood actions of those genes to carry their processes on to their natural end.

Since experimentation advances the human condition, science must go on and on with the use of animals. Although the public's level of consciousness regarding the humane treatment of experimental animals has been elevated with time, the essence of the debate has not changed. It is the same argument Huxley made 140 years ago when he stated, "I would sacrifice a hecatomb of dogs tomorrow if I thought I could thereby cure a single epileptic or paralytic man."[48] Selecting a few animals to sacrifice for science propels society forward by eradicating disease and minimizing pain and suffering throughout the animal kingdom.

Will experimental scientists and animal rights activists ever come to an understanding — some sort of truce? If the ARAs are successful in their drive, animal experimentation will cease, along with much of medical progress. If science can be allowed to evolve further, a better, more natural solution will be realized. Consider how far medicine has progressed in 200 years, resulting almost entirely from animal experimentation. In the early 1800s, scientists, still clinging in the humoral theory, sought answers primarily through dissection of the dead body. They then progressed to the study of function in the living animal, establishing both germ and cell theories in the process. Scientists were still bound to that microscopic cell for explaining vital phenomena until late in the 19th century. Although molecular biology and genome science date back to the late 1800s, for all practical purposes both came of age in the latter half of the 20th century. The focus on disease is already changing from organs and cells to events occurring on a molecular basis. Disease causation and progression is even now viewed more and more on a molecular or atomic basis. In the emerging field of nanoscience Heinrich Rohrer and Gerd Binning have recently developed the scanning probe microscope which allows control of atom-sized particles by the human hand.[49] Manipulation of the atom is thus becoming a feasible act.

The union of several evolving scientific fields, such as molecular medicine and nanotechnology, is already changing how scientists investigate and treat human illness. That old tension between animal exploitation and scientific discovery, something that Darwin felt so acutely, will likely become an archaic remnant of the past. Diseases and their treatment will be understood and manipulated, not per organ systems, but along molecular or atomic lines, changing the paradigm of animal experimentation, rendering much of contemporary methods superfluous. Only in limited areas such as basic physiological research would it remain necessary. With the emphasis shifting to the cell nucleus, simply drawing blood or biopsying the tissue in question will likely represent the next iteration of "vivisection." Such developments will hopefully bring animal experimentation of the past and present to a natural terminus, and with it, a well-deserved end to the confrontation between animal rights activists and experimentalists.

# Epilogue

"More lives could be saved and suffering stopped by educating people on the importance of avoiding fat and cholesterol, the dangers of smoking, reducing alcohol and other drug consumption, exercising regularly, and cleaning up the environment than by all the animal tests in the world."[1] This quote appeared on an August 2011 PETA website posing the question, "Does Animal Experimentation Save Human Lives?" However well-intentioned, the statement not only misses the point about animal experimentation entirely, it is also misleading for a number of reasons. It suggests that animal testing, whether aimed at basic experimentation or toxicological testing, is unnecessary if only we carried out all of the listed preventive measures properly, ignoring the fact that the knowledge behind these preventive measures was gained principally through animal experimentation. The statement also implies that the two health measures, prevention and experimentation, are mutually exclusive — we can perform one or the other, but not both. Similarly misleading, overtly untrue or inaccurate statements are made by such advocates on the internet, in newspapers and in broadcast media on a regular basis.

It is not surprising that a certain amount of ambivalence or confusion about the animal welfare debate exists with the public at large. Readers cannot possibly know what goes on behind closed laboratory doors, nor can they possess reliable means to verify the claims made by partisans from the scientific or animal welfare side. To those interested in seeing animals treated humanely, it is useful to have a credo built upon facts rather than half-truths and emotion — a working set of beliefs concerning a debate that has raged on for nearly 200 years.

Stating the obvious: Many animals are sentient beings. Their sentience varies in accordance with their position within the evolutionary spectrum — from near-vegetative in the lowest forms to highly sensate in sub-human primates (SHPs). Such sensitivity applies not only to what animals perceive generally, but also how they experience pleasure or endure pain and suffering.

Even among the highest SHPs, mental capacities of animals fall far below that of humans. Animal rights activists (ARAs) should not struggle to elevate animals to the same level as humans, just to fit some preconceived scheme of inter-species fairness. Animals should be appreciated for what they are in their own right, intelligent beings entitled to respect. In the distant past, they were undeniably treated badly, not only by scientists but by the general public — a reflection of general human attitudes of the time.

Experimental scientists have just as much right to explore natural phenomena of the biological world, to pursue their own *telos*, as do astronomers, geologists, or chemists who study the physical sciences. Such a right includes the pursuit of basic physiological principles, the application of those principles to treat diseases, as well as the right to teach the principles to others. Because of the sensitivity of their subjects, however, biological scientists do have one additional burden: To carry out their work without causing undue suffering, to both maximize pleasure, and reasonably minimize pain and suffering in their subjects.

I side with the traditional Western philosophical scheme regarding the human/animal relationship. Shank's triad of self-consciousness, feeling-consciousness and facility with language is a collection of traits that defines cognition. It represents a qualitative difference existing between man and animal.[2] That triad serves as the broadest and most reliable criterion for determining whether or not a being belongs to the moral community. For full membership in that community, a being must be capable of satisfying all of the rights and responsibilities expected by that group. Only man belongs unequivocally to that moral community. Even the most intellectually blighted of human beings, whether their conditions are consequent to infancy, injury or congenital defect, belong to that same moral community, based upon the physical qualities of their species, in essence, their DNA.[3] Such individuals cannot be purged from their group just because of impaired sentience. Such defects are anomalous conditions which exclude them from the usual considerations of their group. They cannot be used, for polemical or any other purpose, as representatives of their species.

When considering the moral relevance of any being within the animal kingdom, Shank's principle of charity warrants respect. It appropriately recognizes man's imperfection in quantifying such factors as sentience and consciousness — both feeling and self. Some might assert that the most highly developed sub-human primates could therefore, in accordance with Jeremy Bentham's ideas of sentience and moral relevance, be charitably considered quasi-members of the moral community.[4] However, since no other species possesses facility with language and few clearly possess self-consciousness, accepting that assertion is not a necessity. Still that does not mean that animals can be treated in any manner other than humane.

Rollin is right. Humans must respect animals for what they are in their own right, unique beings, deserving to pursue their own fulfillment regardless of their level of sentience. Such an obligation includes not only a reasonable maximization of their pleasure, but also the minimization of any potential pain and suffering. Every experimenter, at one time or another in his career, faces that paradox of causing an animal some level of pain in expectation for some perceived good. That tension is not a negative. In fact, it is desirable since it serves as the most important determinant limiting pain and suffering during the experiment. Furthermore, they are not being philosophically inconsistent in considering animals morally relevant but still using them in scientific experiments. Such acts are morally defensible so long as they treat their subjects with respect and avoid wanton cruelty at all times.

My own views of animal experimentation are admittedly speciesist, consequentialist and utilitarian. I am a speciesist because man, by Western ethical and legal standards, cannot experiment upon his own kind. Other species serve admirably as templates for human disease. I am a consequentialist because the alternative is so bleak. If one were to suddenly erase all of the progress gained through experimental science over the last 150 years, the consequences would be enormous. Devoid of assertive experimentation, medical advances would have come about only through performing autopsies and passively observing diseases. I am utilitarian because, if one were to sum up the good versus the bad consequences of scientific experimentation, the net positive lies clearly on the side of science.

Despite the animal advocates' penchant for pejorative labels such as "speciesist," one need not apologize for bringing common sense to the animal rights argument. Using "speciesist," like "racist" and "sexist," is an attempt to brand adversaries as ethically challenged when, in fact, their position is highly principled. Taking the advice of the animal rights theorists mentioned above, effectively stopping all animal experimentation and regulation in the name of animal rights would be a reversion back to 1840, when diseases flourished in a sea of medical ignorance. Pasteur and Koch had to first lay a foundation of bacteriological knowledge, including germ theory, before they could intelligently combat the scourge of infectious disease. That same principle still holds true today in relation to an entirely new array of diseases that were undreamed of in Victorian times. Even public health measures, which ARAs still tout as the best answer to disease, are virtually all based upon scientific facts gathered principally through animal experimentation.[5] Good health is not just a simple matter of being "clean" or living a virtuous life as advocated by Cobbe.

Using animals as templates of human disease, in essence pursuing experimental science by the concept of analogy, is a valid scientific method. For hundreds of years, experimental scientists have drawn conclusions based upon such analogies. It is still appropriate in these modern times, despite being applied in a vastly more disparate and sophisticated manner. Contrary to the opinion of Regan, extrapolation of data gathered through analogy is an eminently reliable method of experimentation. If the degree of analogy is weak, it is scientists who are the best equipped to not only recognize it but to correct it as well.

Experimental scientists should follow Russell and Burch's three Rs principles throughout their careers. They should *replace* test animals with the least sensitive subjects possible, ranging from tissue culture methods to perhaps the least sentient species available. Scientists should *reduce* the number of animals to as few as possible through careful planning of all experiments. Finally, *refinement*: The scientist should aspire to perform at the highest level possible, including his experimental technique, use of medications and instrumentation.

Efforts to pass legislation dedicated to improving the industry should be ongoing, addressing further improvements in animal housing, nutrition, and veterinary operative care, both before and after surgery. All such improvements should be effected without interfering with the scientists' ability to pursue their interests.

Society should not accede to misguided legal or philosophical movements aimed at terminating experimental science. With time and further progress, any painful experimentation that might now exist will ideally become superfluous. "Vivisection" may consist of little more than using a needle to withdraw blood or to biopsy suspect tissue.

Finally, as someone who has had some exposure to the experimental side of this debate and has spent time studying and reflecting upon the subject, I offer the following points of argumentation, to be accepted or rejected, partially or completely, by the reader.

- Consistent with the Western philosophical position — only man is clearly a member of the moral community.
- Animals can be morally relevant and still not belong completely to the moral community. The two are not mutually inclusive.
- Even the most blighted of humans belong to the moral community by virtue of their species, their humanity and their DNA. They cannot be purged from the community merely because of impaired sentience.
- Since animals serve well as templates of disease, they validate the concept of argument by analogy.
- Terminating all scientific experimentation would have catastrophic consequences for society.

- Humans, including experimental scientists, must not only respect animals as unique beings, they must also maximize their pleasure while minimizing their pain and suffering.
- It is not philosophically inconsistent to consider animals as morally relevant and still use them in scientific experimentation.
- Biological scientists have as much right to explore the living world as their counterparts do in studying physical phenomena.
- Scientists face a paradox of potentially causing pain while pursuing a putative good. That is a positive factor and the prime determinant of how an animal will be treated during the experiment.
- One need not apologize for being a speciesist, a consequentialist and a utilitarian. All are reasoned ideological positions.
- Experimental scientists should follow the three Rs: Replace, Reduce and Refine.
- Ongoing legislation aimed at protecting animals subject to experimentation is a laudable goal as long as it is pursued in a prudent manner.
- Animal rights activists, who work forcibly, whether through civil or criminal means, to terminate all animal experimentation should, to be intellectually consistent, refuse all healthcare measures that have been achieved through such scientific methods.

# Chapter Notes

## Introduction

1. Matt Rossell, "Why I Protest Animal Research," *The Oregonian* 1 May 2010.
2. Nathan Nobis, "Response to Balcombe's Commentators, Animal Dissection and Evidence Based Life-Science and Health-Professions Education," *Journal of Applied Animal Welfare Science* 5, no. 29 (2002): 159.
3. Ibid., 159–160.
4. Ibid., 160.
5. Theodore G. Obenchain and W. Eugene Stern, "Continuous Monitoring of Ventricular Pressure in Experimental Hydrocephalus, Part I: The Dynamics of Acute Ventricular Obstruction," *Archives of Neurology* 29 (1973): 287–294; Theodore G. Obenchain and W. Eugene Stern, "Continuous Monitoring of Ventricular Pressure in Experimental Hydrocephalus, Part II: The Origin of Undulating Ventricular Waves and Periodic Respirations," *Archives of Neurology* 29 (1973): 295–298.
6. Theodore G. Obenchain, "Speculum Lumbar Extraforaminal Microdiscectomy," *The Spine Journal* 1, no. 6 (2001): 415–420.

## Part I

1. Frances Power Cobbe, "Zoophily," *Cornhill* 45 (1882): 282. In *Animal Welfare and Anti-Vivisection 1870–1910: Nineteenth-Century Woman's Mission*, vol. 1, ed. Susan Hamilton, (London: Routledge, 2004), 179.

## Chapter 1

1. Louisa May Alcott, "Glimpses of Eminent Persons," *The Independent* (1 Nov 1866): 153.
2. Sally Mitchell, *Frances Power Cobbe: Victorian Feminist, Journalist, Reformer* (Charlottesville: University of Virginia Press, 2004), 1.
3. Charles Adams, "The Anti-Vivisection Movement and Miss Cobbe," *Verulam Review* iii (1892–1893): 201. In *Antivivisection and Medical Science in Victorian Society*, ed. Richard D. French (Princeton: Princeton University Press, 1975), 62.
4. Frances Power Cobbe, *The Life of Frances Power Cobbe: By Herself* 2 (Boston: Houghton Mifflin & Co., 1894), 559.
5. Lori Williamson, *Power and Protest: Frances Power Cobbe and Victorian Society* (London: Rivers Oram Press, 2005), 96.
6. Cobbe, *By Herself* 2, 42.
7. Ibid., 48.
8. Ibid., 55–56.
9. Liza Picard, *Victorian London* (New York: St. Martin's Griffin, 2005), 171.
10. Frances Power Cobbe, "Little Health of Ladies," *Contemporary Review* 38 (1878): 283.
11. The *Abolitionist* 5 (1904–1905): 41. In Williamson, *Power and Protest*, 91. Cobbe sometimes emphasized her own grotesqueness.
12. Picard, *Victorian London*, 101.
13. Lady Paget Walburga, *In My Tower* (Hutchinson, 1924), 187. In Williamson, *Power and Protest*, 91.
14. Cobbe, *By Herself* 1, 62. In Williamson, *Power and Protest*, 14.
15. Ibid., 78.
16. Williamson, *Power and Protest*, 25.
17. James Turner, *Reckoning with the Beast* (Baltimore: Johns Hopkins University Press, 1980), 90.
18. Cobbe, *By Herself* 1, 93.
19. Margaret McFadden, *Golden Cables of Sympathy* (Lexington: The University Press of Kentucky, 1999), 162.
20. Frances Power Cobbe, *An Essay on Intuitive Morals* (Boston: Crosby Nichols and Company, 1859), 25.
21. Ibid., 203.
22. Ibid., 41.

23. Ibid., 62.
24. Ibid., 180.
25. Jo Manton, *Mary Carpenter and the Children of the Streets* (London: Heinemann, 1976), 81.
26. Ibid., 148.
27. Cobbe, *By Herself*, 278. In Williamson, *Power and Protest*, 56.
28. Frances Power Cobbe, "Workhouse Sketches," *Macmillan's Magazine* 3 (1861). In Manton, *Mary Carpenter and the Children of the Streets*, 108.
29. Williamson, *Power and Protest*, 62.
30. Cobbe, *By Herself* 1, 314.
31. Mitchell, *Frances Power Cobbe*, xlix.
32. McFadden, *Golden Cables of Sympathy*, 166.
33. Ibid., 167.
34. Frances Power Cobbe, "The Fitness of Women for the Ministry of Religion," *Peak in Darien* (Boston: George H. Ellis, 1886), 199–200. In *Antivivisection and Medical Science in Victorian Society*, ed. Richard D. French (Princeton: Princeton University Press, 1975), 242.
35. Frances Power Cobbe, "Criminals, Idiots, Women and Minors," *Fraser's Magazine* 78 (Dec 1868): 779.
36. Frances Power Cobbe, "Wife Torture in England," *Contemporary Review* 32 (1878): 56. In Carol Bauer Ritt and Lawrence Ritt, "'A Husband Is a Beating Animal': Frances Power Cobbe Confronts the Wife-Abuse Problem in Victorian England," *International Journal of Women's Studies* 6, no.3 (1983): 195.
37. Edward J. Tilt, *On the Preservation of the Health of Women at the Critical Periods of Life*, 31. In *The Female Malady: Madness and English Culture, 1830–1980*, ed. Elaine Showalter (New York: Pantheon Books, 1985), 75.
38. George M. Beard, *A Practical Treatise on Nervous Exhaustion/Neurasthenia*, 3rd ed. (New York: E. B. Treat, 1894), 34–137.
39. Frances Power Cobbe, "The Little Health of Ladies," *Contemporary Review* 31 (1878): 282.
40. Ibid., 278.
41. Ibid., 291.
42. Ritt and Ritt, "A Husband is a Beating Animal," 99.
43. Carol Bauer Ritt and Lawrence Ritt, "Wife Abuse, Late Victorian English Feminists and the Legacy of Frances Power Cobbe," *International Journal of Women's Studies* 6, no. 3 (1983): 195.

## Chapter 2

1. Sally Mitchell, *Frances Power Cobbe: Victorian Feminist, Journalist, Reformer* (Charlottesville: University of Virginia Press, 2004), 128.
2. Frances Power Cobbe, *The Life of France Power Cobbe: By Herself* 2 (Boston: Houghton Mifflin & Co., 1894), 562.
3. Frances Power Cobbe, "The Rights of Man and the Claims of Brutes," *Frasers* 68 (1863): 236. In *Animal Welfare and Anti-Vivisection 1870–1910: Nineteenth-Century Woman's Studies* 1, ed. Susan Hamilton (London: Routledge, 2004), 28.
4. Ibid., 45.
5. Ibid., 107.
6. Cobbe, *By Herself* 1 (London: Swan Sonnenschein and Co, 1904), 708.
7. Ibid., 710.
8. Cobbe, *By Herself* 2, 563.
9. Sheryl R. Ginn and Joel A. Vilensky, "Thyroid History: Experimental Confirmation by Sir Victor Horsley of the Relationship between Thyroid Gland Dysfunction and Myxedema," *Thyroid* 16, no. 8 (2006): 743–747.
10. Patrizia Guarnieri, "Moritz Schiff (1823–96): Experimental Physiology and Noble Sentiment in Florence." In *Vivisection in Historical Perspective*, ed. Nicolaas Rupke (London: Routledge, 1987), 110.
11. Ibid., 106.
12. Ibid., 110.
13. Ibid., 115.
14. "Animal," *Encyclopedia Cattolica* 1 (Vatican City: Ente. Per l' Encic. Catt., 1948). In Rupke, *Vivisection in Historical Perspective*, 116. ("Vivisection" as an entry does not exist.)
15. Ibid., 119.
16. G. Capanni's letters of 30 Jan and 5 Feb 1874, together with the entire report, are in M. Schiff, *Sopra il Metodo*, 2nd ed., v-vii and 72–76. In Rupke, *Vivisection in Historical Perspective*, 119.
17. Cobbe, *By Herself* 2, 623.
18. Claude Bernard, *An Introduction to the Study of Experimental Medicine* (Paris: Henry Shuman, 1949), 111. Cited by Hugh La Follette and Niall Shanks, "Two Models of Models in Biomedical Research," *Philosophical Quarterly* 45, no. 179 (Apr 1995): 148.
19. William A. Locy, *The Growth of Biology* (New York: Henry Holt and Company, 1925), 437.
20. John E. Lesch, *Science and Medicine in France: The Emergence of Experimental Physiology, 1790–1855* (Cambridge: Harvard University Press, 1984), 27.
21. *St. Thomas Hospital Manuscript* 55, 182 verso. In Ruth Richardson (ed.), *Death, Dissection and the Destitute*, 2nd ed. (Chicago: The University of Chicago Press, 2000), 31.
22. Kathryn Shevelow, *For the Love of Animals: The Rise of the Animal Protection Movement* (New York: Henry Holt and Company, 2008), 49.

23. Stephen Greenblatt, *Will in the World: How Shakespeare Became Shakespeare* (New York: W.W. Norton & Company, 2004), 177.
24. Charles D. Niven, *History of the Humane Movement* (New York: Transatlantic Arts, Inc., 1967), 43.
25. Ibid.
26. Harriet Ritvo, *The Animal Estate: The English and Other Cultures in the Victorian Age* (Cambridge: Harvard University Press, 1987), 126.
27. Niven, *Humane Movement*, 47.
28. Humphry Primatt, *The Duty of Mercy and the Sin of Cruelty to Brute Animals*, ed. Richard D. Ryder (Fontwell, Sussex: Centaur Press, 1992), 22.
29. Ibid., 21.
30. Ibid., 125.
31. Ibid., 36.
32. Liza Picard, *Victorian London: The Life of a City, 1840–1870* (New York: St. Martin's Griffin, 2005), 24–25.
33. Adam Hochschild, *Bury the Chains: Prophets and Rebels in the Fight to Free an Empire's Slaves* (Boston: Houghton Mifflin Company, 2005), 3.
34. Ibid., 128.
35. Shevelow, *For the Love of Animals*, 14.
36. Ibid., 212–213.
37. James Turner, *Reckoning with the Beast: Animals, Pain and Humanity in the Victorian Mind* (Baltimore: Johns Hopkins University Press, 1980), 40–45.
38. Ritvo, *Animal Estate*. 143.
39. Ibid., 145.
40. Richard D. French, *Antivivisection and Medical Science in Victorian Society* (Princeton: Princeton University Press, 1975), 28. Cited in Ritvo, *Animal Estate*, 158.
41. Ritvo, *Animal Estate*. 158.

# Part II

1. Frances Power Cobbe, "The Rights of Man and the Claims of Brutes," *Frasers* 68 (1863): 36–37. In *Animal Welfare and Anti-Vivisection 1870–1910: Nineteenth-Century Woman's Mission*, vol. 1, ed. Susan Hamilton (London: Routledge, 2004), 244–245.

# Chapter 3

1. Richard B. Fisher, *Joseph Lister, 1827–1912* (New York: Stein and Day, 1977), 47.
2. Rickman J. Godlee, *Lord Lister (1918)* (London: Macmillan and Co., 1918), 17.
3. W. J. O'Connor, *Founders of British Physiology: A Biographical Dictionary, 1820–1885* (Manchester: Manchester University Press, 1988), 78, http://googlebooks.com.

4. John C. Brougher, "William Sharpey (1802–1880)," *Annals of Medical History* 1 (1829): 125.
5. D. W. Taylor, "The Life and Teaching of William Sharpey (1802–1880), 'Father of Modern Physiology' in Britain," part II, *Medical History* 3 (15 Jul 1971): 255.
6. Ibid., 255.
7. Michael Foster, *Claude Bernard* (New York: Longmanns, Green and Company, 1975), 40.
8. J. M. D. Olmsted, *Francois Magendie: Pioneer in Experimental Physiology and Scientific Medicine in XIX Century France* (Schuman's, 1945), 212–222.
9. Albert Leffingwell, *An Ethical Problem or Sidelights Upon Scientific Experimentation on Man and Animals*, 2nd ed. (New York: G. Bell & Sons, 1916), 19–20.
10. John E. Lesch, *Science and Medicine in France: The Emergence of Experimental Physiology, 1790–1855* (Cambridge: Harvard University Press, 198), 100–103.
11. Ibid., 91.
12. Jerome Tarshis, *Claude Bernard: Father of Experimental Medicine* (New York: The Dial Press, 1968), 3–5.
13. Claude Bernard, *An Introduction to the Study of Experimental Medicine* (Paris: Henry Schuman, 1949), 148. In Niall Shanks, *Animals and Science: A Guide to the Debates* (Santa Barbara: ABC CLIO, 2002), 103.
14. Claude Bernard, *An Introduction to the Study of Experimental Medicine* (New York: Macmillan, 1927). 11.
15. Tarshis, *Claude Bernard: Father of Experimental Medicine*, 66.
16. Frederic L. Holmes, *Claude Bernard and Animal Chemistry: The Emergence of a Scientist* (Cambridge: Harvard University Press, 1974), 377.
17. Eugene Debs Robin (ed.). *Claude Bernard and the Internal Environment: A Memorial Symposium* (New York: Marcel Dekker, Inc., 1979), 13.
18. Roger H. Ungar, "Concepts of Glucoregulation: From 1878 through 1978." In Robin, *Claude Bernard and the Internal Environment*, 51–53.
19. Roger Guillemin, "Hypothalamus, Hormones and Physiological Regulation," In *Robin, Claude Bernard and the Internal Environment*.
20. James J. Walsh, "Claude Bernard, the Physiologist." *Catholic World* 71, no. 421 (Apr 1900): 524.
21. Albert Leffingwell, *An Ethical Problem or Sidelight Upon Scientific Experiments on Man and Animals*, 2nd ed. (New York: G. Bell & Sons, 1916), 75.
22. Tarshis, *Claude Bernard*, 111.

23. Claude Bernard, *An Introduction to the Study of Experimental Medicine* (New York: Macmillan, 1927), 102.
24. Ernst von Weber, *The Torture Chamber of Science* (London: Victoria Street Society, 1879), 25.
25. George Hoggan, "Vivisection," *Fraser's Magazine* 11 (1875): 162, In *Animal Welfare and Anti-Vivisection* 2, ed. Susan Hamilton (London: Routledge, 2004), 522.
26. Leffingwell, *An Ethical Problem*, 20.

## Part III

1. John Erichsen, *Lancet* 1 (1874): 338. In Godlee, *Lord Lister*, 135. Editors of *Lancet* suggest that a scientific trial of Lister's antiseptic method be tried in London hospitals.

## Chapter 4

1. Edward A. Sharpey-Schafer, "Lister as Physiologist, 1927." In *Founders of British Physiology*. Ed. W. J. O'Connor (Manchester: Manchester University Press, 1988), 90–92.
2. Richard B. Fisher, *Joseph Lister, 1827–1912* (New York: Stein and Day, 1977), 122.
3. Rickman J. Godlee, *Lord Lister (1918)* (London: Macmillan and Co., 1918), 53.
4. Ibid., 44.
5. *Transactions Royal Society of Edinburgh* 21 (1857): 549. In Ibid., 45.
6. Godlee, *Lord Lister*, 43–49.
7. Ibid., 82.
8. Michael Worboys, *Spreading Germs: Disease Theories and Medical Practice in Britain, 1865–1900* (Cambridge: Cambridge University Press, 2000), 77.
9. Godlee, *Lord Lister*, 132.
10. See Part III note 1 above.
11. Fisher, *Joseph Lister*, 126.
12. Godlee, *Lord Lister*, 132.
13. Ibid., 560.
14. John Erichsen, "Fisher," *Lancet* 1 (1874): 338. In Godlee, *Lord Lister*, 135.
15. Godlee, *Lord Lister*, 561.
16. René Vallery-Radot, *The Life of Pasteur*, trans. Mrs. R. L. Devonshire (New York: McClure, Phillips and Co., 1902), 102. The Cornell University Library Digital Collections.
17. Fisher, *Joseph Lister*, 121.
18. Godlee, *Lord Lister*, 162.

## Chapter 5

1. Rickman J. Godlee, *Lord Lister (1819)* (London: Macmillan and Co., 1819), 172.
2. Pasteur Vallery-Radot, *Louis Pasteur: A Great Life in Brief* (New York: Alfred A. Knopf, 1958), 50.
3. Gerald L. Geison, *The Private Science of Louis Pasteur* (Princeton: Princeton University Press, 1995), 95–100.
4. Godlee, *Lord Lister*, 173.
5. Richard B. Fisher, *Joseph Lister, 1827–1912* (New York: Stein and Day, 1977), 132.
6. Justus von Leibig, *Organic Chemistry in its Applications to Agriculture and Physiology* (London: Taylor and Walton, 1840). In *Sparks of Life: Darwinism and the Victorian Debates over Spontaneous Generation*, ed. James E. Strick (Cambridge: Harvard University Press, 2000), 26.
7. Patrice Debré, *Louis Pasteur*, trans. Elborg Forster (Baltimore: Johns Hopkins University Press, 1998), 505–506.
8. Godlee, *Lord Lister*, 174–175.
9. Ibid., 177.
10. Ferdinand Cohn, "Untersuchungen über Bacterien," vol. 4, *Beitrage zur Biologie der Pflanzen*, 2, no. 2 (1876): 249–276. In Strick, *Sparks of Life*, 28.
11. Ibid., 88.
12. Debré, *Louis Pasteur*, 185.
13. Ibid., 209–211.
14. Ibid., 507.
15. Vallery-Radot, *Louis Pasteur*, 113–114.
16. Ibid., 113–114.

## Chapter 6

1. Richard B. Fisher, *Joseph Lister, 1827–1912* (New York: Stein and Day, 1977), 90–91.
2. Rickman J. Godlee, *Lord Lister, 1827–1912* (London: Macmillan and Co., 1819), 182.
3. Fisher, *Joseph Lister*, 124.
4. Godlee, *Lord Lister*, 187.
5. Ibid., 189.
6. Ibid., 191–192.
7. Ibid., 198.
8. Ibid.
9. Joseph Lister, "On a New Method of Treating Compound Fractures, Abscess, Etc.," *The Lancet* (16 Mar 1867): 326–329. In Godlee, *Lord Lister*, 318.
10. *The Lancet* 1 (1870): 91. In Godlee, *Lord Lister*, 319.
11. *Zoophilist* 3, no. 15 (1 Feb 1884): 246.
12. O. Mosciucci, "Science of Women," 227–252. Cited in Mary Ann Elston, "Women and Anti-vivisection in Victorian England, 1870–1900." In *Vivisection in Historical Perspective*, ed. Nicolaas A. Rupke (London: Routledge, 1990), 279.
13. Frances Power Cobbe, *The Study of Physiology as a Branch of Education* (London: Victoria Street Society pamphlet reprinted from *Zoophilist* (15 Jul 1893), 2. In Ibid., 279.
14. Mosciucci, "Science of Women," 279.
15. Lawson Tait, *Zoophilist* 7, no. 6 (1 Oct 1887): 101.

16. Lawson Tait, *Zoophilist* 7, no. 7 (1 Nov 1887): 117.

## Part IV

1. Rickman J. Godlee, *Lord Lister (1918)* (London: Macmillan and Co., 1918), 377.

## Chapter 7

1. Doris Lanier, *Absinthe: The Cocaine of the Nineteenth Century* (Jefferson, NC: McFarland & Company, Inc., 1995), 1.
2. Ibid., 25
3. Ibid., 12.
4. Ibid., 69–70.
5. Ibid., 35.
6. Ibid., 2.
7. Ibid., 33.
8. Editorial, "Prosecution at Norwich," *British Medical Journal* (12 Dec 1874): 751–754.
9. Richard D. French, *Antivivisection and Medical Science in Victorian Society* (Princeton: Princeton University Press, 1975), 58.
10. Sally Mitchell, *Frances Power Cobbe: Victorian Feminist, Journalist, Reformer* (Charlottesville: University of Virginia Press, 2004), 228.
11. Frances Power Cobbe, *The Life of France Power Cobbe: By Herself* 2 (Boston: Houghton Mifflin & Co., 1894), 576.
12. Ibid., 447.
13. Ibid.
14. Rebecca Stott, *Darwin and the Barnacle* (London: Faber and Faber, 2003), 171.
15. Ibid., 167.
16. Francis Darwin (ed.). *The Life and Letters of Charles Darwin* (London: John Murray, 1887), 200.
17. Cobbe, *Her Life* 2, 449.
18. Mitchell, *Frances Power Cobbe*, 235.
19. French, *Antivivisection and Medical Science*, 66.
20. Cobbe, *Her Life* 2, 66.
21. George Hoggan, "Vivisection," *Fraser's Magazine* 11 (1875): 521–528. In *Animal Welfare and Antivivisection 1870–1910: Nineteenth-Century Woman's Mission* 2, ed. Susan Hamilton (London: Routledge, 2004), 155–162.
22. Cobbe, *Her Life*, 579.
23. French, *Antivivisection and Medical Science*, 69–70.
24. Bernard Lightman, ed. *Victorian Science in Context* (Chicago: University of Chicago Press, 1997), 130.
25. Thomas H. Huxley to Charles Darwin, 22 Jan 1875, In *Life and Letters of Thomas Henry Huxley* 1 (London: Macmillan & Co., 1900), 470. In Mitchell, *Frances Power Cobbe*, 230.
26. Rene Dubos, *Louis Pasteur: Free Lance of Science* (New York: Charles Scribner's Sons, 1976), 76.
27. Thomas H. Huxley, *Who's Who in British History* 1, general ed. Geoffrey Treasure (London: Fitzroy Dearborn Publishers, 1998), 686.
28. Helen Rappaport, *Queen Victoria: A Biographical Companion* (Santa Barbara: ABC CLIO, 2000), 37.
29. Hansard, 3rd series (1875), CCXXIV. 794. In French, *Antivivisection and Medical Science*, 79.
30. Cobbe, *Her Life*, 584.
31. Hansard, 3rd series, In French, *Antivivisection and Medical Science*, 97–98.

## Chapter 8

1. Richard B. Fisher, *Joseph Lister: 1827–1912* (New York: Stein and Day, 1977), 194.
2. Rickman J. Godlee, *Lord Lister (1918)* (London: Macmillan and Company, 1918), reprinted by Cornell University Library Digital Collections, 377.
3. Ibid., 380–381.
4. Ibid., 382.
5. Godlee, *Lord Lister*, 382–383.
6. Report of the Royal Commission, Q. 3562 and 3538ff. In Richard D. French, *Antivivisection and Medical Science* (Princeton: Princeton University Press, 1975), 104.
7. Leonard Huxley, *Life and Letters of Thomas Henry Huxley* 1 (London: Macmillan & Co., 1900), 440. In French, *Antivivisection and Medical Science*, 105.
8. Frances Power Cobbe, *Public Money: An Enquiry Concerning an Item of Its Expenditure* (London: Victoria Street Society. 1892), 3–11. In *Animal Welfare and Anti-Vivisection 1870–1910: Nineteenth-Century Woman's Mission* 1, ed. Susan Hamilton, 375–383.
9. Frances Power Cobbe, *The Life of Frances Power Cobbe: By Herself* 2 (Boston: Houghton Mifflin & Co., 1894), 585.
10. Ibid., 586.
11. Ibid., 587.
12. Anthony Astley Cooper, Lord Shaftsbury, *Encyclopedia of World Biography*, 2nd ed., vol. 14, sr. ed. Paula Byers (Detroit: Gale, 1998), 137–138.
13. James Turner, *Reckoning with the Beast: Animals, Pain, and Humanity in the Victorian Mind* (Baltimore: Johns Hopkins University Press, 1980), 91.
14. Cobbe, *Her Life*, 589.
15. Richard D. French, *Antivivisection and Medical Science in Victorian Society* (Princeton: Princeton University Press, 1975), 114.
16. Ibid., 116.

17. Cobbe, *Her Life*, 594. In French, *Antivivisection and Medical Science*, 117.
18. Harrowby to Carnarvon and Colam to Carnarvon (23 May 1876), P.R.O., *Carnarvon Papers* 30/6/19/3, 4. In French, *Antivivisection and Medical Science*, 118.
19. Godlee, *Lord Lister*, 383.
20. E. Hodder, *The Life and Work of the Seventh Earl of Shaftesbury* (London: 1886), iii, 373. In French, *Antivivisection and Medical Science*, 130.
21. French, *Antivivisection and Medical Science*, 130–136.
22. Cross to Carnarvon (18 Jul 1875), *Carnarvon Papers*, 30/6/9/24. In French, *Antivivisection and Medical Science*, 137.
23. French, *Antivivisection and Medical Science*, 146.
24. Robert Lowe, "The Vivisection Act," *Contemporary Review* 28 (1876): 297–308. In Hamilton, *Animal Welfare and Anti-Vivisection*, 714.
25. Lowe, "The Vivisection Act," 301; Hamilton, *Animal Welfare and Anti-Vivisection*, 717.
26. Lowe, "The Vivisection Act," 299. Hamilton, *Animal Welfare and Anti-Vivisection*, 715.
27. Frances Power Cobbe, "Mr. Lowe and the Vivisection Act," *Contemporary Review* 29 (1876): 337. In Hamilton, *Animal Welfare and Anti-Vivisection* 2, 129.
28. Ibid., 345/137.
29. Ibid., 338/130.
30. Godlee, *Lord Lister*, 387.
31. Frances Power Cobbe, "The Policy of the Future," *Home Chronicler* (16 Sep, 1876). In Sally Mitchell, *Frances Power Cobbe: Victorian Feminist, Journalist, Reformer* (Charlottesville: University of Virginia Press, 2004), 245.
32. Ibid., 246.
33. Ibid., 247. Robert Lowe, "The Vivisection Act," *Contemporary Review* 27 (Oct 1876), 85.
34. Cobbe, *Her Life*, 599.
35. Mitchell, *Frances Power Cobbe*, 251.
36. Shaftesbury to Frances Power Cobbe (17 Sep 1878). In Mitchell, *Frances Power Cobbe*, 264.
37. Frances Power Cobbe, *Light in Dark Places* (London: Victoria Street Society, 1883), 293.
38. Ibid.
39. Turner, *Reckoning with the Beast*, 111.
40. John Cleland, *Experiments on Animals* (London: J. W. Kolckmann, 1883), 5–6. In Turner, *Reckoning With the Beast*, 112.
41. Pasteur Vallery-Radot, *Vie de Pasteur* (Hachette, 1900), 434. In Patrice Debré, *Louis Pasteur*, trans. Elborg Forster (Baltimore, Johns Hopkins University Press, 1994), 432.

## Part V

1. Christoph Gradmann, *Robert Koch's Medical Bacteriology* (Baltimore: Johns Hopkins University Press, 2009), 115. This is a quote from Koch's "Über bakteriologische Forschung," 659.

## Chapter 9

1. Rickman J. Godlee, *Lord Lister (1918)* (London: Macmillan and Co. 1918), 434.
2. Brock, *Robert Koch: A Life in Medicine and Bacteriology* (Madison: Science Tech Publishers, 1988), 11.
3. C. Barlow and P. Barlow, *Robert Koch: The Great Nobel Prizes* (Geneva: Heron Books, 1971), 32–33.
4. Stephen Badsey, *The Franco-Prussian War 1870–1871* (Oxford: Osprey Publishing, 2003), 86.
5. Gertrud Pfuhl, "Robert Koch in Wollstein," *Erinnerungenseiner Tochter Gertrud Pfuhl. Deutsche Medizinische Wochenschrift*, 66 (1940): 355–57. In Brock, *Robert Koch: A Life*, 24.
6. Barlow and Barlow, *Robert Koch*, 22–23.
7. Rene J. Dubose, *Louis Pasteur: Free Lance of Science* (Boston: Little, Brown and Company, 1950), 239.
8. Henry Harris, *Things Come to Life: Spontaneous Generation Revisited* (Oxford: Oxford University Press, 2002), 128.
9. Brock, *Robert Koch*, 31.
10. Ibid., 44.
11. Dubose, *Louis Pasteur*, 51.
12. Brock, *Robert Koch*, 46–47.
13. Ibid., 49.
14. Barlow and Barlow, *Robert Koch*, 52.
15. Brock, *Robert Koch*, 73–74.
16. Robert Koch, Neue Untersuchungen über die Mikroorganismen bei infectiosen Wundkrankheiten, *Mitteilungen 51 deutschen Naturforscherversammlung zu Cassel. Deutsche medizinische Wochenschrift* (26 Oct 1878): 531. In Brock, *Robert Koch*, 76.
17. Barlow and Barlow, *Robert Koch*, 52–53.
18. Ibid., 54.
19. Ibid., 59.
20. Barlow and Barlow, *Robert Koch*, 60.
21. Brock, *Robert Koch*, 98.
22. Knight, *Robert Koch*, 71.
23. Ibid., 96.
24. Brock, *Robert Koch*, 97.
25. Robert Koch, "The Etiology of Tuberculosis." In *Milestones in Microbiology*, ed. Thomas D. Brock (Englewood Cliffs: Prentice-Hall, Inc., 1961), 117.
26. Brock, *Milestones in Microbiology*, Comment, 108.
27. Brock, *Robert Koch*, 104.

## Chapter 10

1. D. R. Dunlop, "The Life and Work of Louis Pasteur," *The Canadian Medical Association Journal* (1928): 297–300.
2. Rene J. Dubose, *Louis Pasteur: Free Lance of Science* (Boston: Little, Brown and Company, 1950), 243–244.
3. Pasteur Vallery-Radot, *Louis Pasteur: A Great Life in Brief*, trans. Alfred Joseph (New York: Alfred A. Knopf, 1958), 124–125.
4. Dubose, *Louis Pasteur*, 261–262.
5. Vallery-Radot, *Louis Pasteur: A Great Life in Brief*, 139–140.
6. Ibid., 139.
7. Frances Power Cobbe, "Experimental Pathology," *Zoophilist* 11 (1 Oct 1883): 191–193.
8. Rickman J. Godlee, *Lord Lister (1918)* (London: Macmillan and Co. 1918), 435.
9. Patrice Debré, *Louis Pasteur*, trans. Elborg Forster (Baltimore: Johns Hopkins University Press, 1994), 386–388.
10. Rene Vallery-Radot, *Life of Pasteur*, trans., Mrs. R. L. Devonshire (New York: Doubleday, Page & Company, 1915), 313–314. http://books.google.com/books?id=.
11. Ibid., 316.
12. Ibid., 315.

## Chapter 11

1. Patrice Debré, *Louis Pasteur*, trans. Elborg Forster (Baltimore: Johns Hopkins University Press, 1998), 396.
2. Ibid., 395.
3. Gerald L. Geison, *The Private Science of Louis Pasteur* (Princeton: Princeton University Press, 1995), 151.
4. Debré, *Louis Pasteur*, 398.
5. Rene J. Dubose, *Louis Pasteur: Free Lance of Science* (Boston: Little Brown and Company, 1950), 339.
6. Debré, *Louis Pasteur*, 400.
7. Dubose, *Louis Pasteur*, 339.
8. Debré, *Louis Pasteur*, 400.
9. Ibid., 401.
10. Dubose, *Louis Pasteur*, 341.
11. Ibid., 343.
12. Benjamin Bryan, "M. Pasteur and the System of Inoculation," *Zoophilist* 6 (1 May 1886): 9.
13. Pasteur Vallery-Radot, *Vie de Pasteur* (Hachette, 1900), 475. In Debré, *Louis Pasteur*, 411.
14. Vallery-Radot, *Vie de Pasteur*, 459; Debré, *Louis Pasteur*, 412.

## Part VI

1. William MacCormac, *Transactions of the Seventh Session of the International Medical Congress* 1 (London: J. W. Kolckman, 1881), 101.

## Chapter 12

1. W. F. Bynum, *Science and the Practice of Medicine in the Nineteenth Century* (Cambridge: Cambridge University Press, 1994), 144–145.
2. Jurgen Thorwald, *The Triumph of Surgery*, trans. Richard Winston and Clara Winston (New York: Pantheon Books, 1960), 22.
3. Rene Vallery-Radot, *Life of Pasteur*, trans., Mrs. R. L. Devonshire (New York: Doubleday, Page & Company, 1915), 332.
4. Ibid., 333.
5. Rickman J. Godlee, *Lord Lister (1918)* (London: Macmillan and Co., 1918), 442.
6. Ibid., 445.
7. Robert Koch, "Die Atiologie der Milzbrand-Krankheit, begrundet auf die entwicklungsgeschichte des Bacillus Anthracis." *Beitrage zur Biologie der Pflantzen* 2: 277–310. Also in *Gesammelte Werke von Robert Koch*. (Leipzig: Thieme, 1912) 1: 5–26.
8. Ibid., 52.
9. *Maladies virulentes, virus-vaccins et prophylaxie de la rage*. 404, 426. In Patrice Debré, *Louis Pasteur*, trans. Elsborg Forster (Baltimore: Johns Hopkins University Press, 1998), 407.
10. Ibid., 408.
11. Agnes Ullmann, "Pasteur-Koch: Distinctive Ways of Thinking about Infectious Diseases," *Microbe Magazine: American Society for Microbiology* 4 (2007). http://forms.asm.org/microbe/index.asp?bid=52099.
12. Debré, *Louis Pasteur*, 408.
13. Thomas D. Brock, *Robert Koch. A Life in Medicine and Bacteriology* (Madison: Science Tech Publishers, 1988), 175.
14. Pasteur Vallery-Radot, *Vie de Pasteur* (Hachette, 1900), 475. In Debré, *Louis Pasteur*, 409.
15. Brock, *Robert Koch: A Life*, 141.
16. Ibid.
17. Robert M. Frank and D. Wrotonoska (eds. and trans.). *Correspondence of Pasteur and Thuillier* (Tuscaloosa: University of Alabama Press, 1968), 217. In Brock, *Robert Koch*, 154.
18. Brock, *Robert Koch*, 160.
19. "Dr. Koch's Sixth Cholera Report," *British Medical Journal* (22 Mar 1884): 568–569. In Brock, *Robert Koch*, 160–162.
20. Rene J. Dubose, *Louis Pasteur: Free Lance of Science* (Boston: Little, Brown and Company, 1950), 270–271.
21. Brock, *Robert Koch*, 167.
22. Pasteur Vallery-Radot, ed. *Pasteur Correspondence* (Paris: Flammarion, 1951), 430–531. In Thomas D. Brock, *Robert Koch* (Madison: Science Tech Publishers, 1988), 176.
23. Ibid., 176–177.

24. Frances Power Cobbe, "Science and Cholera," *Zoophilist*, 4, no. 4 (1 Aug 1884): 80, 86.
25. "Lister Abandons AntiSepic Spray," *Zoophilist* 3, no. 15 (1 Feb 1884): 246.

## Chapter 13

1. Jurgen Thorwald, *The Triumph of Surgery*, trans. Richard Winston and Clara Winston (New York: Pantheon Books, 1960), 16–20.
2. Gustav Fritz and Eduard Hitzig, *On the Electrical Excitability of the Cerebrum*, trans. G. von Bonin, 76. In *Some Papers on the Central Cortex* (Springfield: Thomas, 1960); also in Robert M. Young, *Mind Brain and Adaptation in the Nineteenth Century* (Oxford: Clarendon Press, 1970), 226.
3. Francois J. Gall, *Sur les Fonctions du Cerveau et sur Celles de Chacune de ses Parties*. 6 vols. Bailliere, Paris: 1822–1825. In Young, *Mind Brain and Adaptation*, 136.
4. Fritz and Hitzig, *On the Electrical Excitability of the Cerebrum*, 78.
5. Gerhardt Von Bonin, *Some Papers on the Cerebral Cortex* XII (Springfield: Thomas, 1960). In Young, *Mind, Brain and Adaptation*, 225.
6. Webb Haymaker, ed. *The Founders of Neurology: One Hundred and Thirty Three Biographical Sketches* (Springfield: Thomas, 1953). In Young, *Mind, Brain and Adaptation in the Nineteenth Century*, 225.
7. Young, *Mind Brain and Adaptation*, 224.
8. Ibid., 239.
9. Stephen Coleridge, *Vivisection, a Heartless Science* (London: John Lane, 1916), 64. In Julie M. Fenster, *Mavericks, Miracles and Medicine* (New York: Carroll and Graf Publishers, 2003), 221.
10. William Rutherford, "Address to the Department of Anatomy and Physiology," *Report of the Forty-Third Meeting of the British Association for the Advancement of Science*, transactions 119–123 (London: Murray, 1874). In Young, *Mind, Brain and Adaptation*, 239.
11. Ibid., 235–236.
12. Thorwald, *The Triumph of Surgery*, 25–26.
13. Ibid., 27.
14. Ibid., 30–31.
15. Ibid., 15.
16. Ibid., 35.
17. Ibid., 37–40.
18. Frances Power Cobbe, "A Reply to Sir James Paget on Vivisection," *The Modern Rack* (London: Swan Sonnenschein & Co., 1889), 97.
19. "The Value of Experimentation on the Brain," *Zoophilist* 3, no. 16 (1 Mar 1884): 268.
20. James Paget, "Vivisection: its Pains and its Uses — I," *Nineteenth Century* 10 (1881): 923. In *Animal Welfare and Anti-Vivisection 1870–1910: Nineteenth-Century Woman's Mission* 3, ed. Susan Hamilton (New York: Routledge, 2004), 131.
21. Ibid., 137.
22. Samuel Wilks, "Vivisection: Its Pains and its Uses — III," *Nineteenth Century* 10 (1881), 943–944. In *Animal Welfare and Anti-Vivisection* 3, ed. Hamilton, 152–153.
23. Frances Power Cobbe, "Vivisection: Four Replies," *Fortnightly Review* 31 (1882): 103. In Hamilton, *Animal Welfare and Anti-Vivisection*, 201.
24. Lorie Williamson, *Power and Protest: Frances Power Cobbe and Victorian Society* (London: Rivers Oram Press, 2005), 141–142.
25. *British Medical Journal* (19 Nov 1881): 836–842.
26. Frances Power Cobbe, *Her Life* 2 (Boston: Houghton Mifflin & Co., 1894), 617.
27. James Turner, *Reckoning with the Beast: Animals, Pain and Humanity in the Victorian Mind* (Baltimore: Johns Hopkins University Press, 1980), 108.
28. G. M. Humphry, *Vivisection: What Good Has It Done?* (London: J. W. Kolckmann, 1882), 4–8. In Hamilton, *Animal Welfare and Anti-Vivisection*, 300–304.
29. Jurgen Thorwald, *The Triumph of Surgery*, trans. Richard Winston and Clara Winston (New York: Pantheon Books, 1960), 102–103.
30. Ibid., 109.
31. Ibid., 112.
32. Douglas Kirkpatrick, "The First Primary Brain-Tumor Operation," *Journal of Neurosurgery* 61 (1984): 811.
33. Ibid.
34. Editorial, *London Times*, 28 Nov 1934, 15. In Kirkpatrick, "The First Primary Brain-Tumor Operation," 15.

## Chapter 14

1. Rene J. Dubose and Jean Dubose, *The White Plague: Tuberculosis, Man and Society* (Boston: Little Brown and Company, 1952), 14.
2. Ibid., 17.
3. Ibid., 8.
4. Thomas Dormandy, *The White Death: A History of Tuberculosis* (New York: New York University Press, 1999), 2.
5. *In de causis et signis dikurnorum morborum* or the *Causes and Symptoms of Chronic Diseases* (London: Sydenham Society, 1856). In Dormandy, *White Death*, 2–3.
6. Friedrich Engels, *The Condition of the Working Class in England*, trans. and ed. W. O. Henderson and W. H. Chaloner (1844; New York: The Macmillan Company, 1958), 111.

7. Dormandy, *White Death*, 91.
8. Dubose and Dubose, *White Plague*, 45.
9. Ibid., 46.
10. S. Jaccoud, *The Curability and Treatment of Pulmonary Phthisis*, trans. M. Lubbock. London, 1855. In Dormandy, *White Plague*, 47.
11. J. D. Rolleston, "The Folklore of Pulmonary Tuberculosis," *Tubercle* 55 (1941): 3. In Dormandy, *White Plague*, 48.
12. Dubose and Dubose, *White Plague*, 97.
13. Erwin H. Ackerknecht, "Anticontagionism between 1821 and 1867," *Bulletin of the History of Medicine* 22 (1948): 566.
14. Robert Koch, "The Etiology of Tuberculosis," in Thomas D. Brock, *Milestones in Microbiology* (Englewood Cliffs: Prentice-Hall, Inc., 1961), 109.
15. Irwin W. Sherman, *The Power of Plagues* (Washington DC: ASM Press, 2006), 286–287.
16. Dubose and Dubose, *White Plague*, 98.
17. C. Barlow and P. Barlow, *Robert Koch: The Great Nobel Prizes* (Heron Books, 1971), 74.
18. Dubose and Dubose, *White Plague*, 103.
19. Thomas D. Brock, *Robert Koch: A Life in Medicine and Bacteriology* (Madison: Science Tech Publishers, 1988), 119–120.
20. Paul Ehrlich, "Modification der von Koch angegebenen Methode der Färbung von Tuberkelbacillen," *Deutsche Medizinische Wochenschrift* 8 (1882): 269–270, in Brock, *Robert Koch*, 121.
21. Brock, *Robert Koch*, 124–125.
22. Barlow and Barlow, *Robert Koch*, 74.
23. Brock, *Robert Koch*, 126–127.
24. Ibid., 127–129.
25. Bernhard Mollers, *Robert Koch: Personlichkeit und Lebenswerk 1843–1910*, in Brock, *Robert Koch*, 129.
26. Barlow and Barlow, *Robert Koch*, 76–77.
27. *London Times*, 22 Apr 1882, cited in Brock, *Robert Koch*, 130.
28. Brock, *Robert Koch*, 133.
29. *Lancet* 2 (1899): 379–381. In Lloyd G. Stevenson, "Science down the Drain," *Bulletin of the History of Medicine* 29, no. 1 (1955): 16. Sanitationist G. Wilson addresses the "fallacy" of vaccination science and bacteriological research.
30. Frances Power Cobbe, "Koch and Tuberculosis," *Zoophilist* 8, no. 21 (1 Jun 1888): 17–18.
31. Brock, *Robert Koch*, 138.

## Part VII

1. Frances Power Cobbe, "The Town Mouse and the Country Mouse," *The Scientific Spirit of the Age and Other Pleas and Discussions* (Boston: George H. Ellis, 1888), 188.

## Chapter 15

1. Frances Power Cobbe, *The Life of Frances Power Cobbe as Told by Herself* (London: Swan Sonnenschein & Co., 1904), 697.
2. Frances Power Cobbe, *The Life of Frances Power Cobbe: By Herself* 2 (Boston: Houghton Mifflin, 1894), 635.
3. Sally Mitchell, *Frances Power Cobbe: Victorian Feminist, Journalist, Reformer* (Charlottesville: University of Virginia Press, 2004), 301.
4. Cobbe, *By Herself*, 706.
5. *The Times* (24 Nov 1886). In Lori Williamson, *Power and Protest: Frances Power Cobbe and Victorian Society* (London: Rivers Oram Press, 2005), 178.
6. HSP, Wister Family Papers, box 4. Frances Power Cobbe to Sarah Wister (22 Nov 1882): in Williamson, *Power and Protest*, 179.
7. Williamson, *Power and Protest*, 182.
8. M.P.G. Martyn to Frances Power Cobbe (27 Jun 1885). In envelope marked "Warnings to Miss Cobbe against Mr. Coleridge." BUAV Archives, Miscellaneous: 1885–1992, DBV 35/2. In Williamson, *Power and Protest*, 182.
9. Frances Power Cobbe, *The Fallacy of Restriction Applied to Vivisection* (London, 1886), 4. In *Animal Welfare and Anti-Vivisection 1870–1910: Nineteenth-Century Woman's Mission* I. Ed. Susan Hamilton (London: Routledge, 2004), 325–326.
10. Ibid., 328.
11. Ibid., 331.
12. *Jewish Chronicle* (27 Feb 1891). In Williamson, *Power and Protest*, 186–187.
13. Williamson, *Power and Protest*, 188.
14. George Tyrell, "Jesuit Philosophy," *Contemporary Review* 68 (1895): 713–714. In Williamson, *Power and Protest*, 188.
15. Frances Power Cobbe, *The Nine Circles of the Tortures of the Innocent*, 3rd (revised) ed., Society for the Prevention of Animals from Vivisection, Victoria Street (London: Swan Sonnenschein & Co., 1893), v–vii.
16. *Zoophilist* 12 (1892–1893): 77. In Williamson, *Power and Protest*, 189. Canon Wilberforce's pronouncement of the upcoming book *Nine Circles*.
17. F. S. Arnold, *Do the Interests of Humanity Require Experiments on Living Animals? And If So, Up to What Point Are They Justifiable?* (London: Reprinted by the Victoria Street Society, 1893), 8–9.
18. Ibid., 13.
19. Ibid., 14.
20. John H. Clarke, *Our Meanest Crime* (London: Reprinted by the Victoria Street Society, 1894), 10.
21. Alfred Barry, *Do the Interests of Mankind*

*Require Experiments on Living Animals? If So, Up to What Point Are They Justifiable?* (London: Reprinted by the Victoria Street Society, 1895), 8.
22. Mitchell, *Frances Power Cobbe*, 339.
23. Ibid.
24. *Zoophilist* 12 (1892–1893): 186–187. In Williamson, *Power and Protest*, 190. Horsley's reply to Cobbe following his confrontation at Folkestone.
25. *The Times*, 11–18 Oct 1892. Horsley's upbraiding of clergy at Folkestone. In Mitchell, *Frances Power Cobbe*, 339. Horsley's upbraiding of clergy at Folkestone.
26. *The Times*, 20–25 Oct 1892. Horsley's ongoing grievances against Cobbe in the *Nine Circles*. In Mitchell, *Frances Power Cobbe*, 339. Horsley's ongoing grievances against Cobbe in the *Nine Circles*.
27. Ernest Hart, "Women, Clergymen and Doctors," *New Review* 7 (1892): 711. In Williamson, *Power and Protest*, 191.
28. Georgine Rhodes, *The Nine Circles*, 143. In Williamson, *Power and Protest*, 193.
29. Armand M. Ruffer, "The Morality of Vivisection," *Nineteenth Century* 32 (1892): 814. In Hamilton, *Animal Welfare and Vivisection* 3, 247.
30. Ibid., 249.
31. Ibid., 250.
32. Victor Horsley, "The Morality of Vivisection," *Nineteenth Century* 32 (1892): 804. In Hamilton, *Animal Welfare and Vivisection* 3, 237.
33. Ibid., 241–242.
34. Ibid., 243.
35. Ibid.

## Part VIII

1. Frances Power Cobbe, "The Medical Profession and Its Morality," *Modern Review* (1881): 35. In *Animal Welfare and Anti-Vivisection 1870–1910: Nineteenth-Century Woman's Mission* I, ed. Susan Hamilton (London: Routledge, 2004): 168.

## Chapter 16

1. Frances Power Cobbe, "Mad Dog!" *Modern Rack: Papers on Vivisection* (London: Swan Sonnenschein & Co., 1889), 227–233. Also, Edward Mayhew and A. J. Sewell, *Dogs, Their Management* (London: George Routledge & Co., 1854), 157–163.
2. Ibid., 233.
3. Patrice Debré, *Louis Pasteur*, trans. Elborg Forster (Baltimore: Johns Hopkins University Press, 1998), 416.
4. Rickman J. Godlee, *Lord Lister (1918)* (London: Macmillan and Co., 1918), 439.
5. Pasteur, *Ouevres* 6, 619. In Gerald L. Gieson, "Pasteur's Work on Rabies: Reexamining the Ethical Issues," *The Hastings Center Report* 8, no. 2. (Apr 1978): 27. http://www.jstor.org/stable/3560403.
6. Lee Goldman and J. Claude Bennett, *Cecil Textbook of Medicine* 2, 21st ed. (Philadelphia: W.B. Saunders Company, 2000), 2132.
7. Alan C. Jackson and William H. Wunner, *Rabies* (Amsterdam: Academic Press, 2002), 221.
8. Debré, *Louis Pasteur*, 416.
9. Godlee, *Lord Lister*, 491.
10. Émile Roux, "L'Oeuvre medicale de Pasteur," *Agena du chemiste* (1896): 76. In Debré, *Louis Pasteur*, 417.
11. Pasteur, *Ouevres* IV, 258. In Gerald L. Gieson, *The Private Science of Louis Pasteur* (Princeton: Princeton University Press, 1995), 178.
12. Ibid., 420.
13. Jackson and Wunner, *Rabies*, 421.
14. Gieson, *The Private Science of Louis Pasteur*, 184.
15. Ibid., 190.
16. Ibid., 184–185.
17. Rene J. Dubose, *Louis Pasteur: Free Lance of Science* (Boston: Little Brown and Company, 1950), 265.
18. Anita Guerrini, *Experimenting with Humans and Animals: From Galen to Animal Rights* (Baltimore: Johns Hopkins University Press, 2003), 98.
19. Debré, *Louis Pasteur*, 423.
20. Ibid., 425.
21. Adrian Loir, *L'Ombre de Pasteur*, 66. In Debré, *Louis Pasteur*, 426–427.
22. Ibid., 428.
23. Ibid., 430–431.
24. F. Rosset, *Pasteur et la rage* (Paris: Foundation Merieux, 1985), 55. In Debré, *Louis Pasteur*, 429.
25. Ibid., 430.
26. Frances Power Cobbe, "No More than a Prick of a Needle," *Zoophilist* 9, no. 38 (1889): 176.
27. Louis Pasteur, *The Manchester Guardian*, 14 Dec 1886, in Frances Power Cobbe, *An Institute of Preventive Medicine at Work in France*, 6th ed. (London: Victoria Street Society for the Protection of Animals from Vivisection, 1891), 8.
28. Cobbe, *An Institute of Preventive Medicine*, 7.
29. Ibid., 2–10.
30. Pasteur, *Oeuvres* 6, 605. In Gerald L. Gieson, *The Hastings Center Report* 8, no. 2 (Apr 1978): 31.
31. Ibid., 32.
32. Ibid.
33. Debré, *Louis Pasteur*, 439–440.
34. Ibid., 440.

## Chapter 17

1. Pasteur, *Ouevres* VI, 603. In Gerald L. Gieson, *The Private Science of Louis Pasteur* (Princeton: Princeton University Press, 1995), 213.
2. Pasteur, *Ouevres* VI, 611. Gieson, *The Private Science of Louis Pasteur*, 217.
3. Patrice Debré, *Louis Pasteur* (Baltimore: Johns Hopkins University Press, 1998), 446.
4. Pasteur Vallery-Radot, *Vie de Pasteur* (Hachette, 1900), 434; Debré, *Louis Pasteur*, 432.
5. Ibid., 433.
6. R. Rosset, *Pasteur et la rage* (Paris: Foundation Merieux, 1985), 76. In Debré, *Louis Pasteur*, 433.
7. Ibid.
8. Ibid., 432.
9. *Monsieur Pasteur's Treatment for the Prevention of Hydrophobia*. Exeter, 1886. In James Turner, *Reckoning with the Beast: Animals, Pain and Humanity in the Victorian Mind* (Baltimore: Johns Hopkins University Press, 1980), 99.
10. Frances Power Cobbe to Mr. White, 4 Apr 1886. National Library of Wales, Aberystwyth. In Sally Mitchell, *Frances Power Cobbe: Victorian Feminist, Journalist, Reformer* (Charlottesville: University of Virginia Press, 2004), 318.
11. Frances Power Cobbe, "The Janus of Science," *Modern Rack: Papers on Vivisection* (London: Swan Sonnenschein & Co., 1889), 121.
12. Mitchell, *Frances Power Cobbe*, 278.
13. Frances Power Cobbe, *Dawning Lights: An Enquiry Concerning the Secular Results of the New Reformation* (London: E. T. Whitfield, 1868), 174. In Lori Williamson, *Power and Protest: Frances Power Cobbe and Victorian Society* (London: Rivers Oram Press, 2005), 172.
14. Frances Power Cobbe, "Science down the Drain," 9. In Lloyd Stevenson, "Science down the Drain: On the Hostility of Certain Sanitarians to Animal Experimental Bacteriology and Immunology," *Bulletin of the History of Medicine* 29 (1955): 1–26.
15. Ibid., 24.
16. Frances Power Cobbe, "Medical Profession and Its Morality," 927. In Williamson, *Power and Protest*, 172.
17. *Liverpool Daily Post*, 27 Feb 1892. Reprinted in the *Zoophilist* (1891–1892): 278. In Williamson, *Power and Protest*, 172.
18. Frances Power Cobbe, *Controversy in a Nutshell* (London: Victoria Street Society, n.d., c.1895), 173.
19. Debré, *Louis Pasteur*, 453–457.
20. Gieson, *The Private Science of Louis Pasteur*, 254.
21. Debré, *Louis Pasteur*, 461.
22. Richard B. Fisher, *Joseph Lister, 1827–1912* (London: Stein and Day, 1977), 294.
23. Rickman J. Godlee, *Lord Lister (1918)* (London: Macmillan and Co., 1918), 521–522.
24. Rene J. Dubose, *Louis Pasteur: Free Lance of Science* (Boston: Little, Brown and Company, 1950), 56.
25. Ibid., 57.
26. Ibid., 496.

## Chapter 18

1. Robert Koch, "Über bacteriologische Forschung," *Verhandlungen des X Internationalen Medizinischen Kongresses*, Berlin 1 (1890): (Aug Kirschwald, Berlin, 1891), in Thomas D. Brock, *Robert Koch, A Life in Medicine and Bacteriology* (Madison: Science Tech Publishers, 1988), 196.
2. Christoph Gradmann, *Laboratory Disease: Robert Koch's Medical Bacteriology*, trans. Elborg Forster (Baltimore: Johns Hopkins University Press, 2009), 99.
3. Robert Koch, "Weitere Mitteilungen über ein Heilmittel gegen Tuberculose" 1890. Also in *Gesammelte Werke von Robert Koch* 1, (Leipzig: Thieme, 1912), 679.
4. Gradmann, *Laboratory Disease*, 122–123.
5. Ibid., 124.
6. Rickman Godlee, *Lord Lister (1918)* (London: Macmillan and Co., 1918), 562–563.
7. Brock, *Robert Koch*, 195–196.
8. Editorial. *Lancet* 2 (1890): 118. Unsigned editorial commenting on Koch's premature release of tuberculin, implying that he must have been pressured to do so by governmental superiors. In Thomas Dormandy, *The White Death: A History of Tuberculosis* (New York: New York University Press, 1999), 140.
9. Arthur Conan Doyle, *Review of Reviews*, A Monthly, December, "Dr. Koch and His Cure" ed. William T. Stead, (London: Mowbray House, 1890), 557. In Dormandy, *White Death*, 140–41.
10. Rudolf Virchow, "Über die Wirkung des Koch'schen Mittels." In Gradmann, *Laboratory Disease*, 102.
11. "Summary of Early Berlin Treatment with Tuberculin." *Lancet* (14 Mar 1891): 631. Cited in Brock, *Robert Koch: A Life*, 210.
12. "Summary of Early Berlin Treatment," 631. In Brock, *Robert Koch: A Life*, 210.
13. Benjamin Bryan, "Kochism: Experiment not Discovery," *Zoophilist*, 178–180. In Lori Williamson, *Power and Protest: Frances Power Cobbe and Victorian Society* (London: Rivers Oram Press, 2005), 163.
14. "Vivisection and the New Treatment of Myxedema," *Zoophilist* 13, no. 2 (1 Jun 1891): 24.
15. Williamson, *Power and Protest*, 164.

16. Frances Power Cobbe, *Zoophilist* 13 (1893–1894): 300. In Williamson, *Power and Protest*, 164. Editorial asserting that patients had become prisoners within hospitals.
17. David Newman, "The History and Prevention of Venereal Diseases," *Glasgow Medical Journal* 81 (1914): 88–100. In Judith R. Walkowitz, *Prostitution and Victorian Society: Women, Class, and the State* (Cambridge: Cambridge University Press, 1980), 55.
18. Cobbe, 300. In Williamson, *Power and Protest*, 164.
19. Frances Power Cobbe, *The Age of Science: A Newspaper of the Twentieth Century* (London: J. Ogden and Co., reprinted by University of Michigan Library, 2010), 20.
20. Ibid., 42.
21. Ibid., 47.
22. Ibid., 48.
23. Ibid., 49.

## Part IX

1. Frances Power Cobbe, "The Scientific Spirit of the Age," *The Contemporary Review* 54 (1888): 127. In *Animal Welfare and Anti-Vivisection 1870–1910: Nineteenth-Century Woman's Mission* II, ed. Susan Hamilton (London: Routledge, 2004), 247.

## Chapter 19

1. Rickman J. Godlee, *Lord Lister (1918)* (London: Macmillan and Co., 1918), 405.
2. Ibid., 402.
3. Ibid., 413–415.
4. Ibid., 414–415.
5. Richard B. Fisher, *Joseph Lister, 1827–1912* (New York: Stein and Day, 1977), 236.
6. Godlee, *Lord Lister (1918)*, 416.
7. Ibid., 420.
8. Ibid., 332.
9. Ibid., 345.
10. Ibid., 336.
11. Ibid., 352–354.
12. Ibid., 357–358.
13. Fisher, *Joseph Lister*, 246–247.
14. Ibid., 250.
15. Ibid., 252.
16. Godlee, *Lord Lister (1918)*, 476.
17. Rene J. Dubose, *Louis Pasteur: Freelance of Science* (Boston: Little, Brown and Company, 1950), 352.
18. Ibid.
19. Benjamin Bryan, *Reasons Why the English Committee's Report Does Not Settle the Question* (London: Victoria Street Society for the Protection of Animals from Vivisection, 1887), 4.
20. Ibid., 5–16.
21. Frances Power Cobbe, "An Institute of Preventive Medicine at Work in France," *Zoophilist* 10 (1 Apr 1891): 236–237.
22. Joseph Lister, *Lancet* (18 May 1891): 1124.
23. Godlee, *Lord Lister (1918)*, 497.
24. Ibid., 499–500.

## Chapter 20

1. Rickman J. Godlee, *Lord Lister (1918)* (London: Macmillan and Co., 1918), 246.
2. Ibid., 535.
3. Walter Hadwen, "The Case Against Vaccination," *Whale*, 25 Jan 1896, http://www.whale.to/a/smallpox77.htm.
4. Patrice Debré, *Louis Pasteur*, trans. Elborg Forster (Baltimore: The Johns Hopkins University Press, 1998), 479–481.
5. Susan E. Lederer, "The Controversy over Animal Experimentation in America, 1880–1914," in *Vivisection in Historical Perspective*, ed. Nicolaas A. Rupke (London: Routledge, 1987), 242.
6. Debré, *Louis Pasteur*, 480.
7. Victor Horsley, "Abstracts of the 'Brown' Lectures," *The Lancet* (27 Dec 1884): 1134.
8. Sheryl R. Ginn and Joel A. Vilensky, "Thyroid History: Experimental Confirmation by Sir Victor Horsley of the Relationship between Thyroid Gland Dysfunction and Myxedema," *Thyroid* 16, no. 8 (2006): 45.
9. "Vivisection and the New Treatment of Myxedema," *Zoophilist* 13, no. 2 (1 Jun 1891): 29–30.
10. "Sir Charles Sherrington's First Use of Diphtheria Antitoxin Made in England," *Notes on the Records of the Royal Society of London* 5, no. 2 (Apr 1948): 156–159.
11. Debré, *Louis Pasteur*, 479–481.
12. *U.S. Report and Hearing* (Washington, DC: 1896), 115–118. In James Turner, *Reckoning with the Beast: Animals, Pain and Humanity in the Victorian Mind* (Baltimore: Johns Hopkins University Press, 1980), 115.
13. Frances Power Cobbe, "The Diphtheria Cure," *Zoophilist* 14, no. 8 (1 Dec 1894): 5.
14. Frances Power Cobbe, "The Slump in Antitoxin," *Zoophilist* 20, no. 11 (1 Mar 1901): 259–260.
15. Stephen Coleridge, letter to the editor, *Zoophilist* (2 Jun 1902): 31.
16. Debré, *Louis Pasteur*, 482.
17. Godlee, *Lord Lister (1918)*, 535.
18. Lois N. Magner, *A History of Infectious Disease and the Microbial World* (Westport, CT: Praeger, 2009), 46–47.

## Chapter 21

1. *Liverpool Daily Post* (27 Feb 1892), reprinted in *Zoophilist* 11 (1891–1892), 278. In

Lori Williamson, *Power and Protest: Frances Power Cobbe and Victorian Society* (London: Rivers Oram Press, 2005), 172.

2. Frances Power Cobbe, *Controversy in a Nutshell* (London: Victoria Street Society, n.d. c. 1895), 5. In Williamson, *Power and Protest*, 173.

3. *Zoophilist* 15 (1894), 8. Hutton's statement concerning using medical gains derived from vivisection. In Williamson, *Power and Protest*, 173.

4. Letter to the editor, *Zoophilist* 9 (1889–1890), 166, 262. Letter claiming "old maid, Cobbe" cared more for animals than man. In Williamson, *Power and Protest*, 173–174.

5. E. M. Warner, letter, *The Times* (12 Oct 1892). In Williamson, *Power and Protest*, 174. Letter asserts that antivivisectionists would better understand the value of animal research if they cared for the sick. Evidence of progress over time is undeniable.

6. Frances Power Cobbe to Sarah Wister (24 Mar, 7 Oct 1895), in Mitchell, *Frances Power Cobbe: Victorian Feminist, Journalist, Reformer* (Charlottesville: University of Virginia Press, 2004), 349.

7. Frances Power Cobbe to Fawcett (11 Nov 1896), Autograph Letter Collection, The Women's Library, London. In Mitchell, *Frances Power Cobbe*, 351.

8. Mitchell, *Frances Power Cobbe*, 351.

9. Ibid., 353.

10. Williamson, *Power and Protest*, 197.

11. Victoria Street Society, *Woman's Signal* (21 May 1896); *Zoophilist* (1 Feb 1898): 171. In Mitchell, *Frances Power Cobbe*, 353. Concerns the decision of NAVS to abandon the pursuit of total prohibition of vivisection.

12. "The Honourable Stephen Coleridge's Rejoinder," *Zoophilist* (1 Feb. 1898):171–72; *Zoophilist* (1 March 1898): 209. In Mitchell, *Frances Power Cobbe*, 353.

13. Stephen Coleridge, letter to the editor, *Zoophilist*, 24 Apr 1898.

14. Williamson, *Power and Protest*, 200–201.

15. Frances Power Cobbe, *Why We Have Founded the British Union for the Abolition of Vivisection* (London: The National Anti-Vivisection Society, 1898), 8.

16. Williamson, *Power and Protest*, 175.

17. The *Abolitionist* 3 (1902–1903): 13–14. In Williamson, *Power and Protest*, 209. A total of 346 admirers signed Cobbe's card on the occasion of her eightieth birthday.

18. Beatrice E. Kidd and Edith M. Richards, *Hadwen of Gloucester: Man, Medico, Martyr* (London: John Murray, 1933), 141.

19. Ibid., 159.

20. Ibid., 147.

21. Frances Power Cobbe to Wister, Sarah (9 May c. 1903), Wister Family Papers, Box 4, HSP. In Williamson, *Power and Protest*, 209.

22. Frances Power Cobbe, "Youth and Age," *Spectator* 92 (1904): 771. Posthumous publication by Constance Battersea. In Williamson, *Power and Protest*, 209.

23. John Verschoyle, "Frances Power Cobbe," *The Contemporary Review* 115 (Jan/Jun 1904): 840. In Mitchell, *Frances Power Cobbe*, 366.

24. Kidd and Richards, *Hadwen of Gloucester*, 147.

25. Cobbe's will, Somerset House. Codicil to this will dated 2 Jun 1903. In Williamson, *Power and Protest*, 210.

26. Cobbe's will, Somerset House. In Williamson, *Power and Protest*, 211.

27. Mitchell, *Frances Power Cobbe*, 353.

28. Walter Hadwen, "The Funeral of Frances Power Cobbe." *The Abolitionist*. 5, no. 1 (20 Apr 1904): 2.

29. Verschoyle, "Frances Power Cobbe." *The Contemporary Review* 115 (Jan/Jun 1904): 836.

30. Ibid., 835.

31. Ibid.

## Part X

1. James Peter Warbasse, *The Conquest of Disease Through Animal Experimentation* (New York: D. Appleton and Company, 1910), 145–146.

## Chapter 22

1. Edwin R. Lankester, *Spectator* 47 (1874): 13–14, 46–47. In Richard D. French, *Anti Vivisection and Medical Science in Victorian Society* (Princeton: Princeton University Press, 1975), 51.

2. French, *Antivivisection and Medical Science*, 392.

3. Peter Singer, *Animal Liberation* (New York: Harper Collins, 1975), xxiii.

4. Roger Scruton, *Animal Rights and Wrongs* (London: Metro Publishing Limited, 1998), 68–71.

5. Richard D. Ryder, *Victims of Science: The Use of Animals in Research*, 2nd ed. (London: National Anti-Vivisection Society Limited, 1983), 3.

6. Ibid., 5.

7. Ibid.

8. Richard Dawkins, *The Selfish Gene* (Oxford: Oxford University Press, 1976). In Ryder, *Victims of Science*, 5–6.

9. Ward Clark, *Misplaced Compassion: The Animal Rights Movement Exposed* (San Jose: Writers Club Press, 2001), 13.

10. Singer, *Animal Liberation*, xxiii.

11. Ibid., 2.

12. Richard Sergeant, *The Spectrum of Pain* (London: Hart Davis, 1969), 72. In Singer, *Animal Liberation*, 12.
13. Singer, *Animal Liberation*, 15.
14. Ibid., 16.
15. Carl Cohen and Tom Regan, *The Animal Rights Debate* (Lanham: Rowman & Littlefield Publishers, Inc.), 127.
16. Tom Regan, *The Case for Animal Rights* (Berkeley: University of California Press, 2004), 389.
17. Ibid., 390.
18. Ibid., 384.
19. Cohen and Regan, *Animal Rights Debate*, 199-200.
20. Ibid., 201
21. Ibid., 202.
22. Paola Cavalieri and Peter Singer (eds.), *The Great Ape Project: Equality beyond Humanity* (New York: St. Martin's Griffin, 1994).
23. Gary L. Francione, *Animals as Persons: Essays on the Abolition of Animal Exploitation* (New York: Columbia University Press, 2008), 18.
24. Ibid., 59.
25. Ibid., 178.
26. Niall Shanks, *Animals and Science: A Guide to the Debates* (Santa Barbara: ABC-CLIO, 2002), 264.
27. Ibid., 285-287.
28. Ibid., 257.
29. Ibid., 231.
30. Ibid., 268.
31. Ibid., 243.
32. Ibid., 254-255.
33. L. J. Lafleur (ed.), *Bentham: An Introduction to the Principles of Morals and Legislation* (New York: Haffner Publishing, 1948), 311. In Shanks, *Animals and Science*, 83.
34. Lafluer, *Bentham*, 80-83.
35. Ibid., 82.
36. Bernard E. Rollin, *Putting the Horse before Descartes: My Life's Work on Behalf of Animals* (New York: Temple University Press, 2011), 259-261.
37. Ibid., 74.
38. Ibid., 76.
39. Ibid., 51-52.
40. Gary L. Francione, *Animals as Persons: Essays on the Abolition of Animal Exploitation* (New York: Columbia University Press, 2008), 177.
41. Regan, *Case for Animal Rights*, 384.
42. Eric Kandel, *In Search of Memory: The Emergence of a New Science of Mind* (New York: W.W. Norton & Co., 2006), 59-244.
43. Office of Laboratory Animal Welfare, *Public Health Service Policy on Humane Care and Use of Laboratory Animals* (24 Nov 2010): 6.
44. Ibid., 7.
45. W. M. S. Russell, R. L. Burch, *The Principles of Humane Experimental Technique* (London: Methuen & Co. Ltd., 1959), 64.
46. Ibid., 105.
47. Ibid., 134.
48. T. H. Huxley to Frances Power Cobbe, 16 Nov 1870. Cited in Sally Mitchell, *Frances Power Cobbe: Victorian Feminist, Journalist, Reformer* (Charlottesville: University of Virginia Press, 2004), 202.
49. Roger W. Whatmore, "Nanotechnology Has the Potential to Provide Significant Benefits Despite Concerns" in *Nanotechnology*, ed. Jacquiline Langwith (Detroit: Greenhaven Press, 2009), 27.

# Epilogue

1. "Does Animal Experimentation Save Human Lives?" *PETA*, 22 Aug 2011.
2. Niall Shanks, *Animals and Science: A Guide to the Debates* (Santa Barbara: ABC CLIO, 2002), 386.
3. Ibid., 375.
4. Ibid., 355.
5. Carl Cohen and Tom Regan, *The Animal Rights Debate* (Lanham: Rowman & Littlefield Publishers, 2001), 304.

# Bibliography

*Abolitionist* 3 (1902–1903): 13–14.
*Abolitionist* 5 (1904–1905): 41.
Ackerknecht, Edwin H. "Anticontagionism between 1821 and 1867." *Bulletin of the History of Medicine* 22 (1948): 562–593.
Adams, Charles. "The Anti-Vivisection Movement and Miss Cobbe." *Verulam Review* 3 (1892–1893): 201.
Alcott, Louisa May. "Glimpses of Eminent Persons." The *Independent* (1 Nov 1866).
"Animal." *Encyclopedia Cattolica* 1. Vatican City: Ente. Per l' Encic. Catt., 1948.
Arnold, F. S. *Do the Interests of Humanity Require Experiments on Living Animals? And If So, Up to What Point Are They Justifiable?* London: Reprinted by the VSS, 1893.
Badsey, Stephen. *The Franco-Prussian War 1870–1871.* Oxford: Osprey Publishing, 2003.
Barlow, C., and P. Barlow. *Robert Koch: The Great Nobel Prize.* Geneva: Heron Books, 1971.
Barry, Alfred. *Do the Interests of Mankind Require Experiments on Living Animals? If So, Up to What Point Are They Justifiable?* London: Reprinted by the VSS, 1895.
Beard, George M. *A Practical Treatise on Nervous Exhaustion/Neurasthenia.* 3rd ed. New York: E. B. Treat, 1894.
Bernard, Claude. *An Introduction to the Study of Experimental Medicine.* New York: Macmillan, 1927.
_____. *An Introduction to the Study of Experimental Medicine.* Paris: Henry Shuman, 1949.
Brock, Thomas D. "The Germ Theory of Disease." *Milestones in Microbiology.* Englewood Cliffs: Prentice-Hall, Inc., 1961.

_____. *Robert Koch: A Life in Medicine and Bacteriology.* Madison: Science Tech Publishers, 1988.
Brougher, John C. "William Sharpey (1802–1880)." *Annals of Medical History* 1 (1829): 125.
Bryan, Benjamin. "Kochism: Experiment not Discovery." *Zoophilist.* London: Victoria Street Society, 1890.
_____. "M. Pasteur and the System of Inoculation." *Zoophilist* 6 (1May 1886): 9.
_____. *Reasons Why the English Committee's Report Does Not Settle the Question.* London: Victoria Street Society for the Protection of Animals from Vivisection, 1887.
Bynum, W. F. *Science and the Practice of Medicine in the Nineteenth Century.* Cambridge: Cambridge University Press, 1994.
Capanni, G. Letters of 30 Jan and 5 Feb 1874. In *Sopra il Metodo.* 2nd ed. Ed. M. Schiff, v–vii and 72–76. Cited in *Vivisection in Historical Perspective.* Ed. Nicolaas A. Rupke, 119. London: Routledge, 1987.
"Case against Vaccination," Verbatim report of an address by Walter Hadwen, 25 Jan 1896. http://www.whale.to/a/smallpox77.htm.
Carter, Codel K. "The Koch-Pasteur Dispute on Establishing the Cause of Anthrax." *Bulletin History of Medicine* 62 (1988): 42–57.
Cavalieri, Paola, and Peter Singer, eds. *The Great Ape Project: Equality beyond Humanity.* New York: St. Martin's Griffin, 1994.
"The Charge Against Professor Ferrier Under the Vivisection Act: Dismissal of Summons." *British Medical Journal* (19 Nov 1881): 836–842.

"The Charles Adams–Mildred Coleridge Affair and Subsequent Lawsuit." *Times of London* (24 Nov 1886).

Clarke, John H. "Our Meanest Crime." London: Reprinted by the Victoria Street Society. 1894.

Cleland, John. *Experiments on Animals*. London: J. W. Kolckmann, 1883.

Cobbe, Frances Power. *The Age of Science: A Newspaper of the Twentieth Century*. London: J. Ogden and Co. Reprinted by University of Michigan Library.

———. "Controversy in a Nutshell." London: Victoria Street Society, n.d., c. 1895.

———. "Criminals, Idiots, Women and Minors: Is This Classification Sound?" *Fraser's Magazine* 78 (Dec 1868): 779.

———. *Dawning Lights: An Enquiry Concerning the Secular Results of the New Reformation*. London: E. T. Whitfield, 1868.

———. "The Diphtheria Cure." *Zoophilist* 14, no. 8 (1 Dec 1894).

———. *An Essay on Intuitive Morals*. Boston: Crosby Nichols and Company, 1859.

———. "Experimental Pathology." *Zoophilist* 11 (1 Oct 1883): 191–193.

———. *The Fallacy of Restriction Applied to Vivisection*. London: Victoria Street Society for the Protection of Animals from Vivisection, 1886.

———. "The Fitness of Women for the Ministry of Religion." 199–200. *Peak of Darien*. Boston: 1882.

———. "An Institute of Preventive Medicine at Work in France." *Zoophilist* 10 (1 Apr 1891): 236–237.

———. "The Janus of Science." *Modern Rack: Papers on Vivisection*. London: Swan Sonnenschein & Co., 1889.

———. "Koch and Tuberculosis." *Zoophilist* 8, no. 21 (1 Jun 1888): 17–18.

———. Letter to Fawcett (11 Nov 1896), Autograph Letter Collection, the Women's Library, London.

———. Letter to Mr. White (4 Apr 1886). National Library of Wales, Aberystwyth.

———. Letter to Sarah Wister (24 Mar, 7 Oct 1895).

———. Letter to Wister, Sarah (9 May c. 1903), Wister Family Papers, Box 4, HSP.

———. *The Life of France Power Cobbe: By Herself*. Boston: Houghton Mifflin & Co., 1894. Two vols.

———. *Life of Frances Power Cobbe as Told by Herself*. London: Swan Sonnenschein and Co., 1904.

———. *Light in Dark Places*. London: Victoria Street Society, 1883.

———. "Little Health of Ladies." *Contemporary Review* 31 (Dec 1878): 276–296.

———. "Mad Dog!" *Modern Rack: Papers on Vivisection*. London: Swan Sonnenschein & Co., 1889.

———. "Medical Profession and Its Morality." *Modern Review* (1881): 927. In *Power and Protest: Frances Power Cobbe and Victorian Society*. Ed. Lori Williamson, 140–175. London: Rivers Oram Press, 2005.

———. "Mr. Lowe and the Vivisection Act." *Contemporary Review* 29 (1876): 335–347.

———. *The Nine Circles of the Tortures of the Innocent*. 3rd (revised) ed. Society for the Prevention of Animals from Vivisection, Victoria Street. London: Swan Sonnenschein & Co., 1893.

———. "No More than a Prick of a Needle." *Zoophilist* 9, no. 38 (1889).

———. "The Policy of the Future." *Home Chronicler* (16 Sep 1876).

———. "Power to Sarah Wister." Wister Family Papers, box 4. Historical Society of Pennsylvania. 22 Nov 1882.

———. *Public Money: An Enquiry Concerning an Item of Its Expenditure*. London: Victoria Street Society, 1892.

———. "A Reply to Sir James Paget on Vivisection." *The Modern Rack*. London: Swan Sonnenschein & Co., 1889.

———. "The Rights of Man and the Claims of Brutes." *Frasers* 68 (1863): 586–602.

———. "Science and Cholera." *Zoophilist* 4, no. 4 (1 Aug 1884).

———. "The Scientific Spirit of the Age." *The Contemporary Review* 54 (1888): 126–139.

———. "The Slump in Antitoxin." *Zoophilist* 20, no. 11 (1 Mar 1901): 259–260.

———. *The Study of Physiology as a Branch of Education*. London: VSS pamphlet reprinted from *Zoophilist* (15 Jul 1893).

———. "The Town Mouse and the Country Mouse." *New Quarterly Magazine* 4 (Jul 1875): 474–510.

———. "Vivisection: Four Replies." *Fortnightly Review* 31 (1882).

———. *Why We Have Founded the British Union for the Abolition of Vivisection*. London: The National Anti-Vivisection Society, 1898.

———. "Wife Torture in England." *Contemporary Review* 32 (1878).

———. "Workhouse Sketches." *Macmillan's Magazine* 3 (1861).

———. "Youth and Age." *Spectator* 92 (14 May 1904): 771. Posthumous publication by Constance Battersea.

———. "Zoophily." *Cornhill* 45 (1882): 279–288.

Cobbe's will, Somerset House. Codicil to this will dated 2 Jun 1903.

Cohen, Carl, and Tom Regan. *The Animal Rights Debate*. Lanham: Rowman & Littlefield Publishers, Inc., 2001.

Cohn, Ferdinand. "Untersuchungen über Bacterien." *Beitrage zur Biologie der Pflanzen* 4, no. 2 (1876): 249–276.

Coleridge, Stephen, letter to editor, *Zoophilist*. 2 Jun 1902.

———. Letter to editor, *Zoophilist*. 24 Apr 1898.

———. *Vivisection, a Heartless Science*. London: John Lane, 1916.

Conan Doyle, Arthur. *Review of Reviews*, a Monthly. Editor William T. Stead. London: Mowbray House, 1890.

Cooper, Anthony Astley. Lord Shaftsbury. *Encyclopedia of World Biography*. 2nd ed. Senior editor Paula Byers. 14. Detroit: Gale, 1998.

Cross to Carnarvon. (18 Jul 1875). *Carnarvon Papers*, 30/6/9/24.

Darwin, Francis, ed. *The Life and Letters of Charles Darwin*. London: John Murray, 1887.

Dawkins, Richard. *The Selfish Gene*. Oxford: Oxford University Press, 1976.

Debré, Patrice. *Louis Pasteur*. Trans. Elborg Forster. Baltimore: The Johns Hopkins University Press, 1998.

"Dr. Koch's Sixth Cholera Report." *British Medical Journal* (22 Mar 1884): 568–569.

"Does Animal Experimentation Save Human Lives?" PETA. 22 Aug 2011. www.peta.org/about/faq

Dormandy, Thomas. *The White Death: A History of Tuberculosis*. New York: New York University Press, 1999.

Dubose, Rene, and Jean Dubose. *The White Plague: Tuberculosis, Man, and Society*. Boston: Little Brown and Company, 1952.

Dubose, Rene J. *Louis Pasteur: Free Lance of Science*. Boston: Little, Brown and Company, 1950.

Dunlop, D. R. "The Life and Work of Louis Pasteur." *The Canadian Medical Association Journal*. (1928): 297–300.

Editorial. *Jewish Chronicle*, 27 Feb 1891. Response to Cobbe's allegations that German Jews were some of the worst vivisectors in Europe.

Editorial. *Lancet* 1 (1870): 91.

Editorial. *Lancet* 2 (1890): 118.

Editorial. *London Times*, 28 Nov 1934.

Ehrlich, Paul. "Modification der von Koch angegebenen Methode der Färbung von Tuberkelbacillen." *Deutsche Medizinische Wochenschrift* 8 (1882): 269–270.

Engels, Friedrich. *The Condition of the Working Class in England*. Trans. and ed. W. O. Henderson and W. H. Chaloner. 1844; New York: The Macmillan Company, 1958.

Fenster, Julie M. *Mavericks, Miracles and Medicine*. New York: Carroll and Graf Publishers, 2003.

Fisher, John Erichsen. *Lancet* 1 (1874): 338.

Fisher, Richard B. *Joseph Lister, 1827–1912*. New York: Stein and Day, 1977.

Foster, Michael. *Claude Bernard*. New York: Longmanns, Green and Company, 1975.

Francione, Gary L. *Animals as Persons: Essays on the Abolition of Animal Exploitation*. New York: Columbia University Press, 2008.

Frank, Robert M., and D. Wrotonoska, eds. and trans. *Correspondence of Pasteur and Thuillier*. Tuscaloosa: University of Alabama Press, 1968.

French, Richard D. *Antivivisection and Medical Science in Victorian Society*. Princeton: Princeton University Press, 1975.

Fritz, Gustav, and Eduard Hitzig. *On the Electrical Excitability of the Cerebrum*. Trans. G. von Bonin. 76. *Some Papers on the Central Cortex* (Springfield: Thomas, 1960).

Gall, Francis, J. *Sur les Fonctions du Cerveau et sur Celles de Chacune de ses Parties*. Bailliere, Paris: 1822–1825. 6 vols.

Gieson, Gerald L. "Pasteur's Work on Rabies: Reexamining the Ethical Issues." *The Hastings Center Report* 8, no. 2 (Apr 1978): 27–32. http://www.jstor.org/stable/3560403.

———. *The Private Science of Louis Pasteur*. Princeton: Princeton University Press, 1995.

Ginn, Sheryl R., and Joel A. Vilensky. "Thyroid History: Experimental Confirmation by Sir Victor Horsley of the Relationship between Thyroid Gland Dysfunction and Myxedema." *Thyroid* 16, no. 8 (2006): 743–747.

Godlee, Rickman J. *Lord Lister (1918)*. London: Macmillan and Company, 1918. Reprinted by The Cornell University Library Digital Collections.

Goldman, Lee, and Claude J. Bennett, eds. *Cecil Textbook of Medicine*. 21st ed. Philadelphia: Elsevier — Health Sciences Division 2, 2000.

Gradmann, Christoph. *Laboratory Disease: Robert Koch's Medical Bacteriology*. Trans. Elborg Forster. Baltimore: The Johns Hopkins University Press, 2009.

Greenblatt, Stephen. *Will in the World: How Shakespeare Became Shakespeare*. New York: W. W. Norton & Company, 2004.

Guarnieri, Patrizia. "Moritz Schiff (1823–96): Experimental Physiology and Noble Sentiment in Florence." In *Vivisection in Historical Perspective*, 105–124. Ed. Nicolaas Rupke. London: Routledge, 1987.

Guerrini, Anita. *Experimenting with Humans and Animals: From Galen to Animal Rights*. Baltimore: The Johns Hopkins University Press, 2003.

Guillemin, Roger. "Hypothalamus, Hormones and Physiological Regulation," In *Claude Bernard and the Internal Environment: A Memorial Symposium*. Ed. Robin Eugene Debs. New York: Marcel Dekker, Inc., 1979.

Hadwen, Walter. "The Funeral of Frances Power Cobbe." *The Abolitionist* 5, no. 1 (1904): 2.

Hamilton, Susan, ed. *Animal Welfare and Anti-Vivisection 1870–1910: Nineteenth-Century Woman's Mission*. 3 vols. London: Routledge, 2004.

Hansard Parliamentary Debates, 3d. series, 224 (London: Cornelius Buck Publishing, 1875): 431.

Harris, Henry. *Things Come to Life: Spontaneous Generation Revisited*. Oxford: Oxford University Press, 2002.

Harrowby to Carnarvon and Colam to Carnarvon (23 May 1876), P.R.O., *Carnarvon Papers* 30/6/19/3, 4.

Hart, Ernest. "Women, Clergymen and Doctors." *New Review* 7 (1892).

Haymaker, Webb, ed. *The Founders of Neurology: One Hundred and Thirty Three Biographical Sketches*. Springfield: Thomas, 1953.

Hodder, Edwin. *The Life and Work of the Seventh Earl of Shaftesbury*. London: Irish University Press, 1886.

Hoggan, George. "Vivisection." *Fraser's Magazine* 11 (1875): 521–528.

Holmes, Frederic L. *Claude Bernard and Animal Chemistry: The Emergence of a Scientist*. Cambridge: Harvard University Press, 1974.

Horsley, Victor. "Abstracts of the 'Brown' Lectures." *The Lancet* 124, no. 3200 (27 Dec 1884): 1133–1136.

———. "The Morality of Vivisection." *Nineteenth Century* 32 (1892): 804–811.

Humphry, G. M. *Vivisection: What Good Has It Done?* London: J. W. Kolckmann, 1882.

Huxley, Leonard, ed. *Life and Letters of Thomas Henry Huxley*, 2 vols. London: Macmillan & Co., 1900.

Huxley, Thomas H. Letter to Charles Darwin, 22 Jan 1875. In *Life and Letters of Thomas Henry Huxley*, vol. 1 (London: Macmillan & Co., 1900), 470.

———. Letter to Frances Power Cobbe, 16 Nov 1870. Frances Power Cobbe Papers, Huntington Library, San Marino, California.

———. *Who's Who in British History* 1. General ed. Goeffrey Treasure. London: Fitzroy Dearborn Publishers, 1998.

Jaccoud, S. *The Curability and Treatment of Pulmonary Phthisis*. Trans. M. Lubbock. London: Kegan Paul, Trench & Co., 1885.

"John Tyndall's Summary of Koch's Discovery of the Cause of Tuberculosis." *Times of London* (22 Apr 1882).

Kandel, Eric. *In Search of Memory: The Emergence of a New Science of Mind*. New York: W. W. Norton & Co., 2006.

Kidd, Beatrice E., and Edith M. Richards. *Hadwen of Gloucester: Man, Medico, Martyr*. London: John Murray, 1933.

Kirkpatrick, Douglas. "The First Primary Brain-Tumor Operation." *Journal of Neurosurgery* 61 (1984): 809–813.

Knight, David C. *Robert Koch: Father of Bacteriology*. New York: Franklin Watts, Inc., 1961.

Koch, Robert. "Neue Untersuchungen über die Mikroorganismen bei infectiosen Wundkrankheiten." *Mitteilungen 51 deutschen Naturforscherversammlung zu Cassel. Deutsche medizinische Wochenschrift* (26 Oct 1878): 531.

———. "Über bacteriologische Forschung." *Verhandlungen des X Internationalen Medizinische Kongresse*. 1. Berlin, 1890.

———. "Weitere Mitteilungen über ein

Heilmittel gegen Tuberculose," *Deutsche Medizinisches Wochenschrift* 17 (1891): 1189-92.

———. "Zur Aetiologie des Milzbrandes." Reprinted in *Gesammelte Werke von Robert Koch* 1 ed. Codell Carter (Westport CT: Greenwood Press, 1987).

Lafleur, L. J., ed. *Bentham: An Introduction to the Principles of Morals and Legislation.* New York: Haffner Publishing, 1948.

La Follette, Hugh, and Niall Shanks. "Two Models of Models in Biomedical Research." *Philosophical Quarterly* 45, no. 179 (Apr 1995): 148.

*Lancet* 2 (1899): 379-381.

Lanier, Doris. *Absinthe: The Cocaine of the Nineteenth Century.* Jefferson, NC: McFarland & Company, Inc., 1995.

Lankester, Edwin R. "Biologists on Vivisection." *Spectator* 47 (1874): 13-14.

Lederer, Susan E. "The Controversy over Animal Experimentation in America, 1880-1914." In *Vivisection in Historical Perspective*. Ed. Nicolaas A. Rupke. London: Routledge, 1987.

Leffingwell, Albert. *An Ethical Problem or Sidelights upon Scientific Experimentation on Man and Animals*, 2nd ed. New York: G. Bell & Sons, 1916.

Lesch, John E. *Science and Medicine in France: The Emergence of Experimental Physiology, 1790 1855.* Cambridge: Harvard University Press, 1984.

Lightman, Bernard, ed. *Victorian Science in Context.* Chicago: University of Chicago Press, 1997.

Lister, Joseph. *Lancet* (18 May 1891): 1124. http://www.books.google.com.

———. "On a New Method of Treating Compound Fractures, Abscess, Etc." *The Lancet* (16 Mar 1867): 326-329; (23 Mar 1867): 357-359; (30 Mar 1867): 387-389; (27 Apr 1867): 507-509; (27 Jul 1867): 95-96.

"Lister Abandons Antiseptic Spray." *Zoophilist* 3, no. 15 (1 Feb. 1884): 246.

*Liverpool Daily Post*, 27 Feb 1892. Reprinted in the *Zoophilist* 11 (1891-1892): 278.

Locy, William A. *The Growth of Biology.* New York: Henry Holt and Company, 1925.

Loir, Adrian. *L'Ombre de Pasteur.* Paris: Le Mouvement Sanitaire, 1938.

Lowe, Robert, "The Vivisection Act." *Contemporary Review* 27 (Oct 1876): 85.

———. "The Vivisection Act." *Contemporary Review* 28 (1876): 297-308.

MacCormac, William. *Transactions of the Seventh Session of the International Medical Congress* 1 (London: J. W. Kolckman, 1881).

Magner, Lois N. *A History of Infectious Disease and the Microbial World.* Westport, CT: Praeger, 2009.

Manton, Jo. *Mary Carpenter and the Children of the Streets.* London: Heinemann, 1976.

Martyn, M. P. G. To Frances Power Cobbe (27 Jun 1885). In envelope marked "Warnings to Miss Cobbe against Mr. Coleridge." BUAV Archives, Miscellaneous: 1885-1992, DBV 35/2.

Mayhew, Edward, and A. J. Sewell. *Dogs, Their Management.* London: George Routledge & Co., 1854.

McFadden, Margaret. *Golden Cables of Sympathy.* Lexington: The University Press of Kentucky, 1999.

Mitchell, Sally. *Frances Power Cobbe: Victorian Feminist, Journalist, Reformer.* Charlottesville: University of Virginia Press, 2004.

Mollers, Bernhard. *Robert Koch: Personlichkeit und Lebenswerk 1843-1910.*

Mosciucci, O. "Science of Women." In *Vivisection in Historical Perspective.* Ed. Nicolaas A. Rupke. London: Routledge, 1990.

Newman, David. "The History and Prevention of Venereal Diseases." *Glasgow Medical Journal* 81 (1914): 88-100.

Niven, Charles D. *History of the Humane Movement.* New York: Transatlantic Arts, Inc., 1967.

Nobis, Nathan. "Response to Balcombe's Commentators, Animal Dissection and Evidence Based Life-Science and Health-Professions Education." *Journal of Applied Animal Welfare Science* 5, no. 29 (2002): 159.

Obenchain, Theodore G. "Speculum Lumbar Extraforaminal Microdiscectomy." *The Spine Journal* 1, no. 6 (2001): 415-420.

———, and W. Eugene Stern. "Continuous Pressure Monitoring in Experimental Obstructive Hydrocephalus, Part I: The Dynamics of Acute Ventricular Obstruction." *Archives of Neurology* 29 (Nov 1973): 287-294.

———, and ———. "Continuous Pressure Monitoring in Experimental Obstructive Hydrocephalus, Part II: The Origin of Undulating Ventricular Waves and Periodic Respirations." *Archives of Neurology* 29 (Nov 1973): 295-298.

O'Connor, W. J. *Founders of British Physiol-*

ogy: A Biographical Dictionary, 1820–1885. Manchester: Manchester University Press, 1988. http://googlebooks.com.

Office of Laboratory Animal Welfare. *Public Health Service Policy on Humane Care and Use of Laboratory Animals* 6 (24 Nov 2010): http://grants.nih.gov/grants/olaw/references/phspol.htm?print=yes&.

Olmsted, J. M. D. *Francois Magendie: Pioneer in Experimental Physiology and Scientific Medicine in XIX Century France.* Paris: Schuman's, 1944.

Paget, James. "Vivisection: Its Pains and its Uses — I." *Nineteenth Century* 10 (1881): 920–930.

Pasteur, Louis. *Oeuvres* 4, 258.

_____. *Oeuvres* 6, 603, 605, 619. In *Pasteur's Work on Rabies.* Ed. Gerald L. Gieson, 31. http://www.jstor.org/stable/3560403.

Paton, William. *Man & Mouse: Animals in Medical Research.* Oxford: Oxford University Press, 1993.

Pfuhl, Gertrud. "Robert Koch in Wollstein." *Erinnerungenseiner Tochter Gertrud Pfuhl. Deutsche Medizinische Wochenschrift* 66 (1940): 355–357.

Picard, Liza. *Victorian London.* New York: St. Martin's Griffin, 2005.

"Prosecution at Norwich." Editorial. *British Medical Journal* (12 Dec 1874): 751–754.

Rappaport, Helen. *Queen Victoria: A Biographical Companion.* Santa Barbara: ABC CLIO, 2000.

Regan, Tom. *The Case for Animal Rights.* Berkeley: University of California Press, 2004.

Report of the Royal Commission. Q. 3562 and 3538ff. 1876.

Richardson, Ruth. *Death, Dissection and the Destitute.* 2nd ed. Chicago: The University of Chicago Press, 2000.

Ritt, Carol Bauer, and Lawrence Ritt. "'A Husband is a Beating Animal': Frances Power Cobbe Confronts the Wife-Abuse Problem in Victorian England." *International Journal of Women's Studies* 6, no. 3 (1983): 195.

_____, and _____. "Wife Abuse, Late Victorian English Feminists and the Legacy of Frances Power Cobbe." *International Journal of Women's Studies* 6, no. 3 (1983): 195.

Robin, Eugene Debs, ed. *Claude Bernard and the Internal Environment: A Memorial Symposium.* New York: Marcel Dekker, Inc., 1979.

Rolleston, J. D. "The Folklore of Pulmonary Tuberculosis." *Tubercle* 55 (1941): 3.

Rollin, Bernard E. *Putting the Horse before Descartes: My Life's Work on Behalf of Animals.* Philadelphia: Temple University Press, 2011.

Rossell, Matt. "Why I Protest Animal Research." *Oregonian.* 1 May 2010.

Rosset, F. *Pasteur et la rage.* Paris: Foundation Merieux, 1985.

Roux, Émile. "L'Oeuvre medicale de Pasteur." *Agena du chemiste* 1896.

Ruffer, Armand M. "The Morality of Vivisection." *Nineteenth Century* 32 (1892): 814.

Rupke, Nicolaas A., ed. *Vivisection in Historical Perspective.* London: Routledge, 1987.

Russell, W. M. S., and R. L. Burch. *The Principles of Humane Experimental Technique.* London: Methuen & Co. Ltd., 1959.

Rutherford, William. "Address to the Department of Anatomy and Physiology." *Report of the Forty-Third Meeting of the British Association for the Advancement of Science.* Transactions. London: Murray (1874): 119–123.

Ryder, Richard D. *Victims of Science: The Use of Animals in Research,* 2nd ed. London: National Anti-Vivisection Society Limited, 1983.

St. Thomas Hospital Manuscript, 55, 182 verso. Manuscript in the Library of St. Thomas Hospital Medical School. (1491–1900) Compiled by Julie Tancell. London: D.T. Bird, 1984.

Scruton, Roger. *Animal Rights and Wrongs.* London: Metro Publishing Limited, 1998.

Sergeant, Richard. *The Spectrum of Pain.* London: Hart Davis, 1969.

Shaftesbury to Frances Power Cobbe. 17 Sep 1878. Frances Power Cobbe Papers. Huntington Library, San Marino, California.

Shanks, Niall. *Animals and Science: A Guide to the Debates.* Santa Barbara: ABC-CLIO, 2002.

Sharpey-Schafer, Edward A. Chapter 3, "Lister as a Physiologist" *Joseph Baron Lister: Centenary Volume, 1827-1927.* Ed. A.L. Turner. Edinburgh: Oliver and Boyd, 1927.

Sherman, Irwin W. *The Power of Plagues.* Washington DC: ASM Press, 2006.

Shevelow, Kathryn. *For the Love of Animals: The Rise of the Animal Protection Movement.* New York: Henry Holt and Company, 2008.

Showalter, Elaine. *The Female Malady: Madness and English Culture, 1830–1980,* New York: Pantheon Books, 1985.

Singer, Peter. *Animal Liberation.* New York: Harper Collins, 1975.

"Sir Charles Sherrington's First Use of Diphtheria Antitoxin Made in England." *Notes on the Records of the Royal Society of London* 5, no. 2 (Apr 1948): 156–159. http://www.jstor.org/stable/531311.

Stevenson, Lloyd, "Science down the Drain: On the Hostility of Certain Sanitarians to Animal Experimental Bacteriology and Immunology." *Bulletin of the History of Medicine* 29 (1955): 1–26.

Stott, Rebecca. *Darwin and the Barnacle.* London: Faber and Faber, 2003.

Strick, James E. *Sparks of Life: Darwinism and the Victorian Debates over Spontaneous Generation.* Cambridge: Harvard University Press, 1956.

"Summary of Early Berlin Treatment with Tuberculin." *Lancet* (14 Mar 1891): 631.

Tait, Lawson. *Zoophilist* VII, no. 6 (1 Oct 1887): 101.

———. *Zoophilist* VII, no. 7 (1 Nov 1887): 117.

Tarshis, Jerome. *Claude Bernard: Father of Experimental Medicine.* New York: The Dial Press, 1968.

Taylor, D. W. "The Life and Teaching of William Sharpey (1802–1880), 'Father of Modern Physiology' in Britain." Part II. *Medical History* 3 (15 Jul 1971): 255.

Thorwald, Jurgen. *The Triumph of Surgery.* Trans. Richard Winston and Clara Winston. New York: Pantheon Books, 1960.

*Times of London.* 11–18 Oct 1892.

*Times of London.* 20–25 Oct 1892.

*Transactions Royal Society of Edinburgh* 21 (1857): 549.

Turner, James. *Reckoning with the Beast: Animals, Pain and Humanity in the Victorian Mind.* Baltimore: The Johns Hopkins University Press, 1980.

Tyrell, George. "Jesuit Philosophy." *Contemporary Review* 68 (1895).

*U.S. Report and Hearing.* Washington DC: 1896.

Ullmann, Agnes. "Pasteur-Koch: Distinctive Ways of Thinking about Infectious Diseases." *Microbe Magazine: American Society for Microbiology,* 4 (2007). http://forms.asm.org/microbe/index.asp?bid=52099.

Ungar, Roger H. "Concepts of Glucoregulation: From 1878 through 1978." In *Claude Bernard and the Internal Environment: A Memorial Symposium.* Ed. Eugene Debs Robin, 51–53. New York: Marcel Dekker, Inc., 1979.

Vallery-Radot, Pasteur. *Louis Pasteur: A Great Life in Brief.* Trans. Alfred Joseph. New York: Alfred A. Knopf, 1958.

Vallery-Radot, Pasteur, ed. *Pasteur Correspondence.* Paris: Flammarion, 1951. 430–431.

Vallery-Radot, Rene. *Life of Pasteur.* Trans. Mrs. R. L. Devonshire. New York: Doubleday, Page & Company, 1915.

———. *The Life of Pasteur.* Trans. Mrs. R. L. Devonshire. New York: McClure, Phillips and Co., 1902. The Cornell University Library Digital Collections.

———. *Vie de Pasteur.* Paris: Hachette, 1900.

"The Value of Experimentation on the Brain." *Zoophilist* 3, no. 16 (1 Mar 1884): 268.

Verschoyle, John. "Frances Power Cobbe." *The Contemporary Review* 115 (Jan/Jun 1904): 836.

———. "The Funeral of Frances Power Cobbe." *Abolitionist* 5 (Apr 1904): 1–2.

Victoria Street Society. *Woman's Signal* (21 May 1896).

———. *Zoophilist* (1 Feb 188): 171.

Virchow, Rudolf. "Über die Wirkung des Koch'schen Mittels auf innere Organe Tuberculoser." *Berliner Klinische Wochenschrift* 28: (1891): 49–52.

"Vivisection and the New Treatment of Myxedema." *Zoophilist* 13, no. 2 (1 Jun 1891): 29–30.

Von Bonin, Gerhardt. *Some Papers on the Cerebral Cortex.* Springfield: Thomas, 1960.

Von Leibig, Justus. *Organic Chemistry in its Applications to Agriculture and Physiology.* London: Taylor and Walton, 1840.

Von Weber, Ernst. *The Torture Chamber of Science.* London: Victoria Street Society, 1879.

Walburga, Lady Paget. *In My Tower.* 2 vols. Hutchinson, 1924.

Walkowitz, Judith R. *Prostitution and Victorian Society: Women, Class, and the State.* Cambridge: Cambridge University Press, 1980.

Walsh, James J. "Claude Bernard, the Physiologist." *Catholic World* 71, no. 421 (Apr 1900): 513–526.

Warbasse, James Peter. *The Conquest of Disease through Animal Experimentation.* New York: D. Appleton and Company, 1910.

Ward, Clark. *Misplaced Compassion: The Animal Rights Movement Exposed.* San Jose: Writers Club Press, 2001.

Warner, E. M. Letter. *Times of London.* (12 Oct 1892).

Westacott, E. *A Century of Vivisection and Anti-Vivisection.* Ashingdon: The C. W. Daniel Company, 1949.

Whatmore, Roger W. "Nanotechnology Has the Potential to Provide Significant Benefits Despite Concerns." In Nanotechnology. Ed. Jacquiline Langwith. Detroit: Greenhaven Press, 2009.

Wilks, Samuel. "Vivisection: Its Pains and Its Uses — III." *Nineteenth Century* 10 (1881): 943–944.

Williamson, Lori. *Power and Protest: Frances Power Cobbe and Victorian Society.* London: Rivers Oram Press, 2005.

Worboys, Michael. *Spreading Germs: Disease Theories and Medical Practice in Britain, 1865–1900.* Cambridge: Cambridge University Press, 2000.

Young, Robert M. *Mind, Brain and Adaptation in the Nineteenth Century.* Oxford: Clarendon Press, 1970.

*Zoophilist* (1 Feb 1898): 171–72 and (1 Mar 1898): 209.

*Zoophilist* 15 (1894): 8.

*Zoophilist* 9 (1889–90), 166, 262.

*Zoophilist.* 11, no. 2 (1 Jun 1891): 24.

*Zoophilist* 12 (1892–1893): 77.

*Zoophilist* 12 (1892–1893): 186–187.

# Index

Numbers in **_bold italics_** indicate pages with illustrations

abscess 53
absinthe 75–76
Adams, Charles 9, 13, 14, 169
aerophobia 183
*Age of Science* 207
Alcott, Louisa May 8
Anderson, Thomas 55
animal rights activists 236
Animal Welfare Act of 1985 248, 250
Anthony, Dr. John 47
anthrax (charbon) 101–103, 116
antiseptic principle 66–67
anti-vaccination movement 196
*An Appeal to the Humane Jews of England* 170
Aretaeus of Cappadocia 154
Association for the Advancement of Medical Research (AAMR) **_94_**, 147
Association for the Assessment and Accreditation of Laboratory Animal Care (AAALAC) 250
Atkinson, Blanche 227

bacteria: attenuation 116, 120; speciation 109–110; virulence 115
Beard, George 19
Bell-Magendie Law 40
Bennet, A. Hughes 148–150
Bentham, Jeremy 15, 245–248
Bernard, Claude 24, 27, **_40_**–45, 47, 63, 93, 147, 194
Biot, Jean-Baptiste 57
Blagdon, Isa 16, 23
blood poisoning 53
blood sports: bull-baiting (running) 29–30; cock-throwing 30
British Association 218
British Institute of Preventive Medicine 215–217
British Medical Association 73, 76, 164
British Union for the Abolition of Vivisection (BUAV) 229

Broca, Paul 139
Broome, Rev. Arthur 33; *see also* humane movement
Brouardel, Dr. 197–199
Bryan, Benjamin 124, 167, 206, 216
Burdon, Sanderson, J. 82, 83, 90, 214, 215

"Cancer Experiments on Human Beings" 207
Cannon, Walter B. 44
carbolic acid (creosote) 67, 68, 71, 149
Cardwell, Lord 89
Carnarvon, Lord 88–89
Carpenter, J. Estlin 233
Carpenter, Louisa 93
Carpenter, Mary 16
*Catholic Encyclopedia* 25
cellulitis 53
Chamberland, Charles 115, 117, 119, **_120_**–123, 175
Chambers, Robert 13
Charcot, Jean-Martin 143
Charité Hospital, Berlin 159, 203
chicken cholera 115
Clemenceau, Georges 198–199
Cobbe, Charles 10
Cobbe, Frances Power: *Age of Science* 207; Alcott's depiction 8; ankle sprain 17; anonymous contributions to *Echo* 9; anti-vaccination stance 196–197; *An Appeal to the Humane Jews of England* 170; attitude towards man and disease 226; attitude towards rabies 179; autobiography 23–24, 227; "Cancer Experiments on Human Beings" 207; Charles Adams' description 9; classical education **_12_**–13; comments on tuberculin 206–207; "Controversy in a Nutshell" 226; death 232; early life 10–11; eightieth birthday 231; *Essay on Intuitive Morals* 14–15; *Essay on True Religion* 14; "Experimental Pathology" 114; "The Fal-

lacy of Restriction as Applied to Vivisection" 170; forming BUAV 229; funeral 233; "An Institute of Preventive Medicine at Work in France" 190; "Koch and Tuberculosis" 164; "Light in Dark Places" 93; literary pursuits 17–20; "Mr. Lowe and the Vivisection Act" 91; *Nine Circles of the Hell of the Innocent* 171; "No More Than a Prick of a Needle" 189; Pasteur's double hecatombs 197; personality 9; petition 77–79; ; "The Policy of the Future" 92; "Public Money" 86; reaction to antisepsis 71; reaction to cholera 135; religious views 13–14; resignation from VSS (NAVS) 228; Schiff affair 24–*26*; selecting a successor 231–232; social activist 16–17; views on diphtheria 223; views on myxedema treatment *221*; views on tuberculosis 164; "Vivisection and the New Treatment of Myxedema" 221; "Vivisection, Four Replies" 45, 170; "Whither is Pasteurism to lead us?" 195; *Why We Have Founded the British Union for the Abolition of Vivisection* 230
Cohn, Ferdinand 62, 103–104, 107, 108
Cohnheim, Dr. Julius 51, 103, *107*, 108, 158
Colam, John 76, 77, 83
Coleridge, Lord Chief Justice John 81
Coleridge, Mildred 169
Coleridge, Stephen 140, 167, 223, 228–230
College de France 37, *38*, 40
Conan Doyle, Arthur 203–204
consumption 152–153
"Controversy in a Nutshell" 226
cortical equipotentiality 138
cretins 220
Cross, Richard 82, 88
Cruelty to Animals Act of 1876 90, 127, 146
curare 44, 81, 90

Darwin, Charles 32, 78–80, 194
Debré, Patrice 179, 194
Declaration of Great Apes 242–243
Descartes, René 31
diphtheria 219, 222
Duclaux, Émile 114
Dumas, Jean-Baptiste 57, 63
Duypuytren, Guillaume 37

Eberth, Carl 219
École Normale 61
Ehrlich, Paul 104, 163, 203
Elloit, Margaret 16
Engels, Friedrich 154
enrichment culture *107*
Erichson, Prof. John 52, 83, 85
erysipelas 53
*Essay on Intuitive Morals* 14–15

*Essay on True Religion* 14
"Experimental Pathology" 114

"The Fallacy of Restriction as Applied to Vivisection" 170
Fawcett, Millicent 228
fermentation *58*–61
Ferrier, David 137–144, 149
flask, double neck *186*–188
Flourens, Pierre 138, *141*
Folkestone Church Congress *172–176*
Foster, Michael 144, 147
Francione, Gary 243–245
Fritsch, Gustav 139

Gaffky, George 108, 131
gangrene 53
General Medical Council 89
Godlee, Rickman 149–150
Goltz, Friedrich 137–*144*
Grancher, Joseph 192
Greenlees, James 68

Hadwen, Walter 218–219, 231–232
Haffkine, Waldemar 222
*hamartia* 234
Hart, Ernest 89–90, *174*
Hengwrt 167, 228
Henle, Jacob 98, 101
Henniker, Lord 81
Hervieux, Jacques-François 113
Hicks-Beach, Michael 216
Hitzig, Eduard 139
Hoggan, Dr. George 46, 80, 87, 88, 93, 195
Horsley, Victor 24, 149, 173, 215, 220
hospitalism 50; abscess 53; blood poisoning 53; cellulitis 53; erysipelas 53; gangrene 53
humane movement 30–34; *see also* Broome, Rev. Arthur; Martin, Richard; Primatt, Rev. Humphry; Royal Society for the Prevention of Cruelty to Animals (RSPCA); Society for the Prevention of Cruelty to Animals (SPCA)
Humphry, Sir George 148
Hutton, Richard 80, 83, 89–90, 226
Huxley, Thomas Henry 81–82, 83, 86, 90, 92
hydrophobia 182; *see also* aerophobia

immunity 183, 184
"the infinitely small are infinitely great" 112
Institute for Animal Care and Use Committee (IACUC) 250
"An Institute of Preventive Medicine at Work in France" 190
International Medical Congresses: 1876 (Philadelphia) 214; 1879 (Amsterdam) 215;

1881 (London) 125; 1884 (Copenhagen) 194; 1890 (Berlin) 202
*Introduction to the Study of Experimental Medicine* 44–45

Jackson, Hughlings 139, 149; *see also* Jacksonian march
Jacksonian march 139
Jenner, Edward 195, 218
Jenner, William 127
Jupille, Jean-Baptiste 192

Kant, Immanuel 241, 247
King Henry VIII 29
King John 29
King's College 210
Kinyoun, J.J. 223
Klebs, Edwin 105
Klein, Emmanuel 86
Koch, Robert 125, 128, 153, 173, 219, 255; anthrax encounter 101–103; bacterial speciation 109–110; cholera, Indian campaign 132–133, comma bacillus 133; country doctor 100; criticism of Pasteur 129; early career 98–99; Egypt cholera expedition 131–132; encounter with Virchow 107–108; enrichment culture 105–107; Indian cholera expedition 132–133; infection templates 105; Koch's phenomenon 203; Koch's pronouncement 162–163; postulates 132, *160*–162; pure culture 108–109; purified protein derivative (PPD) 206; trip to Breslau 103; tuberculosis trials 204–*205*; work with tuberculosis 158–162; youth 98; *Zoophilist's* editorial attitude 206–207
"Koch and Tuberculosis" 164
Kocher, Emil 220

Lankester, Prof. Edwin 236
Lankester, Ray 79
Laveran, Charles 224
Leibig, Justus von 60
"Light in Dark Places" 93
Lind, James 204
Lister, Joseph 34, 92, 112, 113, 125, 128, 135, 147, 180, 199, 203, 214, 219, 222; appearance before Commission 85–86; British Association speech 218; British Institute 215; experiments on capillaries 66–69; introduction to Syme 49; letter from Queen Victoria 85; Lister's peerage 224; move to King's College 210; nervous breakdown 36–37; relation to Sharpey 37–*38*; youth 36; *see also* hospitalism
Llanelltyd Church *168*, 228
Lloyd, Mary 23, 167, 227
Loeffler, Friedrich 108, 163, 219
Loir, Adrien 124, 186, 198

Lowe, Robert MP 91
Lucas-Championnière, Just 214
Ludwig, Carl 45
lupus vulgaris 154

Magendie, François *37*–40, 47
Magnan, Valantin 76
Martin, Richard 33, 34; *see also* humane movement
Martin Act of 1822 33, 77, 78
Mayet, Charles 190
Mayhew, Edward 178
Meister, Joseph *191*–192, 201
Melun 117; *see also* Pouilley-le-Fort
Metchnikoff, Elie 224
milieu, internal 43–44
"Mr. Lowe and the Vivisection Act" 91
Murray, George 220

Neisser, Albert 219
neurasthenia 19
Newbridge 10, 168
*Nine Circles of the Hell of the Innocent* 171
"No More Than a Prick of a Needle" 189
Norwich Affair 76–77

Office of Laboratory Animal Welfare (OLAW) 250
ovariotomy 71–73

Paget, Sir James *70*, 127, 145, 215
Parker, Theodore 13, 24
Pasteur, Louis 55, 99, 125, 128, *129*–131, 134, 153, 173, 218, 224, 255; anthrax vaccine 117; antivivisectionist's reaction 124; chicken cholera 116; double necked flask 186; early life 57; early rabies vaccine 183–*186*; elucidation of putrefaction 111–112; fermentation *58*–60; germ theory announcement 60; Joseph Meister *191*–192; journalist Mayet 190; Melun showdown 119; move to Strasbourg *58*; Pasteur's detractors 194–195; Pasteur's jubilee 199–*200*; puerperal fever 113–114; reply to Koch *130*; Rossignol's proposal 117–118; Rouyer affair 197–199; silkworm work 63–64; spontaneous generation 61–*62*; staphylococci 114; stroke 65
Pasteur Institutes 199
People for the Ethical Treatment of Animals (PETA) 253
Peter, Michael 124, 197–198
Petri dish 109, 184
phagocytosis 224
phthisis 154
"The Policy of the Future" 92
Pouchet, Félix-Archimède 61
Pouilley-le-Fort 117, 119, 120–*123*

PPD (purified protein derivative) 206
Primatt, Rev. Humphry 31–32, 237; *see also* humane movement
*Principles of Humane Experimental Technique* 250–251
"Public Money" 86
puerperal fever 113
pure culture 108–110, 133
putrefaction 111

Queen Elizabeth 29
Queen Victoria 82, 85, 224

Raleigh, Sir Walter 44
Red Lodge School 16
Regan, Tom 240–242
Rhodes, Georgine *172*, 173
Rollin, Bernard 248–249, 255
Ross, Ronald 224
Rossignol, Jean-Pierre 117, 119–123
Roux, Émile 115, 117, *120*–123, 125, 135, 184, 191, 192, 196, 198–199, 219–220, 222
Rouyer, Jules 197–199
Royal Commission of Enquiry 83, 88
Royal Society for the Prevention of Cruelty to Animals (RSPCA) 31, 33–34, 78; *see also* humane movement; Society for the Prevention of Cruelty to Animals (SPCA)
Ruffer, Armand 175, *221*
Ryder, Richard 238–239

St. Augustine 30–31
St. Thomas Aquinas 31
Savory, William 214
Schiff, Mauritz 24–*26*, 220
Schroeter, Joseph 108
scrofula 154
Scruton, Roger 237–238
Shaftesbury, Lord (Anthony Ashley Cooper) 87, 88, 90, 92, 93, 146, 170
Shakespeare, William 28
Shanks, Niall 245–247, 254
Sharpy, William 34, 37–*38*, 49
Sherrington, Charles 221–222
silkworm 63–64
Singer, Peter 237, 239–240
small pox epidemic 218
Snow, John 131, 134
Society for the Prevention of Cruelty to Animals (SPCA) 33
Somerville, Mary 23
spontaneous generation 61–*62*, 124
Stanton, Elizabeth Cady 9
staphylococci 114

*Summa Theologica* 25
Syme, Dr. James 49, *51*

Tait, Dr. Lawson 72, 195, 229
templates of infection 105
tetanus 219
Thullier, Louis *120*–122, 125, 129, 132
Tilt, Edward 19
*Torture Chamber of Science* 45–46, 194
tuberculosis 153, 181 *see also* consumption; lupus vulgaris; phthisis; scrofula

vaccine 116
Vallery-Radot, René 188
Verschoyle, Rev. John 232
vibrion septique 111
Victoria Street Society (VSS) 87
Villemin, Jean-Antoine 158
Villeneuve-l'Étang 188, *200*
Virchow, Robert 98, 100, *107*, 127, 135, 145, 147, 157, 158, 162, 194, *205*
"Vivisection and the New Treatment of Myxedema" 221
"Vivisection, Four Replies" 45, 170
von Behring, Emil 219
von Nageli, Carl 104
von Pettenkofer, Max 134
Vulpian, Alfred 192

"weak strong one" *185*
Weber, Ernst von 45
Wedgewood, Josiah 32
Weigert, Carl 104
"Whither is Pasteurism to lead us?" 195
*"Why We Have Founded the British Union for the Abolition of Vivisection* 230
Williamson, Lori 10
Wilson, George 163–164
Wister, Sarah 227

Yeo, Prof. Gerald 143, 147, 156
Yersin, Alexandre 219, 222

*Zoophilist* 88, 167, 169, 197, 229; Cobbe regarding cholera 135; Cobbe versus vivisection 146; Cobbe's view of rabies treatment 194; "experimental pathology" 114; featuring Nine Circles *172*; Koch's use of 4000 guinea pigs in research 206; letter against Cobbe 227; "No More Than a Prick of a Needle *189*; Pasteur's inoculations 124; Prof. Hermann and brain research 145; "Robert Koch and Tuberculosis" 164; tuberculin 207

www.ingramcontent.com/pod-product-compliance
Ingram Content Group UK Ltd.
Pitfield, Milton Keynes, MK11 3LW, UK
UKHW041928140426
5217IPUK00014B/359